FORTY SOMETHING FOREVER

Harold & Arline Brecher

Also by Arline Brecher

Bye-Bye Bypass (audo tape with Harold Brecher)
Bypassing Bypass (First Edition, with Elmer Cranton, M.D.)
Healthsavers Guide to Staying Fit After Chelation Therapy
(with Harold Brecher)
Psychodietetics (with Dr. E. Cheraskin and Dr. W.M. Ringsdorf)

Also By Harold Brecher

Life is Uncertain, Eat Dessert First (with Dr. Sol Gordon)
Brecher's Field Guide to Strange Birds (with Manu Aloha)

FORTY SOMETHING FOREVER

♡

A CONSUMER'S GUIDE
TO

CHELATION
THERAPY
and other
HEART-SAVERS

♡

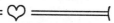
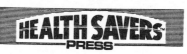

Updated Twenty-Seventh Printing - March, 2000

FORTY-SOMETHING FOREVER
Copyright 2000 by Arline Brecher and Harold Brecher
All rights Reserved, Healthsavers Press
Jacket design by Harold Brecher
Typography Design by Kyle & Chrissy McKibbin
Printed in the United States of America

HEALTHSAVERS PRESS
P.O. Box 683, Herndon, Virginia 20172
(703) 471-4734

ISBN 0927839-46-6

Dedicated to
H. Ray Evers, M.D.,
The Grandfather of Chelation Therapy
1913 - 1990

From 1964 to 1990 Dr. Evers supervised
over 600,000 chelation treatments despite
the continuous harrassment by forces
opposed to his "wholistic" approach.

"ONE DOES NOT HAVE TRUE FREEDOM UNTIL
ONE IS FREE TO CHOOSE HOW HE WISHES TO
BE TREATED MEDICALLY."

H. Ray Evers, M.D.

A HEART FELT THANKS ...

... to all the 'troops'.

If the oft-noted parallel between having a baby and birthing a book is valid - and it is - then *Forty-Something Forever* is the most fortunate of newborns, having been cheered along from conception through gestation and finally to birth by a benevolent band of able labor room assistants and dedicated guardians.

Two visionary physicians, the Gordon orothers, Garry and Ross, helped creation by making it possible for us to be 'in-at-the-beginning' of the chelation story. Although none of us realized it at the time, the germ of the idea for this text took root almost a generation ago when they invited us to the Dr. Frankel meeting.

From that day on, a legion of their colleagues nourished our efforts, helping us keep abreast of chelation-related events: Ray Evers, Harold Harper, Charlie Farr, Dan Roehm, Edward McDonagh, Conrad Maulfair, Maurice Archer, William Mauer, Richard Casdorph, Bruno Crussol, William Goldwag, Bruce Halstead, Ronald Hoffman, James Julian, Warren Levin, Gerald Parker, Ted Rozema, Ricardo Sabates, Charles Rudolph, Murray Susser, Robert Vance plus the "nifty fifty" whom readers will meet in Chapter Twelve.

A tribe of non-physician trustees have also nursed the project along, each contributing specialized wisdom: George Kindness, Henry Belk, Richard Passwater, Jane Heimlich, Stephen Levine, Kurt Greenburg, Ann Cronin, Brian Hirsch, Ed Nettleton, Kay Pierson - to name but a few that come most easily to mind.

A special mention is due the godparents: Joanne Davis of Pleasant Gardens, North Carolina who threatened to punish us in her "pouty house" if we aborted the 'babe'; Ted Dickson, the selfless Canadian chelation advocate who unfortunately did not live to see this long-awaited book in print; Dr. E. Cheraskin, a long-time friend, who thoughtfully 'vetted' critical parts of the manuscript to eliminate bad 'genes' and without whose help we might never have been welcomed into the preventive medicine 'family', and our recently adopted, highly valued "Deepthroat" - the FDA drug expert who made Chapter Six possible.

Finally, our gratitude to Phyllis Hoffman who did double-duty as surrogate mother and midwife, coaching us forward in painful moments, on call for pre-dawn consultations. Her pre-launch efforts eased introducing our infant to a waiting world.

Thanks, guys.

TABLE OF CONTENTS

Truth is like a torch.
The more it's shook,
The more it shines.

Sir William Hamilton
Adaptation from
Discussion on Philosophy

INTRO

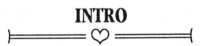

NOT ANOTHER BOOK ON CHELATION!

In 1981, when Arline agreed to co-author a book about chelation (pronounced 'KEY-LAY-SHUN') therapy with Elmer Cranton, M.D., we hoped it would be the definitive work on the subject. Our goal at the time was to describe a valuable, but poorly understood medical treatment so clearly, credibly and completely, there'd be no need to write more - ever.

The work that evolved, *Bypassing Bypass* (Stein and Day, 1984) measured up somewhat. It introduced chelation to countless numbers who never had heard of it, and influenced many to investigate this non-surgical treatment for themselves. Although the book got off to a slow start, it became increasingly popular over time - an astonishing stunt for a text that was the publishing industry equivalent of an orphaned-at-birth child.

THE *BYPASSING BYPASS* SAGA

Bypassing Bypass arrived in the marketplace without fanfare or promotional support. No 'pub' parties, ads, or book reviews marked publication date. There were no talk shows, book signings, or check-out counter displays at retail book outlets. No major distributor stocked it. You get the picture: there was none of the hoopla that celebrates the advent of an important book.

More discouraging yet, within months the publisher ran short of cash. The printer tied up unpaid-for books in his warehouse. When the first edition sold out, reorders went unfilled, and for some three years afterwards, few copies made it to market. Despite all these and other obstacles, the book survived and made its mark. Why? How? We can only assume because it delivered a powerful message, vitally important to many people.

Most of the credit goes to the legion of enthusiastic and diligent chelation supporters who kept the book alive by word-of-mouth recommendations. From 1984 on, rarely a day passed without inquiries from someone advised to get a copy of *BB* for themselves or a loved one. Positive feedback is a real 'high' for a writer. It's always exciting to hear, "I read your book"; better still "I liked your book"; best of all - "Bless you for writing the book, it helped me get well" or ". . .saved my life."

We've heard those wonderful words over and over, the thrill in no way dulled by repetition. On 'dark days', it was cheering to be called by people so grateful for restored health, they'd made a non-profit project of distributing books to friends and relatives. Bernard Smyk of Newport Beach, California, ordered 40 books and asked, "Do you care if I give these away?" Others, angry at the recalcitrant orthodox medical community, passed them out to uninformed or hostile physicians, to legislators, medical societies, to religious counselors or wherever they thought they would do the most good.

One senior citizen, Virgil Brubaker of Haines City, Florida was motivated to call a meeting of his fellow trailer park retirees. He invited his chelation doctor to address the group, and handed out books (at his expense) to all who showed.

"Guess how many people came?" he phoned to gloat. "One hundred and twenty, and it was a stormy night with a hurricane brewing just a few miles off the coast." Happy man. He felt he saved lives.

Since the original work is spreading the word so well, why write another book about chelation? Having said it all, what more is there to say? Quite a bit as it turns out.

BOOKS ARE NOT WINE - THEY *DO NOT* IMPROVE WITH AGE

Medical books have a limited shelf life. Rightly so. Some, like a tasty fruit, develop 'black' spots as the science matures. This is particularly true when writing about chelation, which has 'grown up' a lot in the the last ten years.

We live in fast-moving times. Compare current headlines with yesteryear's and you'll realize how much has changed since 1980. With each day that goes by, there are indications of how radically different today's reading public is: more sophisticated, more health savvy, and more aware of the political influence on medical issues than they were a decade ago. One result is an exploding interest in alternative medicine - the subject of a recent *Time Magazine* front page. Another is the eager reception given to nonconventional voices. Lately, we're asked to speak on more radio programs, at more health seminars, and to more diverse groups than in all previous years. Given those circumstances, an outdated book can be an embarrassment, especially when obliged to discuss or defend it at a public appearance. Let us explain.

- **What was 'new' in 1982 is old hat today.**

  There are an estimated half million or so more chelated patients than a decade ago, and at least two and a half times that number of people bypassed. One consequence is an abundance of new evidence by which to judge the comparative merit of these and other competing therapies.

- **Bypass 'bashing' is out of step with the times.**

  Ten years ago, the dangerous ineffectiveness of bypass surgery had not been exposed or explained. Today. it's no longer big news that this over-prescribed, high-risk procedure is of questionable value and should be avoided more often than not. In the 1980's, it was essential to record how often the 'bypassed' had poor long-range outcomes. In the 1990's, railing against bypass surgery misses the mark. Scads of reputable cardiologists, many from within academia, now voice the same concerns.

- **Angioplasty is NOT the "promising" surgical alternative to bypass we once thought.**

  In 1984, we held out some hope that competitive alternatives to bypass surgery, such as PTCA (percutaneous transluminal coronary angioplasty), would prove significantly safer and more effective than the operations then available to open clogged arteries. Now we know better. Once again, warnings are in order - this time about the newest, equally unproven invasive procedures: balloon angioplasty, atherectomy, laser angioplasty, heart punctures, artery stents and other highly promoted atherosclerotic 'cures'. It's time to restate the reminder: "new" and "good" are not synonymous.

- **The old book told only half the story.**

  Atherosclerosis, (clogged arteries), admittedly a major health problem, is not the *real* cause of most cases of sudden heart attack death. Tachycardia arrhythmia is *the* unaddressed disorder that must be faced. It is difficult to avoid misguided treatment decisions unless you recognize and understand the enemy.

- **Hopes for establishment acceptance of chelation and other alternate therapies have taken a new turn.**

The growth of public enthusiasm for non-invasive treatments has triggered a backlash, intensifying opposition against *all* natural remedies. One state (Arizona) recently 'outlawed' chelation.

Clinicians who challenge orthodoxy routinely face persecution and prosecution, making it more evident than ever that scientific investigation on its own is not likely to set the record straight. Clearly there's a need for consumers, educated as to what's at stake, to work together to protect chelation and other benign therapies from extinction.

- **The much-heralded FDA study of EDTA will NOT be completed as promised.**

The 'Chelation Project' seeking FDA approval of EDTA for arterial disease via controlled double blind clinical trials, begun with such optimism in 1985, has stalled time and again and is now defunct. (See Chapter Twelve.) Contrary to information published in the 'updated second edition' of *Bypassing Bypass*, that study is over.

- **Beneficial as chelation may be, EDTA alone does not assure healthful longevity.**

Contrary to what the over-enthusiastic purport, chelation does not 'cure' old age and its symptoms. It does give the body a reprieve - a chance to regenerate. Health-seekers, chelated or not, need the latest detailed information about diet, exercise, nutritional supplements and all else that makes up a health-promoting lifestyle

Scientific investigation of life extension has shifted into high gear. Impressive research strides have been made in the twin fields of free radical pathology and bio-oxidative medicine. Strategies which boost immune systems and build free radical protection make living happily and usefully to 120 a reasonable goal. Yet most people are confused as to how best to translate findings into practical everyday action that will help them achieve a healthy, indefinitely extended 'middlescence.'

ME, A HEALTH NUT? YOU BETTER BELIEVE IT!

If you're more health-conscious than you were a few years back, you're in step with an important 90's trend. It's clear the tide has turned when former 'hippie' Jerry Rubin, who once advocated political revolution, is now hawking health. Oprah made headlines when she slimmed down. Forty-five year old Cher's newest video is for body-building buffs. Vitamin cocktail bars are in vogue on the west coast. The busiest night spots in trend-setting L.A. feature 'smart drugs' and Vitamin C 'shakes'.

People who once thought it an insult to be called a 'health nut' are flattered instead now that 'health nuts' are in style. Fat-free diets, aerobic exercise and nutritional supplements are fashionable on every Main Street in the USA. Middle America is more willing to consider innovative cures than ever before. Mental imagery, homeopathy, herbal medicinals and natural remedies have attracted countless new followers.

Many suspect the answers to this century's most pressing health problems - cancer, heart disease, AIDS, multiple sclerosis, arthritis, asthma, allergies and other auto-immune diseases may well come from surprising places. Trailblazing investigators are scouring the jungles of Africa, reviewing ancient Far Eastern medicines, and looking into remedies developed by the maverick physicians who dare challenge orthodoxy.

This no-holds-barred approach is paying off. A growing

cadre of tough-minded, independent physicians, including some 200 new chelationists, have abandoned drug and surgery-centered practices and made the switch to non-invasive remedies. They're not hurting for patients. Concerned that many 'cures' have been found to 'kill', a multitude of the ailing seek out holistically-based, natural treatments, immune-boosting therapies and non-toxic healings.

Once we recognized a genuine need for a new book addressing emerging issues, we decided to write it from a fresh point of view - one more in line with consumer perspectives. The person visiting a doctor's office has a totally different slant on health matters than the white-frocked individual sporting a stethoscope. Journalists, accustomed to translating scientific subjects into language non-scientists can grasp, are more familiar with people-oriented issues than physicians temporarily turned scribe.

As every science writer knows, co-authoring a medical book with a doctor is a mixed bag with drawbacks that may outweigh the advantages. On the plus side, the doctor/co-author, well-versed in his or her field of expertise, may be privy to research that will not be public knowledge for some time to come. Teamed up with a skilled writer, the doctor may shed new light on a medical subject and simultaneously do a real public service.

On the downside, the doctor may have a hidden agenda. He may be writing with an eye toward boosting his clinical practice, status among colleagues, standing with medical societies, credibility with licensing authorities. The more eager the doctor is to impress the professional community, the more likely the book will be self-serving. A more grave possibility is the work may fall short of the mark because the doctor/author has something to sell. Business interests may skew editorial contents to promote products in which he has a financial stake. When the author is a practicing clinician, he is wooing not only the book-buyer, but a potential patient and customer as well.

A WORD TO DOCTORS

Some physicians may be offended by a medical book written by nonphysicians, especially when the subjects tackled are highly controversial. Readers who benefited from health books written by Jean Carper (*The Food Pharmacy*), Maureen Salaman (*Foods that Heal*), Jane Heimlich (*What Your Doctor Won't Tell You*), Ann Wigmore (*Be Your Own Doctor*) and Durk Pearson and Sandy Shaw (*Life Extension*) will undoubtedly take a different view.

Those who remember how dramatically Adele Davis in the 1960's and Nathan Pritikin in the 1980's (both nondoctors) changed America's dietary habits for the better, welcome well-researched texts written without a doctor's byline. The public understands journalists have nothing to sell but the truth as they see it. Since they're not part of the medical money stream, they can afford to be totally objective.

While we don't have the credentials of an M.D., (and we certainly insist readers consult a physician before taking any action that will effect their health) we do have a great deal of experience to draw upon. For twenty years, we've crisscrossed the country, covered hundreds of medical conventions both stateside and abroad, to report on research representing wildly diverse points of view. We've filed copy from mainstream gatherings and from some of the more exotic (and interesting) 'fringe' science assemblies.

We're as familiar with the AMA (American Medical Association), AHA (American Heart Association), NCI (National Cancer Institute) - (the full alphabet of prominent associations) - as with the scientific groups you may have never hear much of: the futurists, parapsychologists, dowsers and dreamers. We've investigated and reported on medical breakthroughs and junk science, and hopefully have learned to distinguish between the two.

The result is this book, based on research material and interviews collected over many years, including last-minute news that arrived as the manuscript was on its way to be typeset. We wrote it with the generous help of some hundred or more clinicians, researchers and health authorities from many disciplines, and avoided the onus of giving any one doctor editorial control.

We see our role as translators and intermediaries. *Forty-Something Forever* reflects our personal experience, and is written with the aim of sharing what we've learned over time. As go-betweens, our goals are two-fold: to serve as a bridge between the scientific community and the public-at-large, and to help consumers become more acutely aware of the many behind-the-scenes forces that stand in the way of their achieving optimal health.

While we have no vested interest in promoting chelation therapy or "saving" the chelators, we do want to alert consumers to their vulnerability in the medical marketplace. Anytime doctors and scientists squabble, play politics, or angle for profits, the public is short-changed, medically speaking, and gets hit in the pocketbook. The more that's at stake, the higher the bill. We cannot think of a clearer example than the three decades-old chelation controversy.

Thus, in the pages that follow we'll do our best to address the reader's health concerns. We'll direct our attention to the questions most frequently asked: What's the truth about chelation? Bypass? Angioplasty? Where do I find a good doctor? What does it cost? What's good? What's not? What can I do to regain my health? To live better? Longer? What about oat bran? Margarine? Eggs? What should I eat? What medicines or vitamins are safe to take?

If you are suffering from a degenerative disease, or worried about a loved one whose health is deteriorating, your life and future happiness may well depend on sound answers to such questions. Here goes.

Fear cannot be without hope nor hope without fear.

Benedict Spinoza
Ethics. Definition XIII

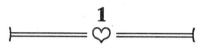

"GOODBYE" BYPASS – "HELLO" CHELATION!

Sixty-two year old Bill Thompson (not his real name) was a newly arrived condo-owner in a Florida retirement community when he began having chest pains.

"It must be something I ate," he assured his wife.

"Since when are you a doctor?" she asked.

"You should have it checked out," advised a neighbor who'd recently had a bypass.

After acknowledging he occasionally had leg cramps and sometimes found it hard to breathe, Mr. T. agreed to see his golf-buddy's cardiologist.

The examining physician ordered a battery of tests before issuing his grim diagnosis: "It's atherosclerosis, all right. You've got hardening of the arteries; there's not enough blood getting through to your heart. Your blood pressure is 154/108; heart function less than fifty percent of normal; there's almost total blockage of the left ventricle arteries leading to the heart and 70% occlusion of the other vessels. It's not good."

"What do you suggest?" Bill asked. "Drugs, diet, no more booze, give up smoking? I'd hate to give up gin rummy and golf."

"You're too far gone," the physician said. "You need a triple bypass and the sooner the better."

Nothing unusual about this tale thus far. Some 40 million men and women suffer symptoms indicating plaque-clogged arteries, and when some 250,000 each year get the bad news, they say "So be it" and agree to surgery.

Mr. T., formerly a University of Minnesota professor of public health, rebelled, aware of an option most people with his condition haven't heard of: chelation therapy.

"Thanks, but no thanks," said the savvy Thompson. "I'm going to try chelation first."

"What?" snapped the horrified doctor. "You can't be serious.

You're making a huge mistake."

"What do you know about chelation?" the professor asked.

"Nothing - except it's no damn good," the doctor sneered, and walked out.

❤ ❤ ❤

The Madison Avenue style 'hard-sell' is usually effective with frightened patients not as knowledgeable as Mr. T.. Surgery by intimidation - "get bypassed today or you might be dead tomorrow" - speeds many a reluctant, but vulnerable individual, on his way to the surgical suite.

Others may be more easily persuaded by the 'soft-sell'. A group of Maryland cardiologists distribute a clever fifty-two page multi-color booklet entitled *Everything You Need to Know About Heart Surgery* to surgical candidates. With more than half the contents devoted to full-page cartoons, and the balance to gushy, light-hearted text, it is clearly designed to be more disarming than informative.

Despite the propaganda, most people would, if they could, avoid surgery. Not many suspect they have a realistic option.

Should one ask, "Is this operation really necessary?", cardiac surgeons respond in a way sure to get the patient on the operating table as quickly as possible.

"You have nothing to worry about. It's a common procedure. We've checked the O.R. schedule, and lucky you - we can fit you right in."

That's precisely what the doctors told Michael Keaton, a 'fictional' bypass patient, in a slice-of-life 1989 episode of NBC's top-rated sit-com *Family Ties.* Bypass surgery has become so commonplace, the media plays it for laughs. In the scene cited, Keaton's surgeons tried to allay his fears by speaking of his operation as a "patient-doctor team effort." Keaton responded with a sure-fire laugh-getter: "Okay. You lie down and I'll do the surgery."

Another bypass patient - this one a retiree - quips: "We expected to travel all over the world - never planned on traveling to the hospital instead." When the man dies on the operating table, the surgeon's black humor: "Transfer him to the ECU - (Eternal Care Unit)."

In another prime-time TV show *Doctor, Doctor,* two surgeons argue over whether they should have warned a patient who died on the operating table of the risks of bypass surgery.

What for?" asks the Rambo-like doc. "If he'd lived, he'd be pain free."

The punch line: "I get it. It's our job to take people out of their misery even if it kills 'em."

Don't be put off guard by the one-liners. Bypass surgery is no laughing matter.

SCARED OF SURGERY? YOU HAVE GOOD REASON!

When you ask people who have opted for chelation what motivated them to bypass their surgeons, most confess, "I was scared to death to be cut up."

"It's perfectly normal to be a little nervous before any operation," the American Heart Association states in their consumer's pamphlet on bypass surgery. Their advice - "A mild sedative can help you relax."

"Relax? Hell! I didn't want to relax - I wanted to get my butt out of there before I got carved up like a Thanksgiving turkey," was one patient's response.

Are people silly to be scared? Contrary to Franklin Delano Roosevelt's history-making assurance, when it comes to bypass surgery, you have more to fear than fear itself.

A HOSPITAL IS NOT A PLACE TO GET WELL

Besides the obvious dangers, there are many unacknowledged perils that present a legitimate cause for concern. For starters, consider the hazards of hospitalization.

In the early days of this century, the famed physician Dr. Henry E. Sigerist called hospitals "temples" of medicine and good health. There's little doubt he'd be distressed to see how his 'temples' have since been defiled.

More than a third of the nation's hospitals fail to meet standards designed to guard patients against a medical calamity, according to a three-year survey of 5,208 facilities conducted by the Joint Commission on Accreditation of Healthcare Organizations that ended in 1988. Among their dismal findings: fifty percent of the facilities did not properly monitor patients in intensive care and coronary care units; thirty-five percent did not supervise blood transfusions properly; fifty-six percent did not properly supervise routine care.

It gets worse.

In the most comprehensive study ever conducted in the U.S., Harvard University researchers concluded that negligence kills thousands of people in hospitals each year and injures many more. What goes wrong? Just about everything. The researchers found frequent mechanical failure of technological marvels: defective defibrillators, anesthesia machines, and cardiac monitors, to name but a few. They found untrained and unqualified technicians operating medical equipment.

Added to the above, there's the risk of anesthesia. Surveys conducted at Harvard Medical School over a fifteen year period have uncovered a long list of chilling errors that occur during anesthesia. While 'only' 10,000 deaths from anesthesia administration are reported each year, investigators suspect the number could easily be three to four times as high.

Among the common errors are syringe swap (wrong drug inadvertently administered), ampule swap (assistant hands over the wrong substance because many different drugs have like-sounding names), drug overdose, wrong choice of drug, wrong choice of administration technique (all due to judgment error by the anesthetist), disconnection of intravenous lines, breathing circuits and other attachments (equipment failure or unfamiliarity of lack of experience with the technology).

There are other 'bugs' in the hospital system - real ones. Of the roughly 35 million Americans hospitalized annually, two million or more get sicker instead of better, according to the Center for Disease Control data. Hospitals are not as zealous about cleanliness as one might presume. Even operating rooms are often not as sterile as required and personnel frequently put patients in jeopardy. There are no fewer than 100,000 hospital-originated infection-related deaths annually in America and some insiders think that's a super-conservative figure reflecting less than one third of the fatalities. This is what we do know: twenty percent of hospital patients leave with a condition they didn't have when they entered the hospital.

None of the above includes the "freak" accidents: surgeons operating on the 'wrong' organ or on the wrong person. Just last year, a 90-year old man burned to death while undergoing ultraviolet light therapy in a hospital treatment room. "They put him in there and forgot to take him out," witnesses testified at the ensuing malpractice trial.

Something else to take into consideration is this: if you have a choice, don't have surgery in July! A long-standing joke in medical circles turns out to be not so funny, because teaching hospitals routinely bring in new interns and residents during the summer. A study at the VA Medical Center in Denver recently found that surgical procedure complications escalate from twenty percent in June to fifty percent in July.

Finally, there are the morbid details you may not have heard about the risks of the bypass itself.

- Death occurs in about 5% of heart-bypass surgeries. That is the official National Heart and Lung Institute statistic and is open to question and upward revision. A new study on 3,500 bypass patients, reported in the August 19, 1991 issue of *JAMA (Journal of the American Medical Association)* finds death rates vary from 1.9 percent to 9.2 percent. A companion study found death rates ranging as high as 9.9 percent. Depending on who does the surgery - and where - your chance of leaving the operating room alive could be as low as one in five.

- The older you are, the worse your chances. There's a ten percent higher mortality, on average, for every year over seventy, so octogenarians should be particularly wary of being told they are considered suitable surgical candidates.

- More to the point, deaths from bypass surgery are increasing, a recent study revealed, perhaps because there are more 'repeaters'. Second and third bypass procedures admittedly expose patients to additional risk.

- Women are 77 percent more likely as men to die as a result of bypass surgery, according to a UCLA School of Medicine study of 2,297 male and female bypass patients. The official explanation is that "The women are sicker than the men when they're operated on." We doubt that's the cause, since statistic-wary surgeons routinely reject patients they fear may be too sick to survive;

- You could survive the operation, but be all the worse off, nonetheless. Some five to ten percent of bypass patients suffer a heart attack immediately following surgery, according to the New York Heart Association. Two percent suffer a stroke and two percent hemorrhage. Heart tissue damage during surgery is common, and usually occurs when the heart suffers oxygen deprivation during the clamping of the aorta. Then when it is resupplied with oxygen-rich blood, the result is a dangerous burst of free radical activity.

- You could pull through a 'changed person'. Neurological damage is one of the least publicized hazards of bypass surgery. It causes memory loss, reduced mental functioning, and temperament alteration. Preliminary results of an international study show that the procedure produces subtle, long-lasting mental impairment in nearly one in five. Seventeen percent experience persistent mental difficulties. Up to twenty percent of patients suffer from serious depression for a year or longer.

How serious? For how long? Ask TV super-star Joan Rivers, whose husband Edgar, committed suicide post-bypass. "He was never the same after his bypasses," she told Phil Donahue in a recent interview. "Before that, he was always able to snap back from adversity. Nothing ever got him down. No matter what went wrong, he was ready to do battle - and then one day in Philadelphia he forgot everything he stood for. Just like that."

Family members puzzled - or alarmed - when the bypass survivor is uncharacteristically rude, hostile, insensitive or noncommunicative, usually blame the undesirable change on the individual's reaction to a traumatic near-death experience. In reality, however, their loved one may be exhibiting the results of oxygen deprivation to the brain during the surgical procedure.

Dr. Thorkel Aberg, a leading heart surgeon at Umea

University Hospital in Umea, Sweden, who is taking part in the new studies, says, "I have no doubt there is subtle brain cell damage during these operations."

When Dr. Maurice Albin, professor of anesthesiology at the University of Texas Health Sciences Center in San Antonio studied post-bypass brain pictures taken by the Trans-Cranial Doppler device, he discovered trapped debris in the brain's blood vessels, meaning a mini-stroke resulting in minor personality changes is a likely aftermath of the surgery.

So much for the risks - how about the benefits?

BYPASS SURGERY - MEDICAL MARVEL OR MEDICAL MALPRACTICE?

According to the American Heart Association, coronary artery bypass surgery is a "common procedure for restoring health and vigor to people suffering from coronary artery disease." There's no argument that it's 'common'. Each year, Americans spend one out of every ten dollars on health care, and treatment of heart disease represents a large chunk of that money. In a typical year, we annually spend $8-$12 billion on some 250,000 coronary bypass operations at a cost of $25,000 to $40,000 each.

What do we get for our money? Not much in the way of the 'health and vigor' promised. Most of the fine results claimed for bypass surgery come from the typewriters of ad agency hacks and not from the halls of science. While the bypass is one of the most widely touted of modern medicine's pricey procedures, a careful look at results reveals it doesn't help the vast majority of those who undergo it.

One of the nation's leading cardiologists, Dr. Thomas A. Preston, professor of medicine at the University of Washington in Seattle, has criticized the operation in very harsh terms. "It's a particularly dramatic and expensive surgery, and scandalously overused."

If you think - or been led to believe - bypass surgery is going to cure your disease, think again. Let's look at survival stats. If a surgical procedure is worthwhile, people who have it ought to live longer. The research does not support this thesis.

Controlled tests beginning with a 1977 Veterans Administration study and capped off with a 1983 published National Institutes of Health survey showed bypass surgery was no better at prolonging life than treatment with prevailing drugs. After spending $24 million to study the subject, government researchers concluded that bypass patients not only did not live longer - they didn't live any better. The nonsurgically treated were just as well off when it came to retaining their jobs, remaining productive and enjoying leisure time activities.

Does the operation prevent future heart attack? Not according to Dr. Preston and others who report: there are NO studies to date that have shown this operation prevents infarction. When it comes to arrhythmia, even the pro-bypass rooting squad admits there is no possibility surgery will prevent arrhythmias. Scads of research reports exhibit little or no beneficial improvement of heart muscle functioning after bypass surgery.

What about symptom relief? As Dr. Preston and others have pointed out, any procedure that reduces anxiety will produce symptomatic improvement. If the patient is convinced the therapy is 'good', he'll report feeling better.

"Think of the patient, who's been told: 'You're a living time bomb'. Then we operate on him and two months later, we tell him 'you're cured' and put him on a treadmill to test his improvement. And does he go to it! He reports 'I'm much better'.

"To what can we attribute his progress? Clearly there's an emotional factor involved. He's been told he's better, he has a vested interest in his operation paying off, and he reports tremendous results as expected. Interestingly enough, there's a study that shows people normally do better on second treadmill tests, even with no intervening therapy or treatment, simply because they are more comfortable with the procedure. They know they won't fall off, drop dead, whatever, etc.. There's a powerful psychological component to this that cannot be lightly dismissed."

An article in *Internal Medicine News* points out that for many patients, symptom relief is distressingly short-term. "Thirty to fifty percent of those who undergo surgery have a recurrence of symptoms within the first year. Even those patients who remain asymptomatic after one year, report a return of angina at a three to five percent rate in subsequent years. Usually the new symptoms are due to a progression of the underlying disease."

The analysis does not surprise, Robert J. Hall, clinical professor of medicine at Baylor College of Medicine, who has commented: "Bypass surgery is not curing the disease. It is "modifying it with a piece of pipe."

Not only is the disease not cured, it almost inevitably returns - only quicker than before. One bypass procedure almost inevitably leads to the need for another, as Dr. Norman Ratlif at the Cleveland Clinic has reported. While coronary artery blockage normally takes about forty years, the grafts implanted during bypass surgery suffer accelerated plaque build-up and usually block again within five to ten years.

What does bypass do best? It bypasses the real problem. It's a patchwork solution to a degenerative disease that effects the entire arterial system, not just one or two replaceable main vessels.

'BYPASS' ON THE DECLINE?

There are signs the bypass procedure is on the wane at long last. The American public is becoming more sophisticated, more learned, more inclined to think for themselves, less disposed to be 'bypassed' merely because "the doctor says so." People are catching on to the profits and politics of the heart disease industry. Articles such as appeared in *Business Week*, hailing Dr. Denton Cooley's new supermarket assembly-line approach to bypass surgery - he's doing six to eight surgeries a day at cut-rate prices to recover from personal bankruptcy - have turned the naive into cynics.

In addition, there's been so much unfavorable publicity about bypass surgery - the darling of the American cardiology business for more than two decades - that even the most trusting individuals suspect that much of the surgery that's prescribed is designed to benefit the surgeon's end-of-the-year balance sheet.

The suspicious are right on target. As the $3 million, five year Rand Corporation study showed, coronary bypass surgery, carotid endarterectomy (the removal of blockages from one or both arteries carrying blood to the brain), and angiography (the pre-surgical x-ray technique to detect blocked arteries) are "significantly overused procedures".

The study's findings: 65% of carotid endarterectomies were done for inappropriate or questionable reasons; 17% of the angiograms were clearly inappropriate; as were an alarming percentage of the bypass procedures. When California researchers looked into this same issue, they found nearly half of the patients who had heart bypass operations in three hospitals either should not have had the procedures or could have done as well without them. Only 56 percent of the coronary bypass operations performed in three randomly chosen hospitals were justified. Thirty percent were done for equivocal reasons - meaning they could be argued either way No wonder many more people are asking questions, getting second and third opinions, seeking alternatives.

Although bypass surgery is still a $6 billion a year industry, and the latest figures show increasing numbers of procedures every year from 1979 on, alternative therapies are becoming more popular, especially in the last five years. That's turning out to be a mixed bag. Knife-happy specialists don't give up a procedure until they've latched on to a profitable substitute. As might be expected, dramatic new high-tech procedures have been introduced. Many of these are equally unproven, ineffective, profit-motivated and risky as the bypass they've replaced. Most are enthusiastically prescribed by the very same physicians who only a short time ago heartily advocated the discredited bypass.

What good is it that more people turn thumbs down to bypass, when they're not offered a more promising substitute? Let's take a look at what happened to Bill Thompson, the heart patient we met at the start of this chapter.

Instead of submitting to surgery, Thompson signed on with a doctor who treats conditions like his with a non-invasive outpatient procedure consisting of a series of intravenous infusions of a synthetic amino acid, ethylene diamine-tetraacetric acid. This man-made protein is popularly called EDTA.

After three months - approximately thirty sessions - Bill's blood pressure read 120/68. Non-invasive testing revealed arterial blockage had been dramatically reduced, heart function was fifty percent better, and Doppler readings showed impressive improvement in circulation throughout his body, especially to his extremities - fingers and toes. His disability rating was reduced to 5%.

More gratifying still, Bill felt more like his pre-diseased self. He could walk the golf course - and carry his bags - instead of needing a golf cart and caddy; he didn't run out of energy at noon; he could out-walk, out-talk and out-distance others his age without breathing hard.

Every day chelation doctors discharge many Bill Thompson treatment-twins - all feel-a-likes when it comes to proving there's a real alternative to bypass and other unnecessarily aggressive procedures. Once you meet someone who's been chelated, you're bound to ask, "How come I never heard about this before?"

We'll save that story for the next chapter.

2

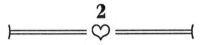

...BUT YOU CAN'T FOOL ALL OF THE PEOPLE ALL OF THE TIME

Although over half a million people have experienced
chelation therapy over the past 30 years, less than one percent
of the population has ever heard of it. How come?

In 1947, a commission formed to investigate the status of
freedom in the press, found the news is "twisted by pressure
groups." Some 45 years later, nothing has changed. *Accuracy
in Media,* a public interest group headed by Reed Irvine, has
documented hundreds of cases in which the news media
manipulated public opinion by distorting the facts.

The average citizen, not privy to the behind-the-scenes
shenanigans of pharmaceutical, medical and food industry
cronies, would be shocked to learn to what extent these
powerhouses are able to distort science news. Few readers
suspect science news is frequently as biased as editorial page
opinions, only not as honestly identified. Take it from journalists
who have fought hard for a more balanced approach, medical

coverage is slanted against the non-orthodox view.

To go back a few years, one of our first important assignments was to discredit non-traditional medicine as quackery. In those days, nutritionally-oriented health professionals were all but ignored. Whenever they condemned nutrient-deficient processed foods, their views were pooh-poohed, as were their expressed concerns that the chemical-laden American diet was potentially carcinogenic. When they suggested that what you ate had something to do with your health, they were ridiculed. The notion that health could be improved by natural means was tantamount to waving a red flag - only communist sympathizers would promote so subversive an idea.

"Find out what those vitamin pushers are up to," our editor ordered. "Get the goods on them. How many people have died because they were diverted from legitimate treatment? Bring me numbers."

WHY TAKE MEDICAL ADVICE FROM A SICK DOCTOR?

The meetings we attended featured such noted mavericks as Linus Pauling, E. Cheraskin, Roger Williams, the Shute brothers and Carlton Fredericks. Instead of uncovering grounds to discredit them, we found cause to convert to their point of view. Why? What they said made sense. Viewed as a group, doctors who allied themselves with the holistic health movement, seemed a heck of a lot healthier than their AMA counterparts. In contrast to other medical meetings, those held by doctors intent on disease prevention did not lead off with a "moment of silence for the recently departed," nor did their program chairmen routinely solicit get-well cards for hospitalized colleagues.

When *Psychodietetics,* co-authored with Dr. E. Cheraskin, made the case for "you are what you eat," it was the first book to establish a scientific link between food and mood.

The psychiatric community considered it heresy and attacked. The *Psychology Today* review which ridiculed the book's thesis, demonstrated how easily the 'in-crowd' can command media clout to undermine the credibility of competitive ideas.

Dr. Cheraskin's scheduled book promotion tour was short-circuited in deference to pressure from anti-nutrition groups. At the very last minute, NBC's *Today Show* canceled him out. Pushed for an explanation, an underling confessed there'd been "so much guff from upstairs," the program manager chickened out. Even small town radio and TV stations were nervous about giving favorable exposure to a nutrition advocate. When invited to appear, Dr. Cheraskin, a world renowned lecturer in great demand, had to share the spotlight with a clique of vocal critics, and was usually outnumbered.

WHO'S LISTENING NOW? EVERYBODY!

Almost twenty years later, the very same nutritional principles hooted off the airwaves in 1974 are the accepted wisdom. The food dyes we deplored are outlawed. In the 1970's, only fanatics read food labels. Today, almost everyone does it. Those were the days when Vitamins E and C were like Rodney Dangerfield. They "got no respect". Now you can stock up on those supplements without hunting through back alley shops. The giant markets that sneered at 'natural' foods now hawk them. Nutritionally-oriented food features are standard fare in every major newspaper and magazine.

How come? The about-face appears to be based more on economic reality than scientific discovery. Now that well-heeled advertisers - the major food manufacturers - have found they can make big bucks selling 'health' foods, they get the editorial support that moves product. The truth is: science news is for sale.

How do we know? We've had more than our fair share of stories blue-penciled for only one reason. They conflicted with editorial policies that were either ad-revenue or AMA-dictated. "Kill this stuff about nutrient-deficient processed foods. Our supermarkets won't like it"; "Why are you quoting these loonies about vitamin cures for depression? Want us barred from the next psychiatric convention?"

Only the naive fail to recognize to what extent advertisers control editorial content. Have you never noticed that you're more apt to get the lowdown on the dangers of smoking from TV (they can't carry cigarette advertising) than from your favorite magazine or newspaper (which still does)?

Editors who personally eat 'lite', pop vitamins and visit holistic doctors, routinely 'kill' medical stories that violate the paper's 'party line'. The American Cancer Society, American Heart Association, and the Arthritis Association are but a few of the powerful self-serving organizations often allowed to 'clear' all stories concerning 'their' disease.

For example: did you ever hear about the prominent official within the National Cancer Institute who spearheaded the drive against 'alternative' therapies? What happened when he discovered HE had cancer? He refused chemotherapy and all NCI-recommended treatments and took off for Europe for the very therapies he'd decried. How come you don't know that?

Sometimes it gets funny. We once did a human interest piece about a couple who lost custody of their two-year old adopted child. The birth mother recanted and took the babe back with the help of an insensitive judge. It was a real tear-jerker. When we described the adoptive parents as "heartbroken," the editor, scanning the copy quickly, underlined the word "heart" and asked, "Did you check this out with the AHA?" Enough said.

What has all this to do with chelation? It's a treatment that has never had a fair hearing.

WHO DECIDES WHICH NEWS IS FIT TO PRINT?

"It's a crime," charges Dr. E. W. McDonagh who has assembled thousands of documented case histories of recovered 'untreatable' patients, "that news of this breakthrough treatment for heart disease, diabetes and stroke has been purposely withheld from the public."

On the few occasions the subject has been addressed by the national media, the coverage has been clearly one-sided. When Dan Rather did a short piece on chelation therapy - *Miracle or Menace?* - on the CBS *Evening News* (December 11th, 1984) - skeptics monopolized the presentation. Requests for equal time were ignored. Censorious newspaper and magazine stories routinely appear in print, with little apparent effort to assure balanced coverage, or scientific fact. NBC's *Hard Copy* recently did a similar 'slash and burn' report with all-too-familiar anti-chelation bias.

An article on chelation which appeared in the September, 1988 issue of *Practical Cardiology* is typical. Entitled "Sham Therapy in Coronary Artery Disease and Atherosclerosis," the item was short on science, long on unsubstantiated attack. It cited 20 year old research, distorted to prove their anti-chelation case. The editors should have been ashamed to print such slander in a publication which is itself a 'sham journal' - a free circulation publication that does not submit articles for peer review.

The copy-cat media periodically publish 'hand-outs' from self-interest groups under the guise of 'news'. Most recently, science editors nationwide ran a story headlined "TOP TEN HEALTH FRAUDS IN THE U.S." as though they'd discovered something newsworthy. It was the same old list that arrives periodically on the science news desk, complements of the FDA. Among those publishing the alleged "hot news" was NBC's medical spokesperson, Dr. Dean Edell, who charges $24.00 for a 10-month subscription for his *Health Letter.*

On this occasion, the item should have proved embarrassing. Chelation therapy was Number Eight on the FDA's official list at the same time that agency was sponsoring clinical trials of the treatment at two VA Hospitals. What happened when the outraged government-approved researchers called this inconsistency to attention? Nothing. The FDA quietly revised its list; now there are only *nine* 'health frauds'. The media, of course, didn't comment on the change, nor have any retracted the original item.

Most papers routinely refuse all pro-chelation stories. The *National Enquirer*, the nation's leading tabloid, once turned down a paid ad for a book favorable to chelation, presumably because the publisher had close ties to the American Heart Association. There's an ironic aftermath: a few months afterwards, Gene Pope, Jr., the *Enquirer's* publisher, suddenly died of a heart attack at a relatively young age (61). The information he denied his readers might have saved his life.

Not even entertainment programs are free of AMA interference. When CBS announced the prime-time medical series, *Island Son,* featuring Richard Chamberlain (best known as TV's Dr. Kildare) - establishment docs demanded, and got, script approval.

"No go," was their decision, after viewing the pilot, which depicted Chamberlain as 'Dr. Daniel Kulani', a Hawaiian-based holistically-oriented, non-mainstream physician. Chastised for making a hero of an off-beat doc, CBS officials kowtowed to clout, and revised the story line.

If the same TV networks that have allowed viewers to witness history in the making - the Chinese students battling the tanks in Tiananmen Square, the destruction of the Berlin Wall, the Senate's inquisition of Clarence Thomas - refuse you a glimpse of the miracles taking place in a chelation clinic, where can you learn about them?

Will a doctor unfamililar with chelation therapy tell you about it? Scant chance. How about the The American Heart

Association? That organization has issued an unsubstantiated anti-chelation statement (see Chapter Twelve) designed to scare people off.

"Our recommendation," AHA officials state, "is this therapy not be widely applied until it has been tested in properly controlled trials." That's a laugh. Only "10 to 20 percent of all procedures currently used in medical practice have been shown to be efficacious (that means 'proven to work') by controlled trial."

Who says so? The U.S. Government, by way of the Office of Technology Assessment, an official watchdog agency commissioned by the U.S. Congress. By contrast, chelation therapy has 'been tested' and 'proven' in the best of all labs - by the many sick people who have taken the treatment and gotten well.

According to Dr. Ross Gordon, one of the founders and a former president of the American College of Advancement in Medicine, "Our group has verifiable medical data on more than 500,000 patients who have received EDTA chelation therapy since the early fifties. Over 85% of those treated received at least some benefit; more than 20% who had been given up for dead by orthodox physicians, are still around and enjoying life. Adverse reactions are practically nonexistent. There have been fewer than 30 EDTA-related deaths in comparison with the more than 18,000 deaths as a direct consequence of bypass surgery in the same period."

IT'S NOT WHAT YOU KNOW BUT WHO YOU KNOW

If knowledge of chelation therapy is so hard to come by, how do people find out about it? When we asked 120 randomly selected chelation patients, "How did you learn of this therapy?", the results of our survey supported suspicions that few got the word the way people usually get news.

Our findings:
- 77% heard of chelation therapy from someone successfully treated or who knew about somebody who'd benefited from chelation;
- 16% read about it in a specialized book, magazine or newsletter that covers the holistic health field;
- 4% were informed by a nutritionally-oriented dentist;
- 2% searched out information in the medical literature;
- Only 1 individual was referred by his doctors and was warned, "Don't use my name or let on that I told you."

Most people learn about chelation therapy over the back fence, by accident, or by word of mouth. Unless you happen to be on good terms with an informed, talkative friend, relative or neighbor, or luck on to this book, you might never hear one good word about it!

Doesn't it say something meaningful about this treatment that despite organized resistance, suppression of the facts, a bad press, and the active hostility of so many professionals, chelation continues to gain ground? Doesn't it prove something strange is going on when each year, chelation grows more popular, attracts more patients and doctors? Isn't it more reasonable to believe the medical monopoly has conspired to distort the truth to maintain their heart disease profits than there's something mentally amiss with the the thousands of patients who claim to have been cured by chelation?

A WORD OF WISDOM FROM HOLLYWOOD

More important, perhaps, is the larger issue: what does this controversy reveal about the way unconventional remedies that compete with traditional modalities are renounced without a fair trial? In the movie *Tucker - The Man, the Car, The Dream* - the hero attempted to produce a car more than forty years ahead of its time. It featured aerodynamic styling, a padded dash, pop-out windows, seat belts, fuel injection, disc brakes and many advances reluctantly adopted by Detroit many years later. Crushed by the big auto makers, Tucker made a dramatic plea for an end to bureaucratic dictatorship over innovative ideas.

This is what he said: "We invented the free enterprise system - that's what this country is all about - where, anybody no matter who he was, where he came from, what class he belonged to, if he came up with a better idea about anything, there was no limit to how far he could go. Now the way the system works, the loner, the dreamer, the crackpot who comes up with a crazy idea that everyone laughs at, that later turns out to revolutionize the world, is squashed from above before he ever gets his head out of the water by bureaucrats ready to kill anyone who might rock the boat."

It's not just a movie. It's not just the automobile business. Tucker's words apply all too well to the medical bureaucracy. His warning, "We're not only closing the door on progress, but sabotaging everything the country stands for," could as easily refer to the demise of U.S. health care leadership as to Detroit's lost clout.

How has it happened? What is this controversial therapy? Where did it come from? What does it do? How does it work? As Golda Meir said to Anwar Sadat when they finally met: "What took you so long?" We thought you'd never ask.

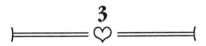

BAD NEWS TRAVELS FAST
GOOD NEWS TRAVELS SLOW

We must go back almost one hundred years to trace the origins of chelation therapy. In 1893, Alfred Werner, a French-Swiss chemist laid the groundwork for modern bio-chemistry by developing the theory of what he called "co-ordination compounds" - now known as "chelates." In 1913, he received the Nobel prize for his monumental work. Like the many chelation-related discoveries since, Werner's prize-winning finding was a serendipitous happening, the first of a series of such occurrences.

"I woke one day at 2 AM, with the entire theory flashing through my consciousness, and by 5 AM worked out all the essential features," Werner said. He was amazed that so complex a method of reclassifying inorganic chemical compounds could have presented itself in this astonishing way. Two textbooks and 150 technical papers later, Werner had established the concepts explaining how metals bind to organic molecules, forming the basis for chelation chemistry.

It was not until the 1920's, however, that the industrial world found practical applications for Werner's theories. Back in those days, heavy metal contamination was less a 'people' problem than a manufacturing concern. The paint, rubber, petroleum, and electroplating industries were all just getting started. Finding some way to purge specific unwanted metals during the production process was an absolute 'must'. A massive search was on for 'chelating' agents that would bind (ala Werner's theories) and eliminate corrupting substances. The leeching process was especially critical to the manufacture of industrial dyes, where an errant metal could stain a fabric and wreck an entire textile print run.

Among the many compounds tried and tested, citric acid earned a top rating. In the mid-1930's, that substance was not satisfactory to German industrialists, many of whom were secretly funding the new Nazi party. Privy to Hitler's militaristic ambitions, magnates of business and industry were uncomfortable with reliance on an import that could only be obtained from potentially unfriendly countries.

SOMETIMES GOOD THINGS COME FROM BAD PEOPLE

As insiders, they knew what the rest of the world was beginning to suspect: the Nazi party was building a powerful war machine. Spurred on by this knowledge and the realization that German industry would soon have to be more self-reliant, industrialists pushed leading scientists to develop "ersatz" products. Among other substitutes given a top priority was something to replace citric acid - they desperately needed a synthetic calcium-binding additive that would keep stains from forming when mineral-hardened water reacted with dyes.

Serendipitous event Number Two.

The urgent project paid off with an unexpected reward: the researchers accomplished their mission, and delivered more than anyone had bargained for. The substance they developed in 1935 - ethylene-diamine-tetra-acetate (EDTA) was more effective and less expensive than the citric acid it was designed to replace. They secured a patent, and began production. At first, distribution was concentrated in Germany, but as its reputation spread, and despite escalating international tensions, Germany began shipping this high-profit substance all over the world.

As EDTA's unique properties became better known, commercial uses expanded both in the U.S. and abroad. Eventually it became an essential ingredient in hundreds of familiar consumer products. EDTA was on an industrial 'roll'. More than half a century after its initial discovery, assorted businesses continue to find new manufacturing applications.

EDTA: A NEW HOUSEHOLD WORD

Check the labels in your cupboard, and you'll find it listed as an ingredient in many canned, bottled and packaged foodstuffs requiring a preservative, from muffin mix to mayonnaise. If it were not for EDTA, your laundry detergent would not work nearly as well. Neither would other cleansers, which rely on its chelating action to vanquish unsightly scum and residue from dishes, clothes, and around wash basins and tubs.

EDTA might have remained an industrial agent, were it not for **serendipitous event Number Three.** Call it coincidence, happenstance, or what have you, pure chance brought attention to its potential for medicinal use.

In the early 1930's, only cock-eyed optimists refused to believe World War II was in the offing. Realists, especially those in the military, not only expected a massive confrontation, but feared the impending conflict would include combat with poison gas.

The prospect posed so fearsome a threat, the Allies launched a frantic search for antidotes. Enter chelation. A team of British researchers headed by the brilliant Oxford University professor R. A. Peters, came up with BAL (British Anti-Lewsite) a chelating compound able to drastically diminish the harmful effects of arsenic in poison gas compounds. It was the first time scientists developed a drug for such a purpose. The far-reaching significance of that discovery was not apparent at the time.

The fear of poison gas attack proved groundless. Nevertheless, researchers had readied chelating agents for an entirely new role - removing toxic substances from humans. It marked the beginning of chelation therapy as we know it today.

The war over, the world breathed a sigh of relief and the victors were able to sleep comfortably at night - but not for long. A new and even graver threat soon supplanted the former menace. With the advent of atomic warfare, nuclear destruction was clearly a hazard. All along America's east coast, people scurried to build backyard bomb shelters. Cuban rockets aimed at the Florida coast gave school children nightmares. The rush was on to find a defense against radioactive fallout.

The solution? EDTA: the most effective chelating agent resourceful government scientists could find, was stockpiled in secret locations all across this land. EDTA, the American scientists claimed, was not only more effective than the Brit's BAL, but caused fewer adverse side effects. So far, the therapeutic potential of chelating agents had been only theoretical. There'd been no chemical warfare; no radioactive fallout in the U.S. or elsewhere. No one was eager to find out whether speculation would prove out or not. EDTA for medicinal use, never tested, was put on a back shelf with the hope it would never be needed.

The perception of EDTA as basically an emergency antidote for a wartime horror, held firm until one day in the summer of 1947. Dr. Charles Geschickter at the Georgetown University Medical Center decided it was time to try it out on a patient.

EDTA: A DOCTOR'S FRIEND

"A momentous day," Dr. Martin Rubin, a colleague on the scene at the time, reported. "Back then, you didn't need to fill out a bunch of forms or wade through months or years of red tape for approval to try something new. Once we had the idea, we just grabbed a vial out of the lab, dashed across the street to the hospital, and went to it."

The patient chosen was suffering from advanced breast cancer. The chemotherapy used to treat her contained highly toxic nickel complexes. As is often the case, the drugs designed to stem the disease were causing havoc. The doctors recognized a pressing need to clear the poisonous metals out her system before deadly side effects won out. They knew of nothing other than EDTA worth a try, administered a dose as best they could and held their breath. When tests showed the EDTA had worked as they hoped it might, and the patient was cheerfully unaffected, there was much to cheer.

That was as far as it went. The experiment, albeit successful, seemingly held no great future promise. Not until the gods once again stepped in, bringing us to **serendipitous event Number Four,** was there a further opportunity for chelation to prove itself.

EDTA: THE WORKER'S FRIEND

In the early 1950's, workers in a Michigan battery plant began getting sick - then sicker, and sicker. The problem was soon diagnosed as lead poisoning, a common condition among exposed employees. Management called in Dr. Norman E. Clarke, Sr., a prominent cardiologist at Providence Hospital in Detroit.

He proved to be a lucky choice. After successfully detoxifying all who fell ill, this astute physician recognized EDTA's potential significance thanks to an unexpected consequence.

Not only did the lead-poisoned recover, they also reported relief from chest pains - a symptom associated with athero sclerosis.

Soon afterward, U.S. Navy commanders discovered that sailors detailed to repaint old war ships were evidencing frightening symptoms. They reported memory loss, irritability, an inability to concentrate, disturbed equilibrium, ringing in the ears, leg cramps, and a variety of other health problems usually associated with aging.

"It's lead poisoning," Navy doctors concluded. Once again the treatment of choice was EDTA! As it turned out, they chanced onto a history-making prescription. The treated sailors spontaneously reported unanticipated health benefits. Among the varied improvements were increased endurance, improved stamina, better memory, enhanced vision, hearing and smell, clearer thinking, fewer headaches, less anxiety. Those with early signs of arthritis or atherosclerosis enjoyed even more extraordinary recovery - increased mobility, reduced leg cramps, easier breathing.

With almost identical unanticipated health improvements showing up in two unrelated groups, word of the dramatic results circulated, and prominent cardiologists began to take note. The question buzzing through medical circles: coincidence or concrete evidence of a new cure?

Two Wayne State University heart specialists, Drs. Albert J. Boyle and Gordon B. Myers, determined to put chelation to the test, selected 'basket cases' as guinea pigs. They searched out patients so debilitated by vascular disease, there was no other hope for them. One of the chosen was in a sorry state indeed. He had a heart valve damaged beyond repair, and no physician expected him to live very long. When his name was proposed as a potential chelation candidate, the selection committee scoffed, thinking it ludicrous to include him in the trials.

All chosen patients had one thing in common. They were so sick, it could be truly said: "They've nothing to lose." No one could have predicted the result. All improved - even those with supposedly incurable conditions came back to life. The sickest among them were restored to near-normal function.

Clinicians are by nature a conservative lot. Much as they dislike being first to gamble on an untried therapy, they hate being last! As word spread that a near-miraculous treatment was rescuing patients from almost certain death, the rush was on to duplicate results.

EDTA: EVERYONE'S FRIEND

From 1950 through 1966, U.S. and foreign medical journals were chock full of tweedledee-tweedledum reports. No distinguished scientist wanted to be left behind in the "publish-or-perish" race to research and extol the wonders of chelation therapy for atherosclerosis and related disorders.

In 1964, Dr. Alfred Soffer, then Director of the Cardiopulmonary Laboratory at Rochester General Hospital and an Associate in Medicine at Northwestern University Medical School, published a treatise on chelation therapy in concert with distinguished colleagues Drs. Martin Rubin, Maynard Chenoweth and Herta Spencer among others. Their findings added up to a huge vote of confidence for this treatment for victims of cardiovascular disease. Among the documentation presented in their 163 page report were patients suffering from advanced ulceration and necrosis of the big toes, whose gangrenous feet they saved from amputation.

"In summary," the doctors wrote, sufferers of atherosclerotic peripheral vascular disease appear to be "benefited by repeated administration of chelating agents." They found the process "particularly promising in patients with diabetes whose lower extremities have been effected by reduced circulation."

They cited the case of a sixty-seven year old man with seriously advanced atherosclerosis with ulcerated lower extremities due to loss of circulation. After twenty chelation treatments, they were able to discharge the patient "with ulcers and open sores completely healed."

For more than fifteen years, study after study - (from Belknap, Butler. Spencer, Vankinscott and Lewin in 1952 to Birk and Rupe in 1966) - reported the same remarkable results. In 1975, Drs. Gordon and Harper reviewed all pro-chelation studies to that date, and produced a collection of more than 300 papers, all authored by prestigious and reputable scientists. Their findings were remarkably consistent. Every report described definite improvement in the patient's circulation as evidenced by better skin color, return of normal temperature to the feet, a regained ability to walk long distances, elimination of angina pain, improved memory and mental acuity. Usually, patients could discard pain relievers and other drugs. In many instances, the therapy also improved kidney function, decreased the amount of insulin required by diabetics and produced significant improvement in arthritis. In some instances, Parkinson's disease sufferers improved.

EDTA: NO ONE'S FRIEND?

If you're confused by what you've read thus far, no wonder. Every thoughtful person must marvel that the 'miracle' treatment of the 1960's was assigned "fraud" status not many years later. Welcome to the real world. When things don't make sense, check out the money trail. The chance for megabuck profits is just as apt to decide which treatments are featured and marketed by the medical monopoly as in any competitive arena.

In the late 1960's, a Philadelphia physician, Dr. John G. Gibson, perfected his heart-lung machine, making open heart surgery conceivable. The advent of this technological marvel proved a mixed bag. A remarkable mechanical achievement, it made many otherwise impossible potentially life-saving procedures available. Among them, of course, was the bypass operation, which might have proven a remarkable advantage, had it been held in check and prescribed discretely.

That's not the way it happened. Although historical experience warns that new health measures should be tried and tested before adoption, the bypass operation captured the attention of television journalists. Cardiovascular surgeons found themselves the stars of a dramatic, and wildly profitable procedure.

From 1967 on, bypass operations became increasingly popular, thanks in part to the efforts of charismatic surgeons like Dr. Denton Cooley. He played up the theatrics of the procedure by inviting the TV cameras into the surgical suite. Irresponsible medical reporters didn't bother to note the bypass operation had "passed Go" without scientific scrutiny. Never properly evaluated, it became an overnight sensation, without proving its worth in clinical trials. Exaggerated claims for benefits bombarded the public thanks to the misguided enthusiasm of the popular press, and without objective review.

Few people in those days, from either side of the hospital bed, were asking the 'right' questions. No one demanded proof the operation worked. Cardiac surgeons and the hospitals that geared up for production-line bypasses, hurried to capitalize on the new specialty. They proceeded with the full blessings of the medical establishment, reaped the bonanza of a zillion dollars worth of free publicity, and it's been going on ever since.

Too many health professionals have too much to gain from the bypass industry to call a halt, even in the face of accumulating evidence that many have been duped. Anesthetists, operating team personnel, coronary care unit staff, radiologists, technicians, hospital administrators - some forty-five specialists in all - owe their sizable paychecks to the steady stream of bypass patients coming through their doors. Few are so noble they can afford to look beyond their own interests and protest the advisability of a methodology that's feeding the kids and paying the rent.

On the contrary, self-serving bypass proponents continue to withhold facts, misrepresent and distort benefits, and viciously oppose the one therapy that might doom them to the unemployment lines. When the early glowing reports of chelation therapy are brought to attention, they call the research "inadequate", "faulty", "bad science" or "outright mistakes." They've resorted to massive pro-bypass propaganda to blast the chelation alternative out of the picture.

How blatantly corrupt have the anti-chelation forces been? On April 4, 1991, Kay Pierson, a Washington, D.C. anti-trust lawyer, requested the Federal Trade Commission to investigate the AMA, Federation of State Licensing Boards, Blue Cross/Blue Shield and Health Care Anti-Fraud Association. As basis for her request, Ms. Pierson supplied the FTC with a seventy-five page fact-filled document supporting her allegation that the parties charged are involved in a conspiracy to stop/stymie the growth and development of alternative medicine in the U.S..

Given full particulars, people suffering obstructed blood vessels would be irrational to choose bypass over chelation therapy. The one bypasses a small segment of diseased vessel; the other helps clear the entire arterial system. The one is hazardous, expensive, and requires extensive hospitalization; the other is relatively inexpensive, pain free, safe, effective and convenient. Surgery is traumatic, disruptive, and requires a prolonged hospital stay; chelation is easily available on an outpatient basis in a practitioner's office - no stress, no fuss. What a deal!

Now forty-something years after its introduction, where does chelation therapy stand today? We'll let chelated patients, the people who know best, tell you.

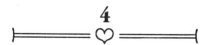

4

BACK IN CIRCULATION

Once American medical practitioners had a reputation as the most honorable in the world. However, that was a long time ago, when New World medicine was one of the great advantages of Colonial life in America, as historians report. In its infancy, this country's medical practice was in the hands of naturalists and botanists. For the most part, they were young, open-minded explorers, eager to discover new cures and treatments among the many unfamiliar plants and animals peculiar to the American continent.

While their European counterparts were bound by dogma, with every eminent professor of medicine seeking prominence by arguing for acceptance for his exotic remedies, things were different in the new land. American physicians relied on simpler, more common-sensical treatments. Instead of the elaborate European concoctions that included human excreta, urine and other abominable preparations, new world healers prescribed good food and enough of it, pure air and water, cleanliness, TLC (tender loving care), and two or three common drugs when needed. They prescribed a glass of good wine when patients needed the very best stimulant. Unlike their European counterparts, American doctors carried on their profession in a most encouraging environment. They were totally free to learn from experience.

Apprenticeship to an older, wiser doctor was the usual path to becoming a physician. The transfer of learning took place quite naturally and was based on simple pragmatism. Their credo: What works, works. What seemed obvious then, is all but outlawed now. Medicine today has become so 'scientific', doctors are no longer permitted to give credence to the testimonials of the cured.

Thus, although hundreds of qualified physicians have practiced chelation safely and effectively in the United States and sixteen foreign countries for more than four decades, traditional medicine continues to scoff. Parrot-like they repeat the monotonous oft-repeated criticism: "It's never been tested or proved."

That's a strange criticism considering, as previously mentioned, so few procedures in current use have passed the stringent review demanded of chelation. We've estimated that several million patients have been successfully chelated over the past forty years. Powerful numbers should speak for themselves. More on this later.

AND NOW A WORD FROM 'REAL PEOPLE'

"Your treatments have turned my life around," Mrs. Ann Checkal told Dr. H. Richard Casdorph. "Before I found you, instead of half over, I felt my life was all over."

Talk about unlikely comebacks, EDTA helped this 46-year old lady overcome so many miseries, she's our nomination for the 1989 Miraculous Recovery of the Year award. When she first enlisted Dr. Casdorph's help, she recited a laundry list of problems that included serious hypertension, diabetes, a variety of circulatory disorders and multiple strokes, and a debilitating weakness of the muscles on her right side, from her face to her legs.

From 1987 on, she'd had episodes of slurred speech - some lasting three weeks at a time - and in December of 1988, an ambulance rushed her to the hospital totally paralyzed and unable to speak. For the next few months, she could not get out of bed for two to three days at a time.

Few would predict a happy ending to so horror-filled a litany. Yet, six months after stepping into Dr. C's office, she was back in circulation, no longer bedridden, with normal blood pressure, free of recurring heart irregularities, blood sugars under control, and off all medications. As you might suspect, both patient and doctor celebrated.

"It's like a miracle. I feel like I did fifteen years ago before I became a basket case," the lady crowed. How does Dr. Casdorph explain such a miracle?

"Not me - the EDTA did it," he modestly reports. "It was nothing unusual. I gave her a series of chelation treatments. While all patients do not respond as dramatically or as quickly, we have seen so many similar results, we expect significant improvement in almost every patient who receives this therapy."

How many doctors could matter-of-factly express such confidence in their treatments? How many physicians have patients who are walking testimonials to their mastery of the healing arts? Hundreds, in fact, can make the same claim and chances are, you've not heard of one of these physicians. They should be famous, but they're not.

That's not surprising, since you won't find chelation doctors in prominent locations. They're not headquartered at big medical centers, in university-affiliated hospitals or research centers, in government-funded clinics or labs.

Most of the more than 1,200 chelationists are in private practice, and keep a low profile, content to let their patients do their advertising for them.

IS YOUR DOCTOR A 'MIRACLE WORKER'?

Ask any run-of-the-mill physician for a case history of a miracle recovery, and he's apt to tell you, "Miracles? I don't think I have any." Pose the same question to any chelation doctor, and he'll rattle off as many detailed tales of near-death recoveries he's overseen as you've patience to hear. In this regard, Dr. Gordon H. Josephs is typical.

"Let me tell you about Wilda, who was eighty years old, and totally dependent on her married daughter. Poor lady - she hated being a burden, but she'd become so frail, she couldn't shop, clean or do much for herself - couldn't even write checks. Worse still, she'd been having episodes that left her unable to move or speak. Her family doctor suspected small strokes, and when tests revealed her carotid artery was 90% blocked, the surgeons wanted to operate as quickly as they could.

"But Wilda didn't want any part of it. A neighbor had told her about chelation therapy and she talked her family into bringing her to me. Three weeks later, after only nine treatments, she was a 'liberated lady'. `I can get to the doctor's office myself,' she told her daughter, and began taking the bus. She's never had another stroke, and is now totally self-sufficient. She walks thirty minutes a day for exercise and the fun of it."

One good tale leads easily to another. Dr. Josephs has other cases to boast about.

"Then there was Blanche. She was 73 and had bypass surgery sometime back before she came to me. The operation hadn't helped. She could not walk the length of her mobile home due to pain in her legs and swollen ankles. Any mild exertion - dusting, fixing dinner, cleaning her parakeet's cage

- left her weak and exhausted. I gave Blanche twenty-six chelation treatments in all. That's all it took to get her back on her feet once more. Last I heard, she was tramping up and down Albany's hilly streets. That's her home town. She's been taking long walks and visiting with old friends."

Without missing a beat, Dr. Josephs insisted on telling us about Richard - " . . . sixty-seven when I first saw him. He was an outdoor enthusiast - a rock hound, a mountain climber and a fresh water fisherman. He'd begun having alarming symptoms - pulsing sensations around his neck and face, ringing in his ears, numbness in his arms and legs. He'd become short of breath and needed a stocking cap to keep his head warm - even indoors. He worried that a stroke lurked in the future.

"Sixteen chelation treatments later, Richard was back in the wilds of the north woods doing his thing. He sent me a postcard that read: Guess what, doc? No more stocking cap needed.'

Dr. Josephs not only has lots of great patients; he also has a remarkable memory. "I'll never forget Don," he continued. "He was forty-five and a football fanatic, utterly distraught because his angina had gotten so bad he could no longer trek up that long hill leading to ASU's Sun Devil stadium to root for his team. Constantly tired, there were days he didn't want to get out of bed.

"Missing football games worried him worse than having to cancel appointments at his hairdressing shop. His biggest worry was his cardiologist found he had four blocked arteries - one 50%, one 60% one 75% and 100% - and insisted he have bypass surgery.

"I've heard a lot of reasons why people don't want to have an operation, but this one took the cake," Dr. Josephs said. "What Don said when he came in to see me was, 'I can't afford to miss the whole football season. So, I'll do what one of my football buddies did - get chelated instead.' He took twenty-six treatments, and after six months, was pain free, full of energy, and could bicycle the seven miles to his shop. He hasn't missed a day of work - or a football game - since.

"Nothing beats Helen, though. If there's anything worse than being old and sick, it's being old, sick AND broke! Having no funds or health insurance turned out to be lucky for this lady, because it saved her from surgery. An angiography at County Hospital revealed three blocked arteries, but because she was too poor to pay for a bypass, they sent her home. She was extremely ill, completely exhausted, unable to stand, and short of breath.

"I heard of her case, took her on and started chelation. Am I glad! After just two treatments - TWO, mind you - she got up from her wheelchair and walked on her own. All the patients in my treatment room cheered!

MORE RUN-OF-THE-MILL EVERYDAY 'MIRACLES'

"Linda was only 37, but the diabetes she'd had since age 19 was causing serious health problems. Despite taking insulin twice daily, the disease was taking its toll. She'd already had several laser eye operations to treat her macular degeneration and progressive blindness. Then she began developing open sores on the tips of her toes - the first signs of circulatory disorders that inevitably lead to gangrene in diabetics.

"Linda learned conventional medicine has nothing to offer but amputation. Her doctors objected to chelation, but Linda felt she had nothing to lose, and came for treatments. After fifteen, her toes had healed. When her ophthalmologist next tested her vision, he was astounded to find it had improved from 20/200 to 20/70, and called it `a real miracle.' Linda never let on to what treatment she'd been taking, but comes in for periodic maintenance shots to make certain her `miracle' doesn't go away.

"Talk about someone nearly dead when they first came in the door, that surely describes Ray who was sixty-nine when he became my patient. This man had everything - everything bad! Peripheral artery disease, coronary artery disease, carotid artery disease - he'd had five bypasses, and had already lost his big toe to gangrene. `Ray's going to die,' his wife wailed. `He just lies there in bed, too sick to move. All his other doctors have given up on him. Can't you do something?'

"I agreed to try. Seven chelation treatments later, Ray was out of bed. One week after that, he went on an overnight hunting trip with his son! Unbelievable? I'll say. If I hadn't seen this myself, I'd swear someone made it up."

Once started, there's no stopping Dr. Josephs. He tells about 80 year old Pauline who'd suffered a stroke and with a paralyzed left arm and left leg, could not get out of her wheelchair. After six chelation treatments, she showed everyone how well she was doing by kicking him in the shin with her once unusable left leg. Then he has to report what happened to Grace, the 68-year old writer who suddenly lost her senses. One day she couldn't think straight, wasn't able to complete a sentence or answer questions appropriately. Her family brought her to Dr. Josephs as an emergency case late one Saturday night. Let him tell what happened.

"After only two chelation treatments, she was completely well and back at work, meeting deadlines as before. How about that? But, you haven't heard about my best cases yet. I'm proud of Jim. He was quite a guy - president and chairman of the board of a mining company, community leader, district governor for the Kiwanis Clubs, church elder, you name it. Vigorous, energetic and forceful, he was a 64-year old dynamo until the day his active life came to a halt. All of a sudden, he had alarming symptoms: forgetfulness, tender gums, marked fatigue - he'd fall asleep at his desk - weakness in the limbs, headaches, leg cramps at night, lightheadedness, and worst of all, he began drooling."

As Dr. Josephs tells it, other doctors shook their heads sadly and said it must be Alzheimer's. Too bad. Poor Jim.

No cure. Dr. Josephs recognized it for what it was - heavy metal poisoning, a result of years of exposure in the mineral labs. Sure enough, testing showed Jim's body was laden with lead, mercury, and aluminum. Twenty chelation treatments over a two month period cleared his system and every symptom vanished!

HEARD ENOUGH? THERE'S MORE.

Hundreds of callers over the past five years have reported equally amazing recoveries. The specifics vary from one story to the next, but parallel the cases recited by chelation doctors for the past forty years. Invariably there's a given-up-for-dead patient, mangled by the medical bureaucracy, who tries chelation as a last resort, and guess what? Cured. It's a classic soap opera script and we hear some version of it every day. Do we believe the callers? You bet we do. Investigative reporters are not pushovers. When offered a hot tip, the first question we ask is: "What's in it for this guy? Why is he telling me this?"

Judged by that standard, what reason to suspect hundreds of people of fabrication? No one's ever tried to sell us anything; we've not found anyone with something to gain from lauding chelation other than the joy of reliving a remarkable recovery. Conspiracy theories to one side, it would be a hoax of monumental proportions if all who called were out to fool us.

Some of the stories we've heard are tear-jerkers. Occasionally, they bring a welcome chuckle. There was the day the caller was a legal secretary from New York City.

"I need a copy of your book - and fast," was the familiar greeting. "For my father," she added. As the caller continued, we learned her sixty-two year old 'dad' (a mob-connected building contractor) was facing a five to ten year jail term but wanted to have his sentence postponed for at least six months . . . to complete a series of chelation treatments!

"The judge never heard of chelation," she explained. "Your book is our only hope he'll grant the request." We couldn't resist a follow-up call which revealed the judge was convinced by what he read. The six month reprieve was granted. The judicial verdict : "Get chelated first, then go to jail. You'll be a healthier prisoner with a better chance for survival."

Perhaps this is the first you've heard of the phenomenal variety of health benefits reported by those who have undergone chelation therapy. If so, chances are you're astonished that this people-proven treatment has been available so long without your being aware of it. Maybe you've caught on that EDTA's biggest problem is it seems 'too good to be true'.

A NEW ROUND OF APPLAUSE FOR AN OLD PERFORMER

The same disdain on the same irrational grounds has haunted other do-a-lot remedies. Take the case of hyperbaric oxygen therapy (HBO). Not too many years go, hyperbaric oxygen, which has been around since the 1600's, was classified a 'quack remedy' and a charlatan inspired rip-off. The main complaint? There were claims it was good for everything from carbon monoxide poisoning to chronic infection. "Impossible," skeptics snorted.

Today, HBO is the latest darling of the scientific community, with experts delightedly claiming. "The miracle of hyperbaric oxygen is that **it's good for everything, from carbon monoxide poisoning to chronic infection.**"

The wonders of hyperbaric oxygen, were explained on *Good Morning, America* in February of 1990 by Dr. Thomas Buzzoto, Director of the Hyperbaric Medicine Division of the Baptist Medical Center, credited by the medical correspondent conducting the interview as being on the "cutting edge" of a "miraculous new medicine."

New? Hardly. Since the mid-19th century, sea divers have known about life-saving hyperbaric oxygen chambers

- the small air-tight rooms filled with oxygen under pressure, in which an overload of blood-borne nitrogen is reduced. The overload, nitrogen narcosis, is more commonly called "the bends."

Since the mid-1960's, new applications for pressurized oxygen have been found. It is currently being used as an adjunct treatment for such life-threatening conditions as sickle-cell ulcers, brain recovery after cardiac arrest, tissue damage resulting from burns and radiated oral cancers, infections, gangrene and carbon monoxide poisoning.

There are many mechanisms by which HBO helps stroke victims, but mainly it restores brain and motor functions by penetrating tissue and force-feeding life-giving oxygen to oxygen-starved cells. The same force-feeding of oxygen aids recovery from migraine headaches, multiple sclerosis, brain and spinal cord injuries, and gangrenous limbs.

In its modern metamorphosis, HBO is usually administered in a transparent acrylic cylindrical chamber in which the patient lies as oxygen pressure is gradually increased to twice the outside pressure (equivalent to being thirty feet under water.) A therapy session usually lasts an hour and is painless. The patient can talk to, and hear, the doctors in attendance, and may have a TV available to help pass the time.

HBO: A STAR ONCE MORE

"The future for oxygen treatments looks bright," Dr. Buzzoto told the TV audience. We'll bet, especially since super-star entertainer Michael Jackson made headlines when he received HBO for burns sustained filming a Pepsi commercial.

What turned HBO's image around? What changed? Not the therapy. Perhaps the old guard who condemned the treatment out-of-hand have at last died off, and new, younger doctors are free to judge it on its merits. Can we expect the same change of heart for chelation therapy? We can only hope so.

There are many similarities in the track records of these two treatments. In both instances, there were thousands of published research documents in the world literature supporting remarkable benefits; for both, historical scientific reviews were overlooked and neglected in the rush to condemn; both treatments were praised by many cured patients, their testimonials cavalierly brushed aside as inconsequential. Perhaps the day will come when chelation will be 'rediscovered' just as hyperbaric oxygen has been. Better still, perhaps we can arrange to have it reinvented in Japan under a new exotic name.

Whenever someone says, "Chelation can't be any damn good because it's been around so long, someone should have proved it out by now," we're reminded of these words by Michel de Montaigne who spoke them in the 16th century:

> *"Whenever a new discovery is reported to the scientific world, they say first, 'It is probably not true.' Thereafter, when the truth of the new proposition has been demonstrated beyond question, they say, 'Yes, it may be true, but it is not important.' Finally, when sufficient time has elapsed to fully evidence its importance, they say, 'Yes, surely it is important, but it is no longer new.'"*

The cause of death in the old?
Veins, which by the thickening of their
tunicles restrict the passage of blood,
and by this lack of nourishment,
destroy their life without any fever,
the old coming to fail little by little
in slow death.

Leonardo da Vinci, 1484

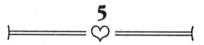

5

UNCLOGGING THE ARTERIES: AN ONGOING STRUGGLE

Arteriosclerosis is not a contemporary plague, unknown prior to recent times. History confirms it's an ancient affliction. Leonardo da Vinci described this disease in explicit and detailed terms eight years before Columbus discovered America. For many centuries afterward, physicians failed to consider it more than an oddity.

Because the early symptoms of arteriosclerosis are difficult to detect and it develops slowly over a lifetime, doctors simply did not recognize the prevalence of this ailment so long as most people died before it turned up. Now that millions are living much longer - thanks in large part to the antibiotics that fight off respiratory killers such as pneumonia and TB - arteriosclerosis is thought to be a thoroughly modern malady, this century's most prevalent 'new' disease.

Ever since its "rediscovery," causes and cures, diagnosis and treatment have come and gone. Well into the 1940's, the treatment of choice was nitroglycerin to relieve pain. Then surgeons devised the "vineberg operation". In this procedure, surgeons shifted, or repositioned, blood vessels in a manner meant to 'force' increased blood flow to the heart. Patients reported dramatic symptom relief and for more than a decade, the technique grew increasingly popular. Despite high mortality, thousands of these surgeries kept operating rooms busy until a group of perceptive investigators thought to take a closer look. When the researchers found that 'sham' operations where patients were prepped for surgery, but not operated upon, resulted in similar - actually many more - 'recoveries', support for the procedure collapsed. In a manner of speaking, the operation withered on the vine.

Medical historians now speculate that the "vineberg" procedure's pain relief resulted from the chest nerves being severed. When that's done, the area becomes numb and angina pain disappears. Scrupulously honest neurologists, recognizing the parallels between the discredited 'vineberg' and bypass surgery, believe the latter could also be classified as 'anesthesia by scalpel'.

BALLOON ANGIOPLASTY - AND OTHER OVER-INFLATED TREATMENTS

Since 1984, 'bypass bashing' has become commonplace, even among tradition-minded specialists.

Duke University's Dr. David Eddy has called for an investigation of the way patients are referred for dangerous procedures. Dr. Eugene Robin, professor of medicine at Stanford University, tells potential surgical patients, "hospitals are very good places to stay out of."

With such blunt criticism coming from within the establishment, skeptics suspected new procedures were in the offing. As medical gadfly Dr. Robert E. Mendelsohn, popularly known as "The People's Doctor", put it, "Remember they never give up a bad operation, until they have a new one to replace it."

High-tech replacements were indeed positioned on the launching pad. The first entry in the bypass substitution sweepstakes was balloon angioplasty (percutaneous transluminal coronary angioplasty is the technically correct name.) It did not take long for PTCA to catch up with bypass surgery's prominence and popularity. Currently, an estimated 300,000 PTCA procedures take place each year in this country alone, outnumbering the bypass by about 50,000 annually.

One major reason for PTCA's phenomenal growth is the intense competition among doctors of different specialties, and among hospitals, for patients. Many cardiologists who formerly had to refer patients to cardiac surgeons for bypass procedures (referral fees may pay the phone bill, but won't cover country club dues or the price of a new Mercedes) can now reap substantial financial rewards by performing PTCAs themselves. As the popularity of angioplasty grows, specialists in the technique are becoming more aggressive.

When an angiogram suggests one or more coronary arteries are badly blocked, the test result is usually followed by a warning to the patient that he is in imminent danger. Alarmed by the (mis)information, most people assume aggressive action is called for, and the sooner the better. No doubt, PTCA appears the more attractive alternative to the patient facing distasteful surgical options. As one 44-year old software consultant put it, "I'd have to be out of my mind to be bypassed and laid up for weeks, maybe months, when with this balloon thing, I can be up and around in a few days."

The way the PTCA is described, it is understandably appealing: "only slight discomfort", "light anesthesia", "nothing to fear", it's a "routine procedure." It is even more tempting when irresistible benefits are dangled: "no more angina", "clog-freed arteries", "no need for bypass surgery."

Promises. Promises. How does PTCA work this magic?

Guided by TV cameras and with the help of special dyes, the cardiologist guides a balloon-tipped catheter up through the femoral (thigh) artery to the site of the blockage. After the guide wire has been snaked through the obstruction, the balloon is inflated with fluid at the site of blockage, hopefully breaking up the plaque and stretching the arterial passageway at the same time.

So far, so good. Right? Wrong. Only the most conscientious cardiologist may warn that after the procedure, the spot the catheter was inserted may remain uncomfortably sore requiring much additional medication, or that there may be an intractable blockage or plaque lodged in a small or inaccessible artery, and should there be unforeseen complications, bypass surgery may still be necessary. That's not the whole story.

WHAT YOUR CARDIOLOGIST MIGHT NOT TELL YOU

The standard depiction of PTCA falls far short of full disclosure. Chances are you won't be told that PTCA increases blood flow mainly by fracturing and creating fissures in stubborn calcified plaque. That's like trying to resolve a traffic jam by sending in a snow plow.

What other disturbing particulars are routinely withheld? That the most troubling problem with angioplasty is restentosis (reblocking), provoked by the procedure itself; that injuries and tears in artery linings caused by wires, catheters and balloons result in restenosis *within 6 months* in approximately thirty-five percent of patients; that when restenosis recurs, angina symptoms reappear and become progressively worse.

Few patients have a clue that in some two to three percent of PTCA procedures, acute complications develop requiring *emergency* surgery - the guide wire jams, or the inflated balloon dislodges a particle of plaque that plugs up a partially occluded artery, or that a guide wire can slice the inner lining of the artery creating a flap that seals off the artery, *or* that a traumatized artery may spasm, causing a heart attack.

Few are briefed on fatality statistics. Although there's not been enough time to compile long-term data on large numbers of patients, early reports are far from encouraging. The most definitive study to date is a five year follow-up of 2,000 patients that showed the incidence of death or myocardial infarction was one to four percent - (for elderly patients, mortality was two to five percent) - with most deaths occurring soon after the PTCA procedure.

The researchers also noted how often PTCAs are prescribed inappropriately. Even though the NHLBI doesn't consider mildly symptomatic patients to be PTCA candidates, an estimated 20 percent of angioplasties involve moderately diseased young-to-middle aged patients, with symptoms that might more easily be controlled with medication, diet and lifestyle changes. Other studies have shown that for clot-induced acute myocardial infarctions (heart attacks), a streptokinase injection is as effective as PTCA for restoring blood flow.

What else do you need to know before signing up for angioplasty? Although both angioplasty and surgery may stop the pain, they only buy time. They don't cure the underlying disease of atherosclerosis. Eventually, unless there are profound life style changes, the blockages will return with a vengeance.

ANGIOPLASTY IS NO SURE-CURE

Most individuals opting for this seemingly 'improved' procedure haven't an inkling that up to thirty-five percent of angioplastied arteries close up within six months, requiring a second or third effort. Nor do they realize there's a good chance the doctor, after repeated failures, will eventually advise bypass surgery. One in three, once they agree to PTCA, are repeat surgical 'customers'. One operation almost invariably leads to another.

Painful as it may be to read so gloomy an assessment, it's far more painful for those for whom the truth becomes known after a dismal personal experience. One such individual, phoned the other morning.

"I wish I'd read your book or bought your tape (*Byebye Bypass* - an audio book) long ago," he began. "At least in time to save my wife's life." Then he explained. His now-deceased mate, diagnosed as suffering from life-threatening arteriosclerosis, had opted for angioplasty, influenced by her cardiologist's assurance that this "modern marvel would do the trick."

What went wrong? The caller couldn't say for sure. He gave a somewhat garbled account of arteries exploding, debris coming loose, clots, trauma, hemmorhage, heart failure. The actual details don't matter that much. The end result does. His wife died on the operating table.

"Now the cardiologist is advising I have the same operation," our caller protested. "It's too late for my wife, but maybe it's not too late for me. Tell me, where can I go to be chelated?"

WHAT ELSE IS 'NEW'?

In an effort to reduce the high rate of restenosis (reblockage), the Achilles heel of balloon angioplasty and bypass surgery, researchers are developing new procedures aimed at actually removing plaque from artery walls. Have you heard about atherectomy? The arterial roto-rooter?

Directional Atherectomy (DA) is one of the freshly minted, highly publicized treatments to come along. This method uses mechanical devices to scrape, cut or pulverize plaque away. Conventional DA shaves plaque with a low speed (2,000 RPM) rotating blade. The device retains plaque shavings within a housing, and periodically removes them. Then the drive wire is reinserted into the catheter and the abrasive device chafes off additional shavings.

DA has obvious drawbacks. It has limited usage due to

the large size of the device. Only the largest, most visible, close-at-hand arterial blockages can be unblocked by directional atherectomy. It is totally useless for smaller heavily calcified arteries.

Nevertheless, DA does hold a few distinctive advantages over other aggressive arterial blockage smashers. Although DA restenosis rates are equivalent to those resulting from balloon angioplasty, reblockage occurs less than half as frequently (14%) when the procedure removes localized plaque in left anterior descending arteries - but only in those NOT previously worked over by balloon angioplasty.

One definite edge of the DA device is the cutter can be directed to eccentric (lopsided) plaque and plaque flap. Currently under development is a smaller device in a more flexible housing.

High Speed Rotational Aretherectomy (HSRA) is a DA upgrade that pulverizes plaque with a high speed (175,000 rpm) rotating granular burr tip. According to reports, 85% of the ground plaque particles are less than 5 microns in size and easily pass through the tiniest arterioles. Since the HSRA device doesn't require cleaning, the procedure is continuous. Early data on HSRA is somewhat encouraging, since success rates of 90% or better are reported, with an 'acceptable' 2% to 3% rate of complications.

HSRA does have limited application, though. It is primarily useful in the smaller sites of calcification, since debris from long lesions have caused small infarctions; also, it is most effective on heavily calcified portions of the coronary artery tree.

Moving right along, there is yet another variation bucking for star billing in the arterial plaque removal sweepstakes: Transluminal Extraction Atherectomy (TEA or TEC). In this procedure, arterial plaque is cut free from the arterial walls, then sucked out of the body through a catheter. Still in the experimental stages, the somewhat inflexible catheter has presented some problems. It is unwieldy around acute vessel bends and thus often requires a PTCA 'cleanup' to achieve a satisfactory result. The inventors claim that the development of a more flexible catheter, now in the works, will eventually make TEA the preferred treatment of choice for large areas of total occlusion. Only time will tell. One more drawback: there are only a few atherectomy facilities now available, making it that much more difficult to comparison shop.

THE STAR WARS TREATMENTS: LASERS AND STENTS

Over the past six years, researchers have developed a dazzling array of high-tech systems for disintegrating plaque in clogged coronary arteries, the most dramatic of which use lasers powerful beams of concentrated light able to destroy solid matter.

The goal in laser angioplasty is to control laser pulses so that they pulverize plaque without disrupting underlying healthy tissue. This has proven so delicate a task, results to date have been mostly disappointing.

Of the 2,000 patients who have undergone laser angioplasty, 40 have suffered a perforated artery; 160 experienced abrupt closure requiring balloon dilation; 60 required emergency bypass operations; 40 suffered heart attacks. If you're not good at math, that means that fifteen percent of the test patients wish they had never heard of the procedure.

More disturbing is a recent report stating that restenosis (reblockage) rates are no better with laser angioplasty than with balloon angioplasty. Considering the laser procedure was developed with the stated purpose of replacing the balloon's disappointing performance, it's hard to understand why it's been called an 'improvement.' The failure of lasers to do better than anticipated is not hard to understand once you realize that lasers leave in their wake segments of heat-traumatized artery walls which resemble crater-pocked moonscapes. Since damaged and roughened artery walls entrap clot-prone blood elements, provoking new plaque deposits, there seems little reason at this time to view laser surgery as optimistically and enthusiastically as prematurely suggested.

SOME STERN WORDS ABOUT STENTS

The most celebrated recent arrival on the Star Wars' cardiovascular scene is the stent, used to prevent damaged arteries from collapsing. Stents are self-expanding doohickeys inserted into compromised blood vessels (such as the leg blood vessels which have undergone angioplasty to unclog them) to prop up blood flow. Examined close hand, stents are best described as an unsatisfactory response to a failed medical procedure.

The stent is supposed to brace the walls of an artery like a scaffold. As matters now stand, the sole rationale for stents is to rectify the unfavorable aftermath of balloon angioplasty and bypass surgery. Their major use is to prop arteries open after angioplasty, or to keep bypass grafts open, improve sub-optimal PTCA results, and repair angioplasty failures.

Even viewed as a 911-style rescue, stents fall short of the mark. One study which analyzed the records of 700 "stented" patients, reported as follows: "The major present limitation of wider stent usage involves the requirement for aggressive systemic coagulation and attending complications. Despite the use of Dextran, intravenous Heparin, Coumadin, aspirin and Dipyridamole, there have been episodes of subacute thrombotic closures (3 to 4 percent) two to ten days after stent placement, In addition, there are significant access site bleeding complications, resulting from the use of large catheters and strict anticoagulation."

If you would like a translation into plain English, here it is. Stents are a disaster. They cause clotting, heart attacks and strokes, and routinely require such heavy doses of blood thinning medications, patients are at risk of bleeding to death!

Dr. Ulrich Sigwart, a Swiss cardiologist and associate professor of medicine, suggests that an "Operator learning curve" may contribute to the problems that have arisen from the use of coronary stents. You can read that apologistic phrase to mean: Most of the practitioners doing stents are indeed 'practicing'.

Dr. Sigwart has had considerable experience with stents, considerably more than most other commentators. He finds a number of built-in difficulties: stents are inelastic, rigid and inflexible, thus intrinsically incompatible with arterial housings. Moreover they have present a high thrombogenic potential, are difficult to implant, and contribute to the problem they are designed to relieve. In language we can all understand: stents breed trouble, by design!

WHO WILL BE FIRST TO SHOOT THIS THEORY FULL OF HOLES?

The latest high-tech wrinkle is a real mouthful: transmyocardial revascularization. In simple lay terms - shooting the heart wall full of holes so that, like a sieve, it will allow blood to 'leak' directly into the heart muscle. This sounds bizarre, we know. But, honest Injun, we didn't make it up.

In this operation, promoted by St. Luke's Hospital and Medical College with experimental approval from the FDA, a tiny laser beam, fired from outside the organ's walls, blasts through the patient's ribs, directly through the beating heart to create up to 20 pin-size holes that, the developer brags, "do not close up." Twenty patients to date have had their hearts turned into pincushions and all that's known about results comes from the American Heart Association that has hailed the procedure "a promising new technique."

A word to the wary: Medical high-tech has an almost

mystical appeal for the uninformed, and excites an unfortunate amount of promotional pizzazz from the anything-for-a-story press. Avoid unproven gee-whiz gimmickry. Remember the x-ray machines once common in stores specializing in children's shoes? They were supposed to prevent cramped toes and foot problems by making sure customers had the benefit of a 'scientific fit'? It took years to expose their potential for harm while the high dose machines zapped salespeople and kids alike.

CONSUMER ADVISORY ON INVASIVE TREATMENTS

Before agreeing to *any* invasive treatment, there are things you should know:

1: Arterial blockage diagnostic exams are apt to be disgracefully inaccurate.

When the cardiologist waltzes in with an angiogram in hand, spouting seemingly precise percentages of arterial closure, it's a set-up. Alternatively termed an arteriogram (or cardiac cathereterization), the procedure is more accurately classified an operation than a diagnostic test. Basically a movie of the heart in action, it should be in the X-rated category.

You may pay a stiff price for your physician's peek into your arteries, since besides the discomfort of lying immobilized for three hours or longer while the injected dye races through blood vessels, you may suffer such minor side effects as nausea, vomiting, coughing or allergic reactions including kidney damage, or the most serious of all - a dislodged piece of plaque that makes its way to the heart or brain causing a heart attack or stroke.

To what benefit? The surgeon's, not yours. Reading the films is more 'guesstimate' than science. The most highly regarded, skilled cardiologists routinely disagree on the meaning of the films they are viewing. In one landmark study, 30 angiograms circulated among first-class ateriographers at three top medical centers. The experts agreed on their significance only 60 percent of the time. Worst still, when the same films recirculated for a second go-around (without warning), the experts agreed with *themselves* only fifty percent of the time!

Will your surgeon admit that the test he's using as the prime reason to rush you to surgery might have been misread, misinterpreted, or could be totally wrong? Not likely, say skeptics such as Dr. Arthur Selzer, cardiopulmonary-lab chief at Presbyterian Hospital in San Francisco, who explains, "There's too much money involved."

2: You're not a legitimate candidate for any invasive treatment (surgery by any name) unless you've had optimal medical management first.

Your doctor should first try to heal you by a variety of relatively benign therapies, including a fine-tuned approach to carefully selected and adjusted medications, diet and lifestyle changes. If he does not take this approach, seek out a more informed doctor.

3: You haven't really given your arteries a chance to recover unless you've stopped smoking, drastically reduced fat and sugar consumption and increased your intake of antioxidants.

Life style changes have proven tremendously effective in reversing atherosclerosis. It is a fact that NO treatment (including chelation therapy) results in long-term benefits unless you clean up your act. Eventually, with or without medical or surgical intervention, you're going to have to change your diet, stop smoking, start exercising - take better care of yourself. Why not do it to start with and skip the hospital trip?

4: Don't let yourself get 'pushed' into the operating room by a super-salesmen doc.

The AMA, in its official journal (*JAMA*), reports that 44 percent of all bypass surgeries are unjustified and/or inappropriately prescribed. A survey of 50 balloon angioplasty operations revealed an incredible 56 percent of patients who undergo PTCA do not fit NHLBI's (admittedly generous) suitable candidate guidelines.

5: Keep it in mind that ALL invasive treatments for atherosclerosis have been (and still are) in the experimental or developmental stage. If the idea of being a guinea pig is appealing, we've no quarrel with that. But in case you've not suspected that's what's going on, here's a recap of some seventy years' worth of once popular 'approved' operations, eventually discarded as worthless:

- In 1922, a French surgeon tried severing the nerve that carried angina pain, and guess what? It worked. Angina pain ceased.

- Eight years later, a team of four physicians conjectured they could eradicate the underlying atherosclerotic disease by removing the thyroid, thereby eliminating the hormones that stimulate the heart. The procedure did as promised. It reduced angina pain - but at a high cost: thyroid deficiency in the treated patients.

- Following World War II, a team of surgeons postulated that tying off two major chest arteries might somehow force tiny mammary arteries to plow their way around the clogged areas and bring blood to the heart. The procedure produced acceptable symptom relief - angina pain stopped and the surgeons claimed great success. Then, one skeptical cardiologist tricked nine patients with angina into thinking they were getting this highly publicized, 'remarkable' operation, while in truth, *NO* operation took place. They were anesthetized and the doctor made only a small incision in their chests. When those deceived were as effectively relieved of angina as patients receiving the full operation, the alarm sounded at last and proponents were forced to admit that this operation was no damn good.

- In the late '50's, an innovative surgeon removed the outer layer of the heart, then scraped the exposed area with asbestos until it was bloody. According to his theory, the heart would obtain additional blood from vessels embedded in the surrounding fibrous sack. In 1958, the surgeon reported that 97 percent of the patients who had undergone this bizarre treatment enjoyed angina pain relief. The Journal of the American Medical Association published this 'scientific' report.
- In 1945, Dr. Arthur Vineberg, a Canadian surgeon, introduced the 'Vineberg procedure', which involved taking a mammary artery and implanting it in the heart. Cardiologists of the day hoped the transplanted artery would spring roots that would eventually increase blood flow by connecting with nearby coronary vessels. Once again, victory was proclaimed before verifiable results were in. The operation was hailed a success based on anecdotal reports that it effectively reduced angina pain. By the time researchers got around to probing results, or thought to ask whether increased blood flow prolonged life, no one within cardiac circles cared. They still don't. Bypass surgery arrived on the scene.
- Bypass surgery - what's left to say? Ever since the first open-heart surgery was performed to bypass blocked coronary arteries like a plumber routing a new section of pipe around a hopelessly corroded conduit, this dramatic operation has benefited from undeserved enthusiasm. For more than two decades, it's been a lucrative business for heart surgeons. Even today, with the Johnny-come-lately adverse publicity, some 250,000 procedures a year take place. We've no doubt that like many of its failed predecessors, it will eventually fade into the history books as one more example of medical folly. It won't be completely discarded, however, until those who profit can replace it with an equally lucrative fad.

If you're getting the idea that white-frocked cardiologists are scrambling for business like Arab rug merchants, willing to go with whatever sells best, you're on the right track. Objective observers who are not part of the money stream are watching on the sidelines and laughing at the way heart specialists are vying to stake claim on whatever new treatment catches public fancy. The in-fighting taking place within cardiology circles is only amusing if you're not a patient.

We know that for many this is painful information to accept. We can hear you now; "Not *my* doctor. He's one of the good guys." Maybe so, maybe not, but chances are you won't enjoy the discovery that the professional you've trusted to watch over you has an eye on his cash flow instead. Nevertheless, that might be the case! For your health's sake, it's better to entertain and investigate that possibility than remain a naive innocent

6: READ THIS CAREFULLY: Compromised blood flow does not *automatically* expose one to the imminent danger of sudden death. Contrary to everything you may be told, atherosclerosis is rarely the no-time-to-think-about-this emergency knife-happy doctors make it out to be!

When your doctor says (explicity or by implication) "Do what I tell you or you're apt to die!", what next? Grim prognostications are sure to provoke a panic, and few patients are strong enough to withstand the pressure of such a dire warning. If you can bring yourself to do it, challenge the doctor to present evidence that he's right.

Ask for published data in books and journals to support his view. Request a balanced research review of studies that show both the pros and cons of suggested procedures. What your doctor comes up with may well determine your course of action - better still, it might help you make up your mind whether he continues as your doctor.

Since early 1948, right through the present time, dozens of reports of postmortem examinations of infarcted hearts have consistently failed to corroborate the clogged coronary artery theory of myocardial infarction. That is, victims of fatal heart attacks frequently have had no evidence whatsoever of coronary occlusion.

A 1980 article in *Circulation* agreed that the data is inconsistent with the idea that removing blockages in coronary arteries is the way to prevent myocardial infarction. In a 1988 editorial published in the *New England Journal of Medicine*, the writer observed no studies have detected a significant benefit to surgical patients over the medically treated. The same holds true for the more recent work investigating angioplasty and anti-thrombolytic agents. In all cases, the verdict is the same: no improvement in survival.

Having lived through a heart attack, try not to be terrorized by a doctor who tells you that you may drop dead any minute if you don't submit to some invasive procedure. Plaqued arteries adjust to reduced blood flow by expanding and through collateral circulation. The April 1, 1988 issue of *The American Journal of Cardiololgy* summing up work completed by Germany's Dr. Berthold Kern that showed this, agreed that bypass grafts are naturally created by the body via the collaterals when a coronary artery becomes blocked. Their most interesting observation was this: the more the coronaries narrow, the less danger there is of infarction. Once that's understood, the surgical bypass becomes redundant to a large degree. The body has beat the surgeon to it.

Usually, you have sufficient time to try a variety of non-surgical treatments (including chelation). In most cases, you can safely put all operations, including bypass and angioplasty, on the back burner as a last resort when diet, drugs, life style changes, stress reduction and all else has failed.

*Some drugs have been appropriately
called "wonder-drugs," inasmuch as
one wonders what they will do next.*

Annals of Internal Medicine

*Half the modern drugs could well be
thrown out the window, except that
the birds might eat them.*

Martin H . Fischer (1879-1962)

6

♡

HEART DRUGS:
THE GOOD, THE BAD, THE UGLY

"What about all those new wonder drugs we're always
hearing about? Are there any that eliminate the need for
surgery?"

Good question. Drug remedies for atherosclerosis have
come and gone - some hailed for a short time, then discarded
when found to do more harm than good.

In the 50's, anticoagulants or 'blood thinners' were the rage,
until a long term study at the University of Oregon Medical
School concluded that anticoagulants increased mortality and
morbidity. Unmedicated controls required less hospitalization
and were more likely to survive. Some hundreds of thousands
of prescriptions were filled before specialists conceded the
drugs were useless and dangerous.

Studies have shown that the decade-old "first-step" therapy
for high blood pressure, Thiazide diuretics (water pills)
elevates `bad fat' levels, increasing the risk of arteriosclerosis,

and coronary heart disease, but these drugs have been popular so long, many physicians are unaware of the latest studies and go right on prescribing them. Beta blockers, one of the newer family of pharmaceuticals supposed to be helpful in treating hypertension, were hyped for a time, until studies showed they, too, made `bad fat'.

Beta blockers, commonly prescribed to prevent recurrence of heart attack and angina, are an example of drugs first hailed as promising, which later research discredited. Dr. Peter Held, at the National Heart, Lung and Blood Institute has investigated and found these drugs actually appear to **increase** the mortality among patients by 7% with no indication they prevented either first or repeated heart attacks or decreased the seriousness of a myocardial infarction.

DO HEART DRUGS KILL OR CURE?

In 1989, two FDA-approved drugs thought to correct heart rhythm irregularity, encainide and flecainide, which since 1987 were prescribed by thousands of physicians across the country, were found instead to increase the risk of death. NIH researchers involved in the Cardiac Arrhythmia Suppression Trial (CAST) studying 2,309 heart attack patients with irregular heartbeat, found patients receiving ecainide and flecainide had a 3.6 times greater chance of dying than those receiving a sugar pill.

Late in November, 1991 came reports that a heart drug - milrinone - designed to help the heart beat more effectively, actually increased the risk of death by 34%. Although it had not yet received FDA approval for general use, the experimental drug had been given to 561 patients, and was said to be responsible for 34 unnecessary deaths in that study group.

Despite many negative reports, medication may be preferable to surgery. One major finding of the latest

NHLBI five year drug study was that people with stable, mild and moderate symptoms of atherosclerosis can receive adequate pain relief with medication AND - in such patients, there was no difference in survival rates between patients on medication and patients who underwent bypass surgery.

The study also found that a small subgroup of patients with an impaired pumping ability of the heart and substantial narrowing of all three major coronary arteries, who opted for bypass surgery, lived longer than similarly afflicted medicated patients. How much longer? After six years, 89 percent of the medicated group had survived as compared with 93 percent of the bypassed group.

The study omitted one extremely important possibility. What if all the medicated patients had been treated with EDTA infusion (chelation therapy was available at the time of the study), and made those life-style changes proven to effect atherosclerosis reversal, and were prescribed fine-tuned medications? Would they have outlived the bypassed group?

"No contest," declares Dr. E. Cheraskin, a noted nutrition and preventive medicine researcher and professor emeritus at the University of Alabama Medical Center. "If the medicated group had undergone a course of EDTA infusions and had embarked on a program of positive life style changes, they'd have outlived the bypass group, with a handful of exceptions - and for the most part could have achieved biochemical homeostasis without any other medications."

A recent NHLBI report supports Dr. Cheraskin. It states: "For many people, medical treatment, rather than surgical treatment, carried out with *carefully* (our emphasis) selected and adjusted medications and specific recommendations for life style changes related to smoking avoidance, weight reduction, lowering blood cholesterol, increased exercise, etc.

- is the best approach."

Put simply: Even when a portion of the patient's heart is blood starved, the NHLBI advises that a doctor must first do his utmost to increase blood flow and relieve symptoms *nonsurgically*.

Good advice. But how is one to know that he's receiving optimal medical management? Are all physicians equally informed about drugs? Do all doctors carefully prescribe only the most appropriate medications? Do all doctors routinely carry out the continual monitoring necessary once drug treatment is initiated? To be certain the desired therapeutic effect is occurring? To note adverse side effects before there is serious harm? To be alert to the possibility of drug overdose and/or underdose?

THE SIMPLE ANSWER IS: "NO"

If you're going to take drugs, you better bone up on the subject and become a drug expert. Resolve to know as much - if not more - about your medication as your doctor (not too difficult). Most physicians get their information from fast-talking pharmaceutical salespersons, or, if they skim through medical journal, from flashy, promise-a-lot, drug ads

We found out how true that was several years ago when Harold's mother was a patient in the ICU of one of New York City's finest hospitals. Diagnosed with a *mild* heart attack, her condition steadily worsened. The third day, nervous about what we were seeing on the high tech monitors, we wrenched her records from the horrified attendants and discovered mama was being medicated with what we considered a totally inappropriate drug. We protested to the nurse, to the intern, to the head of ICU, to the doctor in charge. It took seven hours, in all, to be heard. Soon afterwards, shame-faced doctors revised medication per our suggestion, mama revived in less than 24 hours, was back home in five days, and lived a long time afterwards.

Lucky mama. Lucky us. Could you do the same? Probably not. We've the advantage of many years of close association with the medical community. We are not reluctant to challenge doctors when we suspect they are wrong. Tackling hospital orders is not easy, but challenging your doctor when he writes a prescription ought not to be daunting.

How many do it? Too few, we discovered when we began questioning people taking a variety of drugs to find out if they knew which was for what condition and if they were aware of the contraindications (bad side effects.)

Let's take just one popular heart drug: Inderal - (generic name is Propranolol). Almost every heart patient under a physician's care is prescribed some version of this drug, despite evidence that damaging side effects negate questionable benefits. Yet people who would not think of imbibing from a bottle that says "Drink Me" without knowing what's in it, blithely swallow pills about which they know practically nothing.

WHEN THE DOCTOR SAYS, "TAKE THIS..."

If used properly, drugs can diminish many of the symptoms common to the various cardiovascular diseases. They can, at proper dose levels, bring about a more comfortable life in those afflicted with heart disease - and in some few cases - even prolong life by several years.

More often than not, however, drugs are a far less effective way to improve one's health than appropriate life style changes. An exaggerated example of this is documented by what occurred in Norway during World War II. Prior to hostilities, one Norwegian city hospital annually admitted

400 to 500 heart attack victims. During the German occupation, the same hospital admitted only one or two such patients a year. An identical drastic reduction in heart attacks was matched in a German hospital which, prior to and during the war admitted an average 300 heart attack patients annually. During the first two to three years immediately after the war's end, this same hospital had *no* - that's *zero* - heart attack admissions.

Why? In Norway, food was severely rationed during the war and the average citizen was able to consume only 1500 calories a day. In Germany, for two to three years following World War II, the average person could barely scrape together enough food to consume more than 900 calories a day.

Thus there is dramatic evidence that merely *reducing caloric intake* - just eating less - is a heart-saving strategy. It would seem it matters less which food you eat than how much of it. Losing weight, it appears, is an important life extension strategy.

SMARTEN UP

Before taking any drug, learn all you can about the prescribed medication. A good place to begin your education is with a copy of *Worst Pills, Best Pills* (Public Citizen Health Research Group, 1988) that costs $12.00 and can be ordered from Pills, 2000 P Street, N.W., Suite 700, Washington, D.C. 20036.

If you have pills on your nightstand, that book should be right next to them. The rule is, for each potentially positive benefit from a drug, there are *fifty* - count them, we said *fifty* adverse reactions.

The following rundown of the more commonly prescribed heart medications (listed generically) is an example of what every drug-taker should know.

NITRATES

Nitroglycerine: (*Nitro-Bid, Nitrodisc, Minitran, Transderm-Nitro, Deponit, Nitrocine, Nitro-Dur, Nitrol*)

Isosorbide Dinitrate: (*Isordil, Sorbitrate, Nitrogard, Nitrolingual, Nitrostat, Cardilatae Tiltrate-SR, Nitrospan, Peritrate*)

The nitrates are used to relieve sudden and severe attacks of chest pain (angina pectoris), for which only the sublingual tablets that dissolve under the tongue and specific chewable tablets have proven effective.

Note: Nitrates, when designed to *prevent* attacks, are yet to be proven effective, since the body develops a drug tolerance over the long-term. Many studies have shown that the longer you take this drug, the less benefit.

When used intermittently as *treatment*, nitrates relax blood vessels that in turn increases the supply of blood and oxygen to the heart, reducing its workload, thus relieving anginal discomfort or pain.

ADVERSE EFFECTS: Call your doctor immediately if: your lips, fingernails, or palms turn bluish; you feel pressure in your head; you experience shortness of breath; you become unusually tired or weak; you have an unusually fast heartbeat; your fever rises; you have seizures. Headache, often severe, is the most common adverse effect and should be expected.

PRECAUTIONS: For nitroglycerine products: If pain continues for more than 5 minutes, take a second tablet. If after three tablets in 10 to 15 minutes, you have no relief, go to an emergency room.

For isorbide dinitrate products: If pain is not relieved in 5 to 10 minutes, take a second tablet. If after three tablets in 15 minutes, you have no relief, go to an emergency room. Isorbide dinitrate should *NOT* be used prophylactically (i.e. - to prevent angina attacks.)

Since old tablets lose strength, have your prescription filled at six-month intervals. Effective sublingual nitroglycerine tablets cause a stinging or burning sensation under the tongue.

BETA-BLOCKERS

Timolol: (*Blocadren*)	**Pindolol:** (*Visken*)
Nadolol: (*Corgard*)	**Acebutolol:** (*Sectral*)
Propanolol: (*Inderal*)	**Betaxolol:** (*Kerlone*)
Metoprolol: (*Lopressor*)	**Carteolol:** (*Cartrol*)
Atenolol: (*Tenormin*)	**Penbutolol:** (*Levatol*)
Labetalol: (*TrandateE*)	

Beta-blockers partially minimize angina discomfort by enabling heart and arteries to relax in stressful situations. They do so by interfering with nerve impulse transmissions.

There's formidable evidence that beta-blockers reduce the incidence and intensity of *second* or *third* heart attacks. They have *not* been shown to reduce your chances of suffering a *first* heart attack.

ADVERSE EFFECTS: Call your doctor immediately if you have a headache, difficulty breathing, become anxious and nervous, your skin itches, you get a skin rash, get nauseous, diarrhea, or vomit, become unusually tired or weak, experience heat stress, disturbed sleep and/or nightmares, notice diminished sexual ability, feel numbness or tingling in limbs, cold hands or feet, swelling of ankles, feet or legs, back, joint or chest pain, mental depression, hallucinations, confusion, memory loss, slow pulse, irregular heartbeat, fatigue, malaise. or personality change.

Note: Since adverse effects vary in each of the eleven beta-blockers, talk to your doctor about switching to another if you have problems. One of the eleven choices will cause you less discomfort than the others.

PRECAUTIONS : Do not take double doses. Don't smoke. Smoking practically eliminates the drug's effectiveness. Do not take *any* beta blocker if you have asthma or incipient heart failure.

To avoid "rebound" chest pain (angina) and possible heart attack, do not stop taking this drug without first checking with your doctor. He should titrate the dose downward (i.e. a daily dose reduction for seven days) before stopping the drug entirely.

To avoid heart failure, get immediate medical help if your pulse drops to 50 beats per minute or less, or if you notice shortness of breath and/or a decrease in stamina.

NOTE: Because of its high incidence of side effects, the Public Citizen Health Group designates labetolol a "LIMITED USE" drug. That is probably an overly kind understatement, since the drug's limited benefits come with the heavy baggage of a lifetime of daily malaise. Taking this drug makes you feel more "funky" more often than most of the others, but *all* beta-blockers are almost certain to decrease the quality of your daily life.

CALCIUM-CHANNEL BLOCKERS

Diltiazem: (*Cardizem*)	**Nicardipine:** (*Cardene*)
Nifedipine: (*Procardia, Adalate*)	**Isradipine:** (*Dynacirc*)
Verapamil: (*Calan, Isoptin*)	**Nimodipine:** (*Nimotop*)

Calcium-channel blockers control angina by reducing the flow of calcium into coronary artery cells, relaxing artery muscles, thereby dilating the lumen and increasing the supply of blood and oxygen to the heart while reducing its workload. The eight drugs have different effects on heart rate, heart rhythm, blood pressure and the strength of the heart's contractions any of which could make your heart function worse or negate the "good" effect of increased oxygen.

ADVERSE EFFECTS Call your doctor immediately if you have difficulty breathing, chest pains, irregular missed beats or pounding heartbeat, confusion, sleep disorder, skin rash, ankle, feet or leg swelling, a severe headache, irregular or repetitive jerking movements of limbs (verapamil), slow pulse (diltiazem and verapamil). You may suffer general malaise or just not "feel like yourself."

PRECAUTIONS: To avoid heart failure, get immediate medical help if your pulse slows to 50 beats per minute or less. Because these drugs sometimes cause the heart to pump *less* blood, you may feel shortness of breath, tire easier or develop leg pain while walking.

Try not to miss a dose. Never take double doses. Do not stop taking this drug suddenly. Your doctor must schedule a gradual dosage decrease.

ANTIARRHYTHMICS

Quinidine: (*Duraquin, Quinidex, Cardioquin, Quinaglute, Dura-Tabs*)

Digoxin: (*Lanoxin , Lanoxicaps*)

Disopyramide: (*Norpace*)

Procainamide: (*Pronestyl, Procan SR*)

Tocainide: (*Tonocard*)

Amioderone: (*Cordarone*)

Adenosine: (*Adenocard*)

Encainide: (*Encaid*)

Moricizine: (*Ethmozine*)

Mexiletine: (*Mexitil*)

Flecainide: (*Tambocor*)

Quinidine, by slowing nerve impulses, slows heart rate, decreases irregular heartbeats (arrhythmias) and may relieve angina.

ADVERSE SIDE EFFECTS: Call your doctor immediately if you have blurred vision, feel dizzy or faint, develop a fever, severe headache, ringing in ears or loss of hearing, skin rash, hives or itching, wheezing, shortness of breath, unusual bleeding or bruising, unusually fast heartbeat, unusual tiredness or weakness, confusion.

PRECAUTIONS: Do not miss a dose or take double doses. Wear an ID bracelet or carry a card stating you take this drug (or any other anti-arrhythmic).

♥

Digoxin, usually used to treat heart failure, a condition in which the heart cannot pump enough blood, slows galloping heartbeats. Digoxin is also used to stabilize fast or irregular heartbeats, and it strengthens the contractibility of heart muscle.

ADVERSE SIDE EFFECTS: Because digoxin (digitalis) accumulates in the body and because of the small margin between therapeutic and toxic doses, "digitalis intoxication" is quite common.

PRECAUTIONS: Do not miss a dose. DEFINITELY DO NOT take double doses. Wear an ID bracelet or carry a card stating you take the drug.

Check with your doctor immediately if you exhibit any of the following symptoms of toxicity: loss of appetite, nausea and vomiting, vision problems, bad dreams, nervousness, drowsiness and hallucinations. If you get too much digoxin in your body, you may develop the effects listed above and dignoxin intoxication often results in death. If you get too little, you may develop symptoms of heart failure or a rapid heart rate, but too little is less serious than too much.

NOTE: Before prescribing digoxin for heart failure, your doctor should try giving you an appropriate diuretic (water pill).

♥

Disopyramide, procainamide, encainide, flexainide, miexiletine, ethomozine and tocainide slow the heart rate and stabilize irregular heart beats.

NOTE: Because of their serious side effects, your doctor should first try a safer antiarrhythmic such as quinidine. Procainamide frequently causes lupus erythematosus (a disease ranging from skin to organ disorders). Tocainide causes agranulocytoris (loss of all the white cells in your blood) in one of every 500 patients exposed to it.

NOTE: If you have mild disturbances of heart rhythm and no symptom of heart disease, chances are you don't need any of these drugs, all of which can cause new heart irregularities. High doses can actually *cause* a fatal arrhythmia. Even low (therapeutic) doses can induce a fatal arrhythmia.

VASODILATORS (Blood Vessel Dilators)

Papaverine: (*Cerespan, Pavabid*)	**Nylidrin:** (*Arlidin*)
Cyclandelate: (*Cyclospasmol*)	**Ethaverine:** (*Ethatab*)
Isoxsuprine: (*Vasodilan*)	**Ergoloid mesylate:**
Pentoxifylline: (*Trental*)	(*Hydergine*)

Manufacturer claims that vasodilators improve peripheral circulation of patients with blood vessel disease - and relieve leg pain and improve mental function, but thus far no studies have shown these drugs effective. The one exception is Trental which is the only drug in this group that *may* help because it "softens" red blood cells (increased rheology).

NOTE: You may be wondering why drugs NOT shown to have any benefit are still being marketed with FDA approval. Prior to 1962, the FDA's oversight of new drugs was limited to keeping "dangerous" drugs off the market - they were not authorized to investigate whether or not a drug was 'good' for you - only to make sure it wasn't too 'bad' for you.

All that changed with the passage of the Kefauver Act - a marvelous example of a 'good law gone bad' - that stipulated drug manufacturers had to prove "efficacy" - (the drug has some benefit) before it can be marketed. For the past thirty years, safety issues have taken a back seat while "effectiveness", which is easier to prove with skewed data, has gained ground.

Drugs in use prior to the 1962 law - (they'd only been shown to be 'safe') - were kept on the shelf, and given 6 months to complete research showing they were also "effective". There were so many drugs involved, so much work to be done, so many review panels to be organized, drugs which hadn't complied in six months were given another six months and then *another* six months - and guess what? The vasodilators listed above (they must have been given 60 six month extensions) have *still* not shown they're worthwhile. That's why the Public Citizen Health Group classifies the above vasodilators as "DO NOT USE" drugs, the one exception being pentoxifylline, which is marginally effective.

ANTICOAGULANTS

Warfarin: (*Coumadin*)

Non-steroid anti-inflammatory drugs: (*Aspirin, Motrin, Advil, Anaprox, Ansaid, Climoril, Nuprin, Feldene, Dolobid, Indocin, Meclomen, Naprosyn, Orudis, Tolectin, Voltaren*)

Warfarin, prescribed for people who form abnormal blood clots, reduces the blood's ability to coagulate and prevents blood clots from forming.

ADVERSE SIDE EFFECTS: Call your doctor immediately if you have the following signs of overdose: bleeding gums, nosebleeds, unexplained bruising, heavy bleeding from cuts and wounds, abnormal bleeding, bloody or cloudy stool, abdominal pain or swelling, sudden lightheadedness, weakness, loss of consciousness, backaches, bloody or tarry stool, coughing up blood, vomiting blood or material that looks like coffee grounds - or if you have difficult or painful urination or a decrease in the amount of urine, swelling of ankles, feet or legs, unusual weight gain, blue/purple color of toes, chills, fever, sore throat or unusual tiredness, dark urine, yellow eyes, diarrhea, nausea or vomiting, skin rash, hives or itching, sores or white spots in mouth or throat.

PRECAUTIONS: Do not do the following: Change your diet or take nutritional supplements or vitamins without first checking with your doctor; take double doses; take any other drugs, including nonprescription products.

DOES AN ASPIRIN A DAY KEEP
HEART ATTACKS AWAY?

Let's talk a bit about aspirin. A nonprescription drug, it's said to reduce cardiac events by 50 percent in people with unstable angina (progressively worsening angina discomfort or pain).

According to many published reports, within the year following a heart attack, aspirin has been found to reduce the likelihood of death by 10 percent and the recurrence of a second attack by 20 percent. For people in the midst of a heart attack, aspirin has been found to reduce mortality by 2.6 percent.

All the above benefits are explained by aspirin's well-established ability to reduce blood-platelet clotting. Sounds promising, but before we all rush down to the corner drug store for a lifetime supply of aspirin, read further.

On the down side, another aspirin study you probably won't hear as much about (conducted at Harvard Medical School at that) revealed that while low-dosage aspirin does appear to lower heart attack risks, it also *increased* strokes, many of which result in permanent long-term impairment. Equally disquieting, aspirin can cause macular degeneration - (the leading cause of blindness in the 55-plus crowd), stomach and intestinal bleeding and ulcers. It also blocks the production of certain beneficial prostaglandins. Aspirin has also been linked with kidney damage, liver damage, and most recently Reye's Syndrome - an often fatal condition which affects infants, children, adolescents and young adults.

More than one doctor has pointed out that were aspirin to be introduced as a new drug today. the FDA would be unlikely to approve it. So, let's reevaluate the new jump-on-the-aspirin-bandwagon hoopla with what's known to date. In recent years, aspirin has had a consistently bad press and market share has surely been threatened and diminished by acetaminophen (Tylenol) and ibuprofen (Advil, Medipren, Nuprin and Motrin). That being the case, there is *some* possibility the enthusiastic welcome given the save-your-heart studies might do more to save aspirin sales than people's lives.

There we go again! Suspicious as all get out. It just seems preposterous to believe that man has been born with an aspirin deficiency - just one more of God's little mistakes - that Bayer is prepared to correct.

If blood platelet stickiness is the issue - and it is - surely there are better ways to deal with it than by contributing to aspirin profits. French researchers are crediting red wine - one or two glasses with meals - as the reason the French, despite their rich gourmet diet, suffer far fewer deaths (1/4 as many) from coronary heart disease than Americans. All forms of alcohol beer, wine and distilled liquors - increase blood levels of the 'good' HDL cholesterol, but only red wine, which contains the tannins present in grape skins, decreases blood platelet stickiness (without causing internal bleeding) according to research published in the *Journal of Applied Cardiology*. The French are also high on garlic, which has proven an extremely effective blood thinner, and with no downside, except bad breath. Now, back to aspirin.

ADVERSE SIDE EFFECTS: Call your doctor immediately if you vomit material that looks bloody or like coffee grounds, pass bloody or black, tarry stools (unless you are also taking Pepto-Bismol), wheeze, feel tightness in the chest, or have trouble breathing, develop skin rash, hives or itching, faint or have dizzy spells.

PRECAUTIONS: Don't take aspirin without your doctor's approval. You should not take aspirin if you have ulcers, a severely irritated stomach, gout, severe anemia, hemophilia or other bleeding problems, if you take an anticoagulant drug, or if you are allergic to aspirin or similar painkillers.

In general, one "baby aspirin" per day is all that is required to decrease blood platelet stickiness. The lower the dose, the better.

ANTIHYPERLIPIDEMICS

Gemfibrozol: (*Lopid*)   **Colestipol:** (*Colestid*)

Cholestyramine: (*Cholybar*)   **Mevastatin:** (*Provastatin*)

Clofibrate: (*Atromid-S*)   **Probucol:** (*Lorelco*)

Dextrothyroxine sodium: **Lovastatin:** (*Mevacor*)

(*Choloxin*)   **Nicotinic acid:** (*Nicolar*)

Gemfibrozol is prescribed to lower high blood fat and cholesterol levels. Although this drug does lower blood fat levels, it has little effect on cholesterol levels. It should be used only when there's an *inherited* fat regulating disorder, there's significant risk of heart disease, abdominal pain, or pancreatitis, and you have unsuccessfully tried diet and exercise to control diabetes or thyroid disease.

NOTE: The Public Citizen Health Research Group designates Gemfibrozol a "LIMITED USE" drug. All of the other cholesterol-lowering drugs have effects similar to Gemfibrozol. Many experts believe that the drug-induced decrease in cholesterol (with a few exceptions) is of little or no clinical consequence. None have been shown to retard progressive atherosclerosis, much less reverse the process. Severe toxicity is also seen with this drug category and all cause a high percent of liver damage. After two years on the drug, rats fed lovastatin develop liver cancer.

DRUGS FOR HIGH BLOOD PRESSURE

Hypertension, a major underlying risk factor in atherosclerosis, is commonly medicated with antihypertensives. Once again, let us emphasize drugs are an alternative, *NOT* a substitute, for lifestyle changes. One famous physician was fond of describing diuretic drugs as "the poor man's low-salt diet" - cute, but not very accurate, inasmuch as diuretics are a decidedly unhealthy way to rid the body of excess salt. They tend to increase blood sugar (and sometimes cause diabetes), tend also to increase uric acid in the blood (and sometimes cause gout) and worst of all, decrease potassium which can and *does* cause a variety of unpleasant symptoms, not least of which is cardiac arrhythmias (which in some patients, can be fatal.)

Diuretics, then, can do good by getting rid of the excess salt ingested by many people, but because of the additional drug-induced negative effects, certainly cannot be considered a substitute for a low-salt diet. Although relatively rare, diuretics have been known to kill people. A low salt diet has never been known to kill anyone.

There being so wide a variety of diuretics and other drugs for hypertension, we are simply listing them generically, the 'good', 'bad' and 'ugly' classified according to Public Health Research Group standards.

DIURETICS (Fluid pills)

OKAY:
Hydrochlorothiazide: (*Esidrix, Hydrodiuril*)
Chlorothiazide: (*Diuril*)
VERY LIMITED USE:
Chlorothiazide: (*Diuril*)
Indapamide: (*Lozol*)
Metolazone: (*Diulo, Zaroxolyn*)
USE CAREFULLY:
Chlorthalidone: (*Hygroton*)
Triamterene: (*Dyrenium*)
Methylclothiazide: (*Enduron*)
Trichlormethiazide: (*Metahydrin, Naqua*)

OTHER ANTIHYPERTENSIVES

OKAY:

Atenolol: (*Tenormin*)
Hydralazine: (*Apresoline*)
Metoprolol: (*Lopressor*)
Nadolol: (*Corgard*)
Pindolol: (*Visken*)

Propanolol: (*Inderal*)
Timolol: (*Blocarden*)
Dilitiazem: (*Cardizem*)
Nifedipine: (*Procardia*)
Verapamil: (*Calan, Isoptin*)

LIMITED USE:

Captropril: (*Capoten*)
Hydralazine w/hydrochlorothiazide: (*Apresazide, Apresoline-Esidrex, Lisinopril(Primival)*)
Labetalol: (*Transdate*)
Prazosin: (*Minipress*)
Propanolol w/hydrochlorothiazide: (*Inderide*)
Triamterene w/hydrochlorothiazide: (*Diazide*)
Enalapril: (*Vasotec*)
Furosemide: (*Lasix*)
Methyldopa: (*Aldomet*)
Methyldopa w/hydrochlorothiazide: (*Aldoril*)
Reserpine w/hydralazine and hydrochlorothiazide: (*SER-AP-ES*)
Spironolactone and hydrochlorothiazide: (*Aldactazide*)

DO NOT USE:

Deserpidine w/methyclothiazide: (*Endurinyl*)
Guanabenz: (*Wytensin*)
Reserpine: (*Serpasil, Sandril*)
Reserpine w/hydroflumethiazide: (*Salutensin*)
Reserpine w/chlorothiazide: (*Diupres, Chloroserpine*)
Reserpine w/chlorothalidone: (*Regroton, Demi-Regroton*)

USE AS A LAST RESORT ONLY:

Minoxidil: (*Loniten*)

Once started on blood pressure medication, do you have to keep taking it for the rest of your life? Not necessarily, says a March 1991 JAMA review. If your hypertension is not too severe, you are an excellent candidate for 'step-down therapy'. As the term suggests, this method helps you work down gradually to lower and lower levels of medication while at the same time, you adopt nondrug therapies such as exercise, stress management and diet to achieve acceptable blood pressure levels. (You might also investigate nutritional supple-mentation with potassium and/or magnesium.)

In all cases, the sooner off drugs the better. Long-term drug regimens are not only terribly expensive - more so all the time - toxic buildup can decrease the quality of life and drain your health as well as your retirement savings.

♥ ♥ ♥

The Brechers have always been a non-drug-taking family. We periodically discard the only medication we stock: aspirin. When the bottle on hand is outdated, we throw it away. Usually, it's not been opened. Lucky? Perhaps. Opinionated? No doubt. We come by our anti-drug bias quite naturally. It's in our genes.

Harold's father, God rest his soul, who lived happily and healthily past his 94th birthday, never trusted doctors or drugs. He loved telling how the medical business reminded him of his favorite Charlie Chaplin movie - the one where the lovable tramp was a glazier and drummed up customers by paying a young kid (Jackie Coogan) to throw bricks through store windows. Right behind the rock-thrower came Charlie, tools in hand, ready to repair the damage.

"Doctors work the same way," Pop would say. "The medicine they give you to make you well makes you sicker instead, and you have to keep going back for more medicine. I don't want any part of it."

♥

What use can you make of this information?

Check labels in your medicine chest carefully. Of the 58 prescription drugs for heart disease, high blood pressure and diseases of the blood vessels that the authors of "Worst Pills,

Best Pills" include in their book, 23 are listed as **"Do Not Use"** because of the unnecessary risks they pose. Should you be taking one of them, bringing this report to your doctor's attention might save you much grief.

Anytime your doctor prescribers a medication, ask: "Is this drug necessary?" If the drug *is* necessary, it is equally essential to ascertain the proper dose level for you. The *lowest* dose that produces the desired effect is the *best* dose for the patient receiving it, since the bad things drugs do are dose-related. More often than not, doses that conventional wisdom would assume to be 'too low' to work, are the *optimal* dose. Make certain therefore, before beginning a drug regimen, that the lowest available dose is the one prescribed.

As an example of why this is so: a certain thiazide diuretic will decrease elevated blood pressure just as much whether the dose is 10 mg or 100 mg., but the two doses will have vastly different effects on blood sugar, potassium and other parameters. At the 10 mg dose, less than 5% of patients will suffer drug-induced hypokalemia (low potassium); at the 100 mg dose levels, hypokalemia will result in more than 50% of patients.

It also helps to be aware your doctor has a variety of drug choices in each of the cardiovascular disease categories. As many as 25 different drugs will lower blood pressure and there are just as many marketed to decrease the incidence of angina attacks. Some drugs are better tolerated by some people than by others. One person's "drug X" may well be the next person's "poison X". Rarely, if ever, is there just *one* drug available to treat your particular cardiovascular disease. For drug treatment to be effective, you must stick with your drug regimen, day in, day out. You're not apt to do it if the drugs you're taking make you feel ill all the time. If you are sickened every time you take a prescribed drug, request an alternative - and another - and another. You may have to try two, three, four or more, before finally finding one that you can tolerate.

What else? Read through the long scary lists of adverse side effects that pertain to the drugs your doctor prescribes. Insist on being given the least damaging alternative. Try to avoid multiple medication. Even relatively mild and innocuous drugs can propel you into the "drug-illness" cycle. Forewarned, you might be prompted to seek nondrug treatments. There's good cause, after all, why one after another, chemical medicines, launched with great fanfare, have bit the dust!

With one notable exception: the chelating agent, EDTA. While all other medications, to varying degrees, offer primarily symptom relief, EDTA (the chelation drug) is the only one that both provides symptom relief AND minimizes the disease process, and in some way not yet known, does so with minuscule adverse effects.

No aphorism of Hippocrates holds truer to this day, than that in which he laments the length of time necessary to establish medical truths....

Commentaries on the History and
Cure of Diseases, 1799

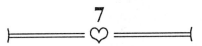

7

WHAT'S NEW ABOUT CHELATION? NOTHING. THAT'S REALLY BIG NEWS!

EDTA has withstood the test of time. Over the years, chelationists have made a few treatment and diagnostic improvements. They are somewhat more knowledgeable about the life style changes required to maintain treatment benefits, but not much else has changed. Reading current chelation literature triggers a sense of deja vu. Much of what's said today matches what was said repeatedly before.

There's a comforting consistency between past and present scientific reports and conclusions. Block out the release dates and author names, and it's almost impossible to distinguish between accounts from early pioneers and present-day clinicians.

STANDING THE TEST OF TIME

Go back twenty years, and read what a doctor said then. Here's what famed Vitamin E researcher Wilfred E. Shute, M.D.

reported in *How To Survive The New Health Catastrophes* in 1973.

"I've searched the medical literature and quickly accumulated more than 200 journal articles on the subject. In every case, the results of the therapy with chelating agents were just short of fantastic."

Nobel prize winner Linus Pauling writing currently says: "EDTA chelation therapy makes good sense to me as a chemist and medical researcher. It has a rational scientific basis and the evidence for clinical benefit seems strong."

Pauling goes on to deplore the harassment of chelating physicians. He places the blame on professional ignorance of the scientific literature and their disregard of the large body of available published documentation that supports what he calls "this emerging nonsurgical treatment for atherosclerosis and related age-associated disease."

In 1979, Dr. Bruce Halstead, in his classic text, *The Scientific Basis of EDTA Chelation Therapy,* explained the chelation concept and documented EDTA's chemical properties in elegant terms. What he said then is valid today.

As Dr. Halstead pointed out at the time, a patient's 'need to know' depends to some extent on his educational background and interest. If you have a B.S. in Biochemistry, the pharmacology of EDTA and its effects on lipid peroxidation, mitrochondria, platelets, and bone structure and a summary of its action on metabolic function could be of great interest.

If, on the other hand, you had trouble passing Chemistry 101, your interest is probably far more pragmatic and limited. Chances are the questions you want answered are far different from those that consume the scientific community. All the same, you cannot make an informed judgment about treatment choices, or participate appropriately in the doctor-patient partnership, without a smattering of knowledge about the complicated scientific issues in which you hold a very large stake.

PLEASE DON'T SKIP THIS

For starters, the basics. The definition of 'chelation' is a grabber - literally. The word comes from the Greek word 'chele' that refers to the claw of a crab or lobster. Picture a claw's pincer-like grip, and you'll have a graphic image of how a chelating agent attracts minerals and metals into its electro-magnetic field. A substance is 'chelated' when it is grabbed, trapped and transformed by a chelating agent.

Scientific purists may find Dr. Halstead's description more acceptable: "Chelation is specifically defined as the incorporation of a metal ion into a heterocyclic ring structure. An example would be a metal or mineral, such as calcium or lead, that comes in contact with a chelating agent, and is imprisoned by the chelating chemical, thereby taking on a new identity."

Ethylene diamine tetra-acetic acid - EDTA is its nickname - is a man-made amino acid, which mimics the action of natural chelates, with a particular affinity for toxic metals such as lead, mercury, cadmium, aluminum. Should EDTA meet up with such named substances in the blood stream and/or cell walls, it unites with the metal atom, forming a closed ring within which the assimilated metal is sequestered. Once that happens, it loses its physiologic and toxic properties, and is later excreted in body wastes.

We have already described the considerable variety of Industrial uses of EDTA - as a water softener, for one example. In nature, chelation is an important process by which plants and animals use inorganic metals. Chlorophyll, the green part of plants, is a chelate of magnesium. Many valuable drugs, among them the antibiotics, are dependent on chelation processes for their effectiveness. There are a number of natural chelators in the human body - amino acids such as histidine and cystine, and vitamins C and E. Therapeutically, EDTA is diluted into about a quart of fluid, slowly fed into the patient a drop at a time via an intravenous drip, over a three to four hour period.

HEARTBEATS AND SKIPPED BEATS

Before you can begin to understand what EDTA accomplishes pharmaceutically, you need to know a little something about what keeps your heart beating - and what makes it stop. Asked to name their number one health fear, people name blindness, a fatal heart attack and cancer, in that order. Thanks to the widespread publicity given to atherosclerosis as *the* high-risk factor leading to myocardial infarctions, cardiophobics believe if they're felled, it will be because of plaque-clogged arteries shutting off blood supply to the heart pump.

That's not likely to happen. The truth is that ventricular arrhythmia (disrupted heart rhythm), the most common of all heart conditions, is the prime culprit in over 500,000 sudden heart deaths each year Electrophysiologists - clinicians and researchers involved in cardiac electrical function - have determined that arrhythmias or failing and disjointed heart rhythms are the most deadly of all heart conditions - responsible for more than two-thirds of all deaths linked to heart disease.

According to J. Thomas Bigger, M.D., Director of the Arrhythmia Control Unit at Columbia-Presbyterian Medical Center in New York, "An American dies suddenly and unexpectedly every minute of every day, causing an incredible emotional burden on society. Nearly all of these cardiac events are due to a severe form of cardiac rhythm disturbance called ventricular fibrillation."

As Dr. Bigger explains, the heart is not merely a vital muscular pump feeding life sustaining blood throughout the vascular system, but is more importantly a "hot-wired organ," dependent on steady and unfailing electrical impulses to function efficiently.

The heart contains four chambers: two blood-collecting chambers at its top, called atria. There are two pumping chambers at its bottom, called ventricles: one oxygenates blood, the other pumps oxygen-enriched blood throughout the body.

What keeps your heart beating? Electrical signals originating within the heart usually start in the sinoatrial (or sinus node) at the top of the right atrium. The sinus node is considered the heart's pacemaker because it is the originating point and control center for normal heartbeats.

Nerve fibers then conduct electrical impulses from the sinus node to the atrioventricular node located between the atrium and ventricle chambers. Among many functions, the atrioventricular node assures that the ventricles do not discharge blood to the lungs and body until they fill up with blood from the atria. The sinus node and atrioventricular nodes transmit the exquisitely timed signals that control heart chamber contraction and expansion.

Cardiac rhythm disturbances - or arrhythmias - are classified according to where they occur in the heart and their effect on heart rhythm. Those arising in the atria are called 'atrial arrhythmias'; 'ventricular arrhythmias' begin in the ventricles, and are generally considered the more serious.

There are further classifications:

- **Sinus arrhythmias** - cyclic changes in the heart rate during breathing, common in children and often found in adults;
- **Sinus tachycardia** - the sinus node sends out electrical signals faster than usual, speeding up the heart rate;
- **Sick sinus syndrome** - the sinus node does not fire its signals properly, so that the heart rate slows down. Sometimes the rate alternates between a slow (bradycardia) and fast (tachycardia) rate;

- **Premature supraventricular contractions** or **premature atrial contractions** (PAC) - a series of early beats in the atria speed up the heart rate. In paroxysmal tachycardia, repeated periods of very fast heartbeats begin and end suddenly;
- **Atrial flutter** - rapidly fired signals cause the muscles in the atria to contract quickly, leading to a very fast steady heartbeat;
- **Atrial fibrillation** - electrical signals in the atria fired in a very fast and uncontrolled manner. Electrical signals arrive in the ventricles in a completely irregular fashion, resulting in a heart beat that is quite erratic;
- **Wolff-Parkinson-White syndrome** - abnormal pathways between the atria and ventricles cause the electrical signal to arrive at the ventricles too soon and to be transmitted back into the atria. Very fast heart rates may develop as the electrical signal ricochets between the atria and ventricles;
- **Premature ventricular complexes** (PVC) - an electrical signal from the ventricles causes an early heart beat that generally goes unnoticed. The heart then seems to pause until the next beat of the ventricle occurs in a regular fashion;
- **Ventricular tachycardia** - the heart beats fast due to electrical signals arising from the ventricles (rather than from the atria);
- **Ventricular fibrillation** - electrical signals in the ventricles - fired in a very fast and uncontrolled manner, causing the heart to quiver rather than beat and pump blood.

What are the underlying causes of cardiac arrhythmias - commonly called the electrical storms of the heart? There's a little we know; a lot we don't.

WHAT KILLED JIM FIXX?

Arrhythmias have frequently occurred in individuals supposedly free of heart or blood vessel damage. Asymptomatic individuals have unpredictably dropped dead. Case in point: Jim Fixx. From 1977 to 1984, this famed best-selling author (*The Complete Book of Running*) promoted running as the high road to health, longevity and well being. He lived by his principles, running 10 to 15 miles each day. When, at 52, he dropped dead while jogging in rural Vermont, his demise seemed a mockery and shook the runners' world.

A celebrity-linked event attracts attention. For years the medical community has ignored similar instances of seemingly healthy individuals who've dropped dead in like fashion. Occasionally, to some doctor's embarrassment, they've just emerged from their annual medical checkup with a clean bill of health. Five minutes later, they're a corpse lying on the sidewalk. Unfortunately, the confusion caused by the Jim Fixx event triggered a national debate on the wrong subject. Experts explored the merit of exercise, instead of concentrating on the causes - and prevention - of sudden, unexplained cardiac death.

As often happens, the medical mirror was reflecting on the wrong issue. Disappointing, but not surprising. Although more people die of arrhythmias in one week than from AIDS since the beginning of the 'epidemic', professionals pay scant attention to the fatal arrhythmias long known to kill more men than any other disease. It's a problem too long ignored.

Physicians have known about electrical malfunction of the heart since 1774, with the successful resuscitation of a boy who had 'died' - stopped breathing after a fall out of a window - by electrical stimulation. By 1820, the fervor for electrical treatment for all manner of illnesses peaked with the appearance of the first 'electric chair'. Ironically, it was designed to 'cure' not 'kill'.

During the first half of this century, cardiologists concentrated on studying the cause, mechanism, prevention and treatment of coronary artery spasm. They had minimal success until the development of electrocardiograms in 1920 aided their investigations. Nothing much transpired until the mid 60's. By that time, it was a well established fact that arrhythmias were the underlying pathology in heart disease. Until the mid-1970's, major medical centers conducted innumerable clinical investigations into the provocation and control of acute myocardial infarction.

Then abruptly, the focus of exploration changed. Frustrated perhaps by their inability to combat arrhythmias effectively, and presented with a highly promotable new technology - bypass surgery - cardiac centers switched the spotlight from the crux concern to the more treatable (and profitable) corollary disease, clogged arteries. A few stalwarts protested.

"Performing surgery on coronary arteries or cardiac valves while ignoring the underlying arrhythmias makes as little sense as treating a patient with diabetes and a cut finger by merely putting a band aid on the injured limb and pronouncing him cured."

Sound familiar? That's a voice from the past making a point truly as applicable today, but widely ignored by America's knife-happy surgeons. In other parts of the world, researchers with unclouded memories recall that sixty years of research supports a need to focus on arrhythmias, not clogged arteries, if we're ever to solve the mystery of myocardial infarctions. From 1948 through 1980, over a dozen studies of infarcted hearts have consistently failed to corroborate the coronary artery thrombosis theory. Thrombosis, the complete obstruction of an artery by a blood clot, so often implicated as the cause of a myocardial infarction (heart attack or coronary), is more apt to occur *AFTER* the heart attack. Thousands of post mortems have shown victims of fatal hearts attacks have had no evidence whatsoever of coronary artery blockage. So why do doctors continue to insist it's clogged arteries that will do us all in?

HAS THE DIAGNOSIS BEEN DESIGNED TO FIT THE TREATMENT?

There could be several reasons for the over-concentration on clogged arteries. For starters, the cornerstone of therapy for treatment and prevention of MI for almost thirty years is the need to remove blockages in coronary arteries under the supposition they are the cause of infarction. No matter the literature persuasively refutes so simplistic a notion. It's been easy to sell the public on clogged-artery disease as the basis for many profitable clean-out-the-arteries-at-all-costs therapies.

Perhaps doctors don't know any better. Possibly. Maybe they think Joe Average patient is not smart enough to comprehend a more sophisticated explanation of what ails him. Perchance it's just too embarrassing to admit they don't have the foggiest notion how to address the *real* issue. Or, because they have nothing better to suggest, cling to an invalid hypothesis so they can pretend patently ineffective therapies may do some good.

One thing for certain, researchers still don't know the precise cause of cardiac arrhythmias. Symptoms are unpredictable and vary greatly from one individual to another. Complicating the picture, they've found a high incidence of coronary vasospasm in persons without underlying heart or blood vessel damage.

One underlying cause of arrhythmia seems to be a lack of oxygen transfer into the heart's left ventricle (the chamber that supplies blood to most of the body.) This can set up a condition called metabolic acidosis, which eats away at heart tissue, causing biochemical lesions. Left unchecked, and subject to continued oxygen radical damage, lesions ulcerate and cause irreparable injury to the heart's nervous system.

In 1986, Drs. Rita Levi-Montalcini and Stanley Cohen shared that year's Nobel Prize for identifying the first two growth factor proteins that control the growth and proliferation of cells. Following up on their finding, a University of Washington cell biologist, Russell Ross, discovered that when a growth factor derived from blood platelets (PDGF) goes out of control, atherosclerosis is the result. This put atherosclerosis in a brand new perspective. According to Ross, this disease is demonstrably different from the common description and "not at all like the sludge buildup in a sewer pipe."

White blood cells, it appears, flock to the site of an injury in an artery or heart wall and secrete PDGF that stimulates the growth of smooth muscle cells. When free radicals disrupt control systems and receptors there is a devastating communication breakdown and smooth muscle cells multiple into what may eventually develop into calcified plaque.

The newest research findings are that communication between the cells takes place via ions, growth factor proteins and growth factor cell receptors. All are subject to free radical attack (more on this later) and may be largely responsible for the disruption of intracellular communication. Two German scientists, Drs. Erwin Neher and Bert Sakmann, received the 1991 Nobel Prize in physiology for their work in measuring how living cells communicate with each other via electrically charged ions. Their trail-blazing research has advanced our understanding of the development of a spectrum of degenerative diseases: diabetes, epilepsy and heart disease.

THE ORDER OF CHAOS

The very unpredictability of the heart's behavior has led some scientists to turn to chaos theory for a better understanding. By this mathematical hypothesis, first applied to the vagaries of weather prediction, a new understanding of the heart's beating pattern is now under investigation.

It's long been supposed that the heart goes from beating regularly to beating chaotically in the most common form of heart attack - ventricular fibrillation. And while it's been known that the heartbeat is not as constant as a metronome, and that the intervals between beats will vary by small but measureable amounts, it's now thought these minute changes in rhythm are not perilous in the way once thought.

According to one group of researchers at Harvard Medical School, the more *chaotic* these tiny fluctuations the better, for the degree of chaos is significantly more pronounced in healthy hearts than in diseased ones. What's more, say these scientists, an early sign that something is about to go wrong is when the interbeat interval becomes too regular and monotonous! As cardiologist Ary Goldberger explains it, true health - physical as well as mental - includes the ability to roll with the punches, react in a flexible way to unexpected environmental changes, and make a rapid adjustment to whatever stresses come along.

Of what use is so exotic a view of the heart's unpredictable behavior? The obvious application is that someday heart patients might wear a tiny monitoring device that would signal an automatic alert when the heartbeat loses too much variability.

Besides metabolic acidosis and disrupted ion and protein growth factor communication, there are many other factors acting singly or in concert that increase the risk of fatal arrhythmia:

- **Plaque-clogged arteries do play a vital role.** Impaired electrical heart function is apt to occur when heart cells - both muscle and nerve cells - are damaged by a severely reduced blood supply.
- **High blood pressure is a factor.** Arrhythmias can be triggered by the enlargement of heart cells due to hypertension.

- **'Sticky' blood is at fault.** Blood platelet aggregation coupled with the release of the artery-constricting prostoglandin, thromboxane A2, are integral to artery spasm - a neurological response. Spasms compromise blood flow to heart muscle and nerve cells.
- **Drug use is a catalyst.** The so-called 'recreational' drugs (cocaine, crack, marijuana) are known to trigger ventricular tachycardia and fibrillation - deadly forms of arrhythmia that often result in death.
- **You can be scared to death.** Terror in the mind, or any highly stressful emotion - anger, passion, excitement, glee or great sorrow - can interrupt the flow of electrical impulses to the heart, causing them to become obstructed and confused. Mayhem may be the result.
- **Overexertion can provoke arrhythmia.** Damage can occur quickly during periods when the heart is under pressure. Like any muscle, the heart needs more oxygen to do more work. If demand exceeds reserve capacity - (the classic case being the middle-aged man with a paunch shoveling snow out of his driveway) - the muscle can starve, developing "dead zones" that short-circuit electrical impulses.
- **Metabolic dysfunction is a primary component**. Research has shown that a magnesium/manganese deficiency or imbalance produces spasms of coronary arteries.
- **Anti-arrhythmia drugs can precipitate attacks - so can remedial surgical procedures.** Many of the therapies (bypass surgery and angioplasty, for two examples) supposedly designed to protect patients from fatal spasms actually trigger them. Two FDA-approved drugs, encainide and flecainide, thought to correct heart rhythm irregularities were found instead to increase the risk of death in certain patients.

- **Heavy metal toxins disrupt neurological pathways.** Our polluted environment poisons the air we breathe, the water we drink and the food we eat with the heavy metals - lead, cadmium, iron, copper, mercury, aluminum. The cardioneurological system is particularly vulnerable to neurotoxic chemicals whether from pesticides, pollutants, cosmetic ingredients or food additives. Lead in particular, has an especially deleterious effect on the gastrointestinal tract, the blood-forming tissues and neurological functioning.

- **The worst culprit may be free radical activity,** the pathological process that not only disrupts every cell in the body, including nerve cells, but as many now believe, is also the underlying cause of all forms of life-shortening sickness. From cancer to AIDS, arthritis to asthma, Alzheimer's to atherosclerosis - there's evidence free radical proliferation is largely responsible for the cell and tissue damage that eventually leads to chronic degenerative disease. (More on free radicals in Chapter Eight.)

ONE SOLUTION? GET THE LEAD OUT

So where does EDTA fit in? EDTA (the chemical used in chelation therapy) removes chromium, iron, mercury, copper, lead, zinc, cadmium, cobalt and aluminum from the body - in that order of affinity - and is also the "treatment of choice" for lead poisoning.

Who says so? The AMA. The FDA. The CDC (Center for Disease Control). Licensed doctors. From first year interns to professors of medicine at Harvard University and equally prestigious medical centers - all will confirm EDTA chelation therapy is the "treatment of choice" for excess lead deposits and will also remove the aforementioned toxic metals from the body.

EDTA's ability to chelate an array of cell-disrupting metallic toxins from the body expands its therapeutic usefulness far beyond the common practice of keeping it on hand as an antidote for lead poisoning. Three of EDTA's lesser known benefits:

- EDTA removes iron and copper, two potent free radical catalysts and will diminish destructive free radical activity by a million-fold, according to Harry B. Demopoulos, M.D., associate professor of pathology at New York University Medical Center, an internationally known cancer researcher.

- EDTA, independent of its effect on blood supply, enhances the heart muscle's phosphorous utilization, thereby improving heart function, according to Drs. C.F. Peng, J.J. Kane, M.L. Murphy and K.D.Straub in a study published in the *Journal of Molecular Cell Cardiology.*

- Many studies have shown that EDTA removes toxic metals that compete with and neutralize nutrients necessary for optimal protective enzymatic function, for example: the cadmium in tobacco smoke that competes with zinc in metalloactivated enzymes.

- EDTA in solution is the substance used to keep the donor's heart alive while awaiting transplant.

How about that?

They (Radicals) form in the liver from all kinds of drugs,
From solvents and nasty things used to kill bugs ...
They'll infarct your heart, even make you grow old,
and they'll mutate your genome is what we've been told.
Their causes, reactions, and guessed repercussions
Are turning up often in Journal discussions.

Kathryn T. Knecht
NIH Institute for Environmental Health

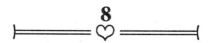

FREE RADICAL DAMAGE
CALLS FOR RADICAL REMEDIES

If a nuclear accident were to rupture a nearby power plant, how quickly would you and your family pack up and leave? What if there was no safe place to flee? Would it surprise you to learn that that *is* your predicament, even if the nearest nuclear threat is a thousand miles away?

Leading scientists say so. The deadly consequences of a utility spewing forth lethal radiation are not all that different except in degree - from the free radical assaults that encircle us every day. We live, as Jimmy Durante was wont to say, " . . . surrounded by assassins."

It makes no matter where we live; we're vulnerable to exposure. Worse yet, we cannot escape. As if we didn't have enough to worry about, we've a new enemy - this one dangerously invisible. Potentially deadly free radicals lurk in ambush, unrelenting and destructive. We only recently got this bad news. Sophisticated detection instruments had to be developed to alert scientists to the free radicals prowling and ricocheting around and throughout our bodies. It took years of investigation - still going on - to grasp their significance and understand how and why free radicals are *the* common denominator in more than sixty of this century's most prevalent degenerative diseases.

Where do free radicals come from?

1: Inhaled toxic chemicals;

2: Drinking contaminated water;

3: Eating chemical additives;

4: Consuming unsaturated processed oils

5: Smoking (and exposure to tobacco fumes);

6: Everyday radiation: X-rays from television, airport security and medical diagnostics; video display terminals, luminous clocks, watches and other dials, cosmic rays, tinted eyeglasses, porcelain dentures, amalgam fillings, smoke detectors - and the list goes on.

Sunlight generates free radicals, as do auto engines, burning wood or paper, radon in your home. Free radicals spew forth when your teeth are x-rayed, or drilled, you file your fingernails, warm up leftover roast beef, barbecue on your backyard grill, consume anything containing rancid oils or fats, drink, breathe polluted air or ingest polluted water. Awake or asleep it goes on. The environment in your office and home may be contributing to free radical attack. And that's just for starters!

Before we go further, be assured nature provides the body with built-in protection. Moreover, you can upgrade defenses with potent fortification against free radical attack. We shall be sharing helpful information on that subject in later chapters, but to make the best use of preventive and restorative techniques requires a working knowledge of free radicals - and how they become your number one health enemy.

IT ALL STARTS (AND ENDS) AT THE CELL

So what are free radicals? At the risk of telling you more than you care to know about the complex field of molecular cell biology, here goes.

A free radical is an impaired or out-of-balance molecule or atom that is the by-product of a chemical interaction. If you studied science in high school, you may recall the basic building blocks of all substances are called elements: oxygen, carbon, hydrogen, sodium, calcium, and so forth. The smallest part of an element to take part in a chemical reaction is an atom.

Atoms are surrounded by "paired" electrons that keep them in balance. When a chemical reaction causes an electron to lose its mate, the atom goes spinning out-of-control. It becomes a highly unstable and promiscuous radical, "free" to latch onto and disrupt any substance in the body. The noted gerontologist, Dr. Alex Comfort, describes a free radical in more down-to-earth terms: "A free radical is like a lecherous convention delegate away from his wife."

Free radicals, particularly oxygen free radicals (oxygen radicals) are also on the prowl. They're "electron-hungry" and have a voracious appetite for cell membranes - the fattier the better. Like many terrorists, they enlist accomplices to help them do their dirty work. In the body, misplaced iron and copper ions serve as catalysts to initiate and accelerate oxygen radical activity.

The interaction between an oxygen radical and its target produces a cascade of free radicals. Left unchecked, they will in turn attack and disrupt nearby cells that will also produce torrents of additional free radicals, and so on and so on. Since uncontrolled free radical activity disrupts the chemistry, viability and very life of cells, it is best described as the human counterpart of the "China Syndrome" - a nuclear plant meltdown.

You can observe free radicals do their dirty work outside the body, too. If you've ever cut apple slices for a pie and saved them for later baking, only to find they've turned an ugly brown , or left your bike out in the rain where it rusted, you've seen it happen. Free radicals strike again.

Ironically, not all free radical generation is destructive. Many biochemical processes which generate free radicals are essential to good health. For example: your cells couldn't breathe - absorb oxygen or emit carbon monoxide - without producing free radicals; your liver couldn't detoxify noxious materials without producing free radicals; defender blood cells couldn't fight off health-destroying organisms without producing free radicals; you couldn't see without the melan in pigment whose production relies on the free radical process. Even more ironic, the most prevalent and destructive are the oxygen radicals, yet without oxygen, we could not survive.

If this is a confusing concept, consider the difference between water and ice. Both are forms of H_2O, yet have different characteristics. You can't skate on an unfrozen pond; you would not dive into an iced-up pool. An oxygen radical is simply a mutated form of oxygen.

So how do we protect ourselves against the objectionable oxygen radicals? Fortunately, cells contain built-in safeguards - highly effective enzyme systems that produce superoxide dismutase (SOD), catalase, and glutathione peroxidase. Like volunteer fire fighters, these powerful substances stand ready to quell oxygen radical brush fires. Serving as a back-up crew are anti-oxidants such as vitamins E and C, beta-carotene, and glutathione. Although not nearly as effective as enzymes, they also function as capable oxygen radical neutralizers.

Like many a well-conceived scheme, it's only great when it works as designed. Unfortunately, our enzymatic shields become less potent as time goes by. Undermined by misplaced metallic ions and subjected to ongoing free-radical disruption, the once orderly apparatus wears out and breaks down. As birthdays add up, no one is spared. We all display subtle as well as obvious signs that free radicals are gumming up our works: fading memory, wrinkled skin, failing eyesight, split nails, 'liver' spots, 'floaters', cold hands and feet, the 'always tired' syndrome, hearing loss, increased sensitivity to pets, fumes, tobacco smoke and other irritants.

If you don't look or feel as young as you'd like, that's understandably disquieting, but not nearly as depressing as when free radicals take over. Once environmental insults clobber our defenses, it can be all down hill. First cells, then tissues, next genetically weakened "target organs" give way. The result is some form of degenerative disease involving the heart (heart disease), joints (arthritis), brains (Alzheimers), lungs (cancer), pancreas (diabetes), immune systems (AIDS), or whatever organ is first to falter. The final affront can result in a near fatal heart attack. Let's zero in on that.

AND NOW TO THE HEART OF THE MATTER

Your heart, no bigger than a clenched fist and weighing about 11 ounces, drives blood through some 60,000 miles of blood vessels (many more miles in the overweight) to nourish trillions of body cells. Working ceaselessly, it beats 100,000 times a day, 2.5 billion times in a lifetime and pumps enough blood to fill the Astrodome.

One would assume that with all this blood coursing through, the heart would have access to plenty of nourishment. Not so. Though constantly flooded with blood, the heart cannot take nourishment from this supply - its walls are too thick and have a water-tight lining. The heart muscle gets its blood supply from three coronary arteries (so named from the Latin word "crown" because they lie over the heart like a lopsided tiara).

When coronary artery lumens (the channels in arteries

through which blood flows to your heart) become encrusted with plaque, blood flow to the heart muscle gradually diminishes. The resulting discomfort feels like a squeezing, constricting, tight or heavy feeling in the chest. This is the scary condition popularly known as angina. It's an indication an area of heart muscle requires more blood than an artery can provide. The pains signal a problem of supply and demand and is your heart's way of warning, "Help, I need more oxygen!"

How does arterial plaque develop? Remember when you were a kid and scraped your knee on the sidewalk and a pesky scab formed over the wound? If you were awkward and kept reinjuring that knee, the scab would grow larger and uglier and seem to take forever to heal. Well, plaque can be likened to an internal scab that develops in response to repeated irritation.

To understand plaque formation, it helps to know that all arteries, including the coronary arteries, are subject to continuous trauma from blood pressure, viral and bacterial assault, biochemical and free radical attack. 'Young' arteries are flexible, springy and supple. As time goes by, arteries harden, thicken, and lose much of their resilience for any of a number of reasons, including age-related cross linkage.

When stresses cause fissures in artery linings, the body's enzymatic defenses normally provide protection. Should fortifications be weakened by genetic defect, or if they're held in check by toxic metals such as mercury and lead, arteries continue to thicken. Roughened by deposits of fatty materials in the damaged walls, tumor-like atheromas (lesions) develop. Under ongoing, progressive free radical assault, small areas harden into calcified plaque.

Arteriosclerosis - the medical term for what many refer to as "hardening of the arteries" - is the precursor to atherosclerosis: plaque-clogged arteries. Now you know the science behind the old axiom, "You're as old as your arteries." That's true.

THE BYPASS OPERATION:
SURGERY BY INTIMIDATION?

Almost every bypassed patient we've talked to over the past eight years has bitter comments on what led up to the "rush to surgery." No matter the event - angina, heart attack, arrhythmia, stress test failure - that brought him to medical attention, there is a predictable pattern to what happens next.

First, the doctor mandates an angiogram (an unscientific, unreliable, questionable, high-risk overused procedure); next comes the sober pronouncement of arterial blockage in precise percentage terms (50%, 65%, 75%, 95%) to support the pretense the figure is precise and accurate, when in fact, the digital read-out on a two dollar kitchen clock is far more accurate. Following that, the suggestion that death is imminent - and finally, the hurried trip to the operating amphitheater. In recent months, we hear the same complaints and scenarios from people who have agreed to angioplasty-type surgeries.

No telling how many hundreds of thousand of patients with atherosclerosis realize too late they're two-time losers: first victimized by their disease and then by the professionals they relied on to treat it. Intimidated by a quasi-scientific diagnosis, combined with the ominous warning their clogged arteries might close up or shut down at any moment, they fall for the fiction that they may drop dead on the spot.

Dr. Robert Mendelsohn, author of *Confessions of a Medical Heretic* said it best when he termed such routine scare tactics the "voodoo curse of modern medicine." When the doctor stares you down and states in his grimmest tight-lipped voice, "I won't be responsible for what happens to you," the most common reaction is to tremble with fear, and 'take your medicine', whatever it is.

You've got to be not just brave, but knowledgeable to resist. The only thing that will save you is some inkling that it's a half-truth at best that the procedure offered is your last chance at life.

How can we say that? Atherosclerosis is not in itself a fatal disease. Arterioles (small coronary arteries) provide collateral circulation between main arteries or segments of a main artery when they need to. When plaque blocks 50% of a coronary artery, the artery enlarges and allows the *same* blood flow as a healthy artery; when plaque clog exceeds 50%, collateral circulation will often compensate for the reduction in blood flow; with a 75% blockage, artery enlargement provides a blood flow equal to that of a 50% blocked artery; and most reassuring - less than a 10% increase in the diameter of a plaqued artery will double blood flow.

These basic teachings have been in the literature since 1971 when the International Association of Infarction Control, in response to a request by the World Health Organization, published their findings. Any doctor that doesn't know this should be sent back to medical school. Any doctor who knows this and pretends otherwise, should be defrocked for malpractice. What was valid about the heart twenty years ago, is just as true today.

Does this mean compromised blood flow is unimportant? Can be ignored? Left untreated? Of course not. Every cell in the body depends on adequate sustenance via unimpeded circulation. To feel your best, maintain vigor and vitality, you must do whatever necessary to improve the status of the entire cardiovascular system.

HEART ATTACKS: A MISNOMER

According to ancient Chinese philosophers, the start of wisdom is to call things by their right name. The term 'heart attack' is both inaccurate and misleading. Your heart would never attack you! It's far more accurate to say, it's **been** attacked - by free radicals. Let's summarize the typical 'heart attack' scenario:

- Oxygen radicals play an integral role in the process called "cross-linkage" - the reduction of elasticity in artery wall tissue (hardening of the arteries). As previously mentioned, inelastic arteries are more vulnerable to viral, chemical and physical damage.

- When lesions in coronary walls ulcerate, small blood vessels in the artery swell and leak red blood cells which rupture and release copper and iron.

- Like sharks frenzied by the smell of blood, oxygen radicals are drawn to the copper and iron ions. They attack cells in the vicinity, disrupting cell membranes, enzyme systems, neurotransmitters, and neuroreceptors. Neuro-systems are particularly susceptible to peroxidative destruction because of their high concentration of fat insulation.

- After a significant number of artery nerve elements suffer impairment or are destroyed, a coronary artery spasm frequently occurs. Coronary artery spasms momentarily cut off blood flow to the heart causing additional minimal disruption of the heart's electrical pathways and control systems.

- In conjunction with a blood clot, a coronary artery spasm causes additional extensive damage to the heart's neurological system. Blood clots can become lodged in arteries free of plaque.

- Many of the same chemical and physical forces that attack artery walls, attack the heart muscle itself - and with equal, if not increased, intensity. Consequently, lesions develop in the heart muscle and they too suffer the damage caused by destructive oxygen radical activity. Lesions and scars are routinely observed in hearts whose coronary arteries were free of atherosclerotic disease. For causes not completely identified yet, the heart's left ventricle is most vulnerable. This is the chamber that receives oxygenated blood, expends the most energy and where blood pressure is greatest, and more apt to suffer serious damage.

- Continued assault by oxygen radicals and other toxic chemicals impact on the heart's electrical system, and is the underlying cause of an often fatal cardiac neurological breakdown. To emphasize the point once more: *the heart can and does become arrhythmic in the absence of atherosclerosis.*

In the event of cardiac arrest, cardio-pulmonary resuscitation can buy time until a defibrillator arrives on the scene to shock the heart's nerve control centers back to life. (See the Appendix for improved CPR procedure). When the heart is revived, the administration of anti-clotting drugs can prevent a recurrence.

The important lessons to be learned from this chapter are that your heart's health and your life depend on: (1) blood platelet stickiness (tendency to form clots); and (2) how well your heart's neuro-systems can withstand electrical malfunction.

Your total health, on the other hand, depends on optimal blood flow. To feel your best, be your best, look your best, you must get oxygen-rich blood flowing throughout your body. Atherosclerosis is a system-wide condition. It diminishes blood flow not just to the heart, but to the tips of your fingers and the tips of your toes, and to your brain as well.

Restoring coronary artery blood-flow with a bypass, angioplasty or any similar procedure, is but a piecemeal panacea to a system-wide problem. EDTA chelation therapy is the *only* known treatment that 'jump starts' biochemical processes back into business. It does this by a number of mechanisms (many still unknown) that increase blood flow throughout the body, reduce blood platelet "stickiness" and at the same time, limit free radical activity from further disrupting the heart's neuro-systems. EDTA does it all by removing misplaced toxic metal ions from the sites where they've accumulated. In so doing, EDTA restores enzyme function, reduces exessive free radical activity, and protects you from a death-dealing heart attack.

WHY SO MUCH FLACK ABOUT PLAQUE?

To quote TV's Church Lady (from NBC's *Saturday Night Live*) it's been "so-o-o convenient" for those who stand to profit to exaggerate the dangers of atherosclerosis. To be more explicit, marketers of sophisticated equipment and procedures designed to repair only reachable placqued sites have consistently overstated treatment benefits and emphasized the perils of occlusion. Deliberately or out of ignorance, they've pinned the tail on the wrong donkey - blood flow in place of system-wide biochemical malfunction - to promote the widespread acceptance of their products and services. To take the cynical view, they've terrorized patients into opting for intrusive, dangerous and ineffective treatments.

Does this mean that atherosclerosis need not be taken seriously? Heck no! Besides lessening the quality of life because of poor circulation, placqued arteries are more likely to spasm and more inclined to entrap blood clots. These are both contributing factors to heart damage. Along with more serious intimate traumatization, when the heart's neurological function is further compromised by such ongoing events, the heart muscle itself may give up and die.

STROKES OF GOOD LUCK:
TIAs (TRANSIENT ISCHEMIC ATTACKS)

Although heart disease is the number one killer, many people fear a stroke more than a heart attack - and rightly so. Why? Strokes raise the possibility of irreversible damage. While many heart attack survivors don't get around as much as they'd like, stroke survivors often suffer a triple whammy: immobility plus impaired face, leg, and arm function and worse still, brain and speech dysfunction.

Stroke presents the scariest scenario: few of us can contemplate the possibility of going on life support, a living 'vegetable', without shuddering. The bad news is, these things do happen; the good news is, there are things you can do to reduce the likelihood it will happen to you.

You stand a better chance of avoiding the disaster of a major stroke by paying attention to transient ischemic attack - ministrokes - better known as TIA's, which are brief neurological deficits lasting from a few minutes to less than 24 hours. Normally, there is complete recovery between attacks. People who have had one or more TIAs are 9.5 times more likely to have a full-blown stroke than people of the same age and sex who have not had a warning episode. Approximately one-third of all who experience one TIA will continue to have them (and continue to be candidates for a full stroke.)

Predisposing factors most apt to lead to TIA's are: emboli; hypotensive (low blood pressure) episodes; temporary occlusion of neck vessels brought on, for example, by sudden turning or twisting of the head and neck; temporary cardiac arrhythmias; arteriosclerotic vessel disease. Simply put, a TIA is most likely to occur when a clot or some debris *momentarily* blocks blood flow to the brain. A stroke occurs when a blood clot or debris gets hung up long enough to cause brain damage and associated physical and mental impairment.

What are the symptoms to watch out for? The most common are: (A) temporary weakness, clumsiness or loss of feeling in an arm, leg or the side of the face (or some combination); (B) temporary loss of vision in one or both eyes or double vision; (C) temporary speech loss or speech difficulty; (D) temporary confusion; (E) temporary dizziness.

Symptoms may materialize individually, or in combination. In either event, should you experience any of these TIA symptoms, view it as a stroke of good luck. You have been given time to get help and ward off a major attack.

To mend the arteries which feed the brain following a TIA, the most desirable treatment is identical to the one that works best with atherosclerotic coronary arteries. A course of EDTA infusions in conjunction with anti-coagulant supplements is applicable for all arteries, and is usually the only procedure which wards off subsequent strokes. (One proviso: This treatment is NOT applicable when there's a thinning or ballooning of a brain artery wall, blood vessel leakage or tumor.)

Can you wait for some small symptom? Don't trust to luck. Since not all strokes are preceded by TIAs, it's essential to have your blood's slipperiness tested periodically by a blood platelet adhesion index. If it's found too sticky, your doctor can prescribe an anticoagulant, EDTA infusions or nutritional supplements - preferably the latter two.

STRIKE BACK AT STROKES

- Seventy to 80 percent of strokes result from clots that plug up one of two carotid arteries that supply blood to the brain. Most TIAs or mini-strokes, are caused by temporary blockages, and have the same underpinnings as full-fledged stroke;
- The most common cause of blockage is atrial fibrillation. When the two small upper chambers of the heart quiver instead of beating effectively, they don't completely divest themselves of blood. Stagnant blood pools form clots that make their way to the carotid arteries.
- The second common denominator is blockage from a blood clot or debris from an atherosclerotic carotid artery - often following a carotid artery spasm.

- A third widespread reason for blockage is clots or debris that have broken away from some blood vessel in the body.

To sum up: atherosclerosis is a system-wide condition that effects ALL arteries equally. Any quick-fix remedy which attends to one artery while ignoring all others is as ineffectual as trying to stop a sieve from leaking by plugging up one hole.

What can be done after a full-blown stroke? Let us tell you about a friend of ours.

A STRIKING RECOVERY

One day Harold came home shaking his head and mumbling to himself. What was wrong?

"Well, you know, I sometimes stop at Ali's (a close-to-home gourmet grocery and cafe) for a can of guava juice," he began. "Well, this morning I did and I'm sorry. Do you remember me telling you about his mother?"

"Yes. Isn't she the lady who had balloon angioplasty after you told Ali everything we knew about it was bad?

"Right. That was only about five months ago. Well, today she was sitting in the back of the store with her right eye half closed, her face and mouth twisted out of shape, drooling and mumbling - sort of like an incoherent Buddy Hackett."

"The poor woman. Why are you so upset?"

"Well, this is what Ali told me. His mother was hospitalized and 'under observation' for a week or so. Then her doctor told him there was nothing more they could do and sent her home."

"That's par for the course. So?"

"So, that joker of a doc said that considering the mother's age - she's 77 - and the number of drugs she's been taking - a bunch - he told Ali he was 'expecting something like this to happen?' 'Expecting' it? What is this - Jeanne Dixon cum stethoscope? If this doc is so bright, why didn't he warn them ahead of time and do something about it?

"I'm through giving advice. I told Ali all about chelation, and when his mother started having chest pains he automatically took her to their doctor who said if she didn't have an angioplasty right away, there was no telling how long she would last.

"When I reminded him that I also warned him angioplasty and bypass surgery didn't do anything for all the rest of the screwed up arteries, he said, 'I know, I know, but the doctor said my mother needed this angioplasty right away, and I didn't want to take any chances. And who am I to argue with a big doctor?'

"So help me - I'm through talking about chelation. From now on, we write about it, and I keep my big mouth shut."

If you believe that, you've never met Harold. On a follow-up visit, he convinced his grocer-friend to have his mother treated by our nutritionally-oriented physician, Dr. Sohini Patel, who is experienced in administering EDTA. Ten days and four chelation treatments later, Ali's mom had full control of her eye, mouth and speech, and her face was back to normal.

How's Ali's mother now, after twenty treatments?

"She's back to normal," says an elated Ali. "Picky, picky, picky. She's right on top of us - pointing out any little thing we do wrong. But I'd rather have her that way than . . . well, you know."

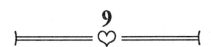

THE EDTA/HEART-SAVER CONNECTION

If you are a 'more science-less hype' person, you have the right mind set for making health decisions. You would probably appreciate rational reasons for considering chelation. You are right to want something more convincing than "we said it's good", before giving it a try.

In times past, chelation doctors didn't have much in the way of justifiable science to offer. They had little objective documentation of treatment benefits. Few considered it necessary or important, given the thousands of testimonials from grateful patients.

"Sick people get better. That's good enough for me," old-timers assured each other. The more scientific-minded took before-and-after pictures of patients whose gangrenous toes had turned from black to pink, people who'd arrived in wheelchairs and later walked out unaided, oldsters whose wrinkles had visibly faded. Almost all first generation chelationists kept albums stuffed full with ecstatic 'thank you' letters from brought-back-from-dead patients.

Before the establishment of a medical society (first AMPS, now ACAM) with a specialized interest in chelation and related therapies, doctors using EDTA for atherosclerosis were pretty much on their own. Most were solo practitioners with none of the research resources available to pacesetters at large medical centers or government-funded universities. With more than enough patients to keep their waiting rooms full, pioneer chelationists had little motivation to seek research funds to undertake formal clinical studies proving chelation's worth. Their prime concern at the time - it seems funny now - was that EDTA treatments would get *too* popular, *too* quickly.

"Don't let the press in on this. Once word gets out that we've latched onto a real CURE, watch out," said Dr. George Frankel, the physician who organized the forerunner to today's professional association. He assembled the very first meeting devoted to the subject. We remember that evening in 1974 very well. As luck would have it, we were on hand, crammed shoulders and knees with about fifty doctors. Most of those crowded into the tiny hotel suite had no more idea than we did why they were there.

THANK GOODNESS DOCTORS MAKE BAD PATIENTS

Frankel, a prominent west coast cardiologist, had suffered a heart attack - then disappeared from sight. The invitation-only meeting marked his first reappearance in more than nine months. He got right to the point.

"I've an experience to share," he told the group - "one you will find hard to believe," he added.

Almost a year earlier, while on the golf course, Dr. F. was felled by a heart attack. Rushed to the hospital where he was on staff, a group of his colleagues examined him. The verdict, as expected was "George, you need a bypass."

"Not me," he objected, a clear case of a doctor not wanting to take his own medicine.

"I admit it," Frankel confessed. "I've bypassed hundreds of patients, but didn't want the same thing done to me."

Objections brushed aside, the doctors overruled him and scheduled surgery. Then fate stepped in.

"It was the week before New Year's, and the Red Cross canceled all elective surgery because they didn't have sufficient blood on hand to cope with emergencies. When my operation was postponed ten days. I took it as a reprieve."

Dr. F. wasted no time. He issued a D.I.D. (doctor in distress) by phone, by letter, by word-of-mouth.

"I need help, guys," he appealed to physician-friends and anyone within the medical community he thought could help. "There must be something other than surgery that will get me back on my feet."

For three days, there was silence. Thus, when a call from New York City brought a small glimmer of hope, he was ready.

"Found something you ought to check out, George. It's called chelation therapy. I never heard of it, but there's a guy in Alabama, by the name of Ray Evers, who knows all about it."

Frankel followed up with a quick trip to the university library, delved into the literature and to his great surprise found hundreds of references. In each instance, the research reports supported the therapeutic benefits of a treatment he had never heard mentioned before.

"I called Evers, arranged to fly to his clinic and checked in," Frankel continued. "Within hours, I was in treatment, and after the first week, was feeling so much better, I started making rounds with the doc."

FOR THIS M.D., SEEING *WAS* BELIEVING

Impressed by his rapid improvement, and from what he observed visiting patients and from scrutinizing their clinical records, Frankel stayed on to learn more. Finally, he made a crucial decision - to stick around long enough to bone up on the therapy.

"How do I look?" Frankel challenged his stunned listeners. "Great, right? Played eighteen holes of golf yesterday. Feel my old self - no, better. Younger. Healthier. More energy. Haven't felt this good in years. I'm seeing patients again - not operating on them. I've started chelating."

The room was silent. It was hard for attendees to reconcile their long-standing aversion to anecdotal testi-monials with their boundless respect for this reputable scientist. How to explain a doctor they admired sounding like an easily-duped patient?

A NEW MEDICAL SOCIETY IS BORN

"This is why I called you together, my friends," he concluded. "As soon as news of this wonder treatment leaks out, there won't be enough trained doctors to handle the mobs. Chelation mills will open on every street corner. Things are going to get out of hand, with people beating the doors down to be chelated, willing to pay anything - go anywhere - for the treatments. We better be ready. It's very important we form a medical association to set standards and guidelines to protect this new lifesaver from its potential success," he warned.

Frankel, whose psychic abilities will never rival Jean Dixon's, was seeing the future through a flawed crystal ball. He didn't come close to identifying the real problems chelation doctors would face in the years ahead.

The early rave reviews of chelation benefits never did reach the public. Instead, that portion of the medical community heavily invested in bypass, beat the drums for surgery. Intolerant of competition from an unwelcome contender, especially one tarnished by its provincial origins and tainted by the "NIH (not invented here) Syndrome," they turned 'thumbs

down' on chelation, and never looked back. They character-
ized chelation practitioners as 'know nothing country docs'.
The battle for recognition of EDTA begun three decades back,
goes on yet.

For these many years, critics have worked overtime to bad
mouth a therapy most of them can't pronounce, much less
explain. To this day, beleaguered chelationists - some bewil-
dered, others outraged - have demanded naysayers heed the
evidence of sheer numbers (more than 5,000,000 successful
treatments at last count). Others, sensitive to the larger issues,
take a more generous view of objections, saying, "They're right
to want better proof. We have an obligation to the scientific
community to validate therapeutic claims."

THEY WANT PROOF? GIVE THEM PROOF!

So a small cadre of the resourceful and research-minded,
have begged and borrowed funds to appease detractors. Many
expended out-of-pocket cash to document sophisticated
treatises with such erudite titles as: *Influence of Ethylene
Diamine Tetraacetic Acid (EDTA) On Activated Partial
Thromboplastin Time (APPT) and Prothrombin Time (PT) in
Human Plasma* and *An Oculocerebrovasculometric Analysis
of the Improvement in Arterial Stenosis Following EDTA Chelation Therapy,* to name but two.

They certified the effects of EDTA on renal function by
measuring creatinine clearance, blood urea nitrogen (the BUN
standard), levels of trace and toxic metals in urine specimens,
creatinine clearance - well, no one can say they haven't tried.

One of the country's most insightful scientists, Bruce
Halstead, M.D., whose credentials run to seventy-three pages,
recognized the credibility gap earlier than most when he wrote
the classic text, *The Scientific Basis for Chelation Therapy,*
(Golden Quill Publishers, Inc., 1979). It is a technical treatise
on EDTA's multiple biochemical actions at cellular level that

seeks to explain the startling variety of perceived benefits.

That's not easily done, for as Dr. Halstead spelled out, the prevalent position within medical circles is anti-holistic. Doctors are trained to seek out and rely upon disease-specific treatments. Recognizing that mindset goes a long way to explain why today's medicine is so patently ineffective when dealing with the interlocking complexities of chronic degenerative disease.

"It is becoming increasingly apparent," Halstead wrote, "that the processes of aging and chronic degenerative disease are not the result of a single cause but a complex of interacting factors."

Tackling this critical issue head on, Dr. Halstead analyzed the bioinorganic properties of EDTA, and summarized actions on a number of biological systems. His aim was to detail all the ways by which EDTA might affect health at the most basic level: the cell. By discussion and illustration, he specified EDTA's effects on lipid peroxidation, mitochondria, platelets, ionic calcium, bone structure, malignant tumor cells, elaborated on its workings on enzyme systems, nerve transmission, and various hormonal activities. This remarkable work, years ahead of its time, provided interested parties with all they needed to know to develop, as he had, a deep appreciation for the clinical value of EDTA. More remarkable still, Dr. Halstead identified and defined what has turned out to be its most potent action when he explained the EDTA/free radical connection.

Those were the days when the public thought 'free radicals' were hippies on the rampage. Only lately has the phrase evolved into the most popular 'buzz' words in scientific circles. Long before others were thinking in such terms, this trailblazing scientist laid the groundwork for current conviction that EDTA maintains cellular health by reducing free radical pathology. EDTA does this, he explained, by removing the metal ions (especially iron and copper) that are the catalysts for lipid peroxidation. Nothing that's been learned since refutes that revelation. Perhaps Halstead's greatest contribution, however, was that he set a new and higher standard for all future scientific discussion of EDTA.

A NEW BREED OF DOCTOR -
A NEW BRAND OF MEDICINE

Efforts to quantify and qualify EDTA's performance in the clinical setting have produced a formidable collection of published papers, many of which first appeared in peer review journals. Over the years, chelation research became more refined, more sophisticated, more elegant, and by all fair-minded standards, equal in quality to studies published in the most prestigious medical journals. Among the many well-referenced contributions establishing the scientific efficacy of EDTA chelation therapy for circulatory and other chronic diseases, the more notable are:

- **Inhibition of platelet aggregation (blood stickiness) in humans within three minutes of EDTA infusion;**
- **12% to 20% improved pulmonary function (as measured by Forced Vital Capacity and Forced Vital Expiration following 30 chelation treatments in 90.5% of 38 patients with independently diagnosed chronic lung disorders;**
- **90% reduction in cancer mortality after chelation therapy with EDTA;**
- **Marked improvement in 91% (and good improvement in 8%) in 1,130 patients with peripheral vascular disease and intermittent claudication over a 28-month treatment period;**
- **Marked improvement in 76.9% (and good improvement in 17%) of 844 patients with ischemic heart disease over a 28-month treatment period;**

- Marked or good improvement in 89% of all 2,870 patients treated over a 28-month period, no matter what their presenting health problem;
- 14% reduction in serum cholesterol levels in 142 patients following two months of EDTA therapy;
- 2% increase in bone density in 25 individuals with early onset osteoporosis after three months of chelation therapy;
- 35% reduction in serious (76.63%) carotid artery blockage and 620% increase in blood flow in 16 men and women after ten months of EDTA infusions;
- Statistical evidence of significantly improved blood flow following EDTA chelation as shown by objective measurement in 17 of 18 patients;
- Documented evidence of the long-term success of EDTA chelation as an alternative to amputation in four patients originally scheduled for surgery. Each had been diagnosed by the referring vascular surgeons as suffering end-stage gangrene in their lower extremities.
- Improved post-chelation EKG scores in a random sample of 28 'healthy' volunteers;
- Prolonged post-chelation improvement of the brain wave patterns of patients with Alzheimers disease as shown by brain mapping done by sophisticated computers;
- EDTA-chelation has completely cleared a totally clogged right coronary artery. Before and after angiograms proved these results in a patient rejected (considered too sick) for bypass surgery;
- 23% to 50% improvement in emotional status in a group of 139 chelation patients (average age 62.5 years) as measured by the Cornell Medical Index Health Questionnaire.

- **Very significant improvement in blood flow to the brain, confirmed independently by duplicate studies by two unaffiliated researchers using different technologies;**

In the fall of 1991, *A Nonsurgical Approach to Obstructive Carotid Stenosis Using EDTA Chelation* - (C.J. Rudolph, DO, PhD, E.W. McDonagh, DO, ACGP, and R.K. Barber, BS, ACSM, ETT) published in the *Journal of Advancement in Medicine*, established chelation's effectiveness in clearing the carotid artery. This research is of particular note in light of the clear evidence that carotid artery blockage is an almost certain precursor to stroke, and two wide-scale studies (the European Carotid Surgery Trial and the National Institute of Neurological Disorders and Stroke Project) confirm that surgery to unclog neck arteries does prevent strokes.

Several of the more recent studies deserve special attention. In 1988, Drs. Hugh Riordan and E. Cheraskin published the first documented proof that chelation with EDTA results in significantly improved myocardial health as gauged by the supersensitive QRS complex measurement of the electrocardiagram. Their work gives credence to the oft-made claims that chelation normalizes irregular heart rhythms.

Dr. E. W. McDonagh, a board certified general practitioner who has practiced and researched chelation for almost thirty years, tells of having thousands of electrocardiogram tracings of patients' heart activity before, during and after chelation with EDTA. What do they show?

"This treatment is remarkably beneficial to cardiac arrhythmias," he states, reporting his clinical records reveal sinus bradycardia, sinus tachycardia, sinoatrial block, atrial extrasystoles, atrial fibrillation and flutter and ventricular tachycardia - forms of arrhythmia - all respond well to EDTA treatment.

"The heartbeat becomes smooth, regular and more efficient," is Dr. McDonagh's summary.

The double-blind study is the only proof-positive research acceptable to prim and rigid scientists. To structure such a study requires two (or more) groups of similarly afflicted patients, but only one group gets the real treatment while the other group gets phony look-alike. Chelation researchers have long resisted such chicanery in the name of science, but finally in 1989 undertook to complete such a study.

PROOF AND MORE PROOF

Ten male patients with hardening of the arteries, randomly assigned to one of two groups were either chelated with EDTA or given an equal number of intravenous slow drips with an innocuous non-biologic substance. No one involved with the project knew who was getting what until after ten 'treatments'.

When half the group showed dramatic improvement - they could walk farther, and scored better on stress tests - the investigators broke the code. Every one of the improved patients had been chelated with the 'real' drug; every one whose condition remained unchanged was part of the unlucky placebo-taking group. To further prove out the validity of the dramatic results, there was a second part to the study. This time, the patients who had shown no improvement (the placebo bunch) had ten infusions with EDTA. In each case, they improved exactly as the initially chelated subjects.

Scientists who place credence on large numbers should be impressed by the chelation study reported in 1988 that involved close to 3,000 patients and spanned two continents. Drs. James Carter of Tulane University and Efrain Olszewer, clinical cardiologist at the Clinica Tuffik Mattar in Sao Paulo, Brazil, chelated 2,870 patients with various types of chronic degenerative disease, including many with blocked arteries. Results? And how. Ninety percent of the patients with peripheral vascular disease and 76.9 percent of the patients with ischemic heart disease showed marked improvement.

Want larger numbers? Try these on for size. The Cypher study (the first of its kind) involved 20,000 patients, all of whom were chelated and given nutritional counseling by the members of the Great Lakes Association of Clinical Medicine (GLACM). Thermographic studies - a standardized noninvasive diagnostic technique for determining circulation throughout the body - conducted before, during and after chelation showed that 79 percent of the 20,000 patients experienced significant circulatory improvement in arms and legs.

What's more, improvement proved to be dose related. Patients receiving twenty chelation treatments showed far more improvement than patients who received five or less. A control group of non-chelated, nutritionally counseled patients showed no improvement at all.

From a humanist's viewpoint, one cured patient is all the proof anyone should need. That's why the following 'study', presented by Dr. Ralph Lev, a Mayo Clinic-trained cardiovascular surgeon, is our favorite.

ONE MIND-CHANGING PATIENT

What did Dr. Lev initially think of chelation?

"It's the bunk," he told anyone who asked.

That was before his father-in-law had a stroke, and nothing in Dr. Lev's bag of medical tricks could return functioning to the once active gentleman, now totally incapacitated. When the best his colleagues could offer was "Put him in a nursing home and let him die," Dr. Lev reached out in desperation. Remembering he'd 'heard' somewhere it helped stroke patients, he bit the bullet and decided to try the last hope: chelation. Just like so many ordinary people in similar circumstances, the skeptical doctor said: "What have we got to lose?"

Thirty-two chelation treatments later, a fully recovered 'dad' was walking, talking, his old lively self. And Dr. Lev? He's now a fully certified chelation specialist. His father's recovery changed his life for the better, too.

The research studies mentioned are but a token sample of the many pro-EDTA works. Counting European, South American, Australian, Mexican and Canadian studies, there are more than 3,000 published articles in the world literature, all supportive of the dramatic and varied therapeutic potential of chelation therapy.

"BUT, WHY HAVE I NEVER HEARD OF IT?"

Good question. If EDTA chelation therapy has been around so long, is so well tested, so proven, so beneficial for so many hundreds of thousands, why is it medicine's best kept secret?

Dr. James P. Carter, Professor and Head of the Nutrition Section at Tulane University School of Public Health and Tropical Medicine, blames "medical politics," and referring to the bypass industry explains, EDTA chelation "threatens the financial well being of a politically powerful and well established branch of the medical profession."

To put Dr. Carter's analysis in more simple terms, the operational word is "greed." The history of medicine has many examples of innovative treatments unreasonably condemned by traditional practitioners. All too often, rejection is based on the fear a new therapy would out-date their skills and result in lost patients, lost revenue and professional obsolescence.

Imagine the frustration of the cardiologist with eight years of specialty training who finds himself in competition with a doctor who completed training in chelation in less than eight weeks. His rival treats the same patients with the same conditions as he does. The chelationist does it cheaper, easier, and with better results. No wonder well entrenched practitioners yelp, "It's not fair."

Cardiac surgeons and the entire bypass-plus-offshoots industry are right to fear comparison with doctors who help patients preserve or regain health without resorting to high-tech surgical procedures. Given a fair hearing chelation's popularity has to zoom, especially in light of growing enthusiasm for natural remedies.

Dr. Carter supports the premise that the public rarely gets the straight scoop from the popular press. Neither do doctors, he's quick to add.

"Special interests have a major influence on lay and professional exposure through the news media," he says.

Good point. The 'news' which reaches doctors is most certainly tainted by unconscionable influences, the most self-serving coming from the pharmaceutical industry. Some 10,000 medical journals appear in the United States every year, and most could not afford to publish were it not for revenue from the drug ads. That holds true for such prestigious journals as *JAMA,* the *New England Journal of Medicine, Post-graduate Medicine* and also their less illustrious state and local limited circulation counterparts.

A sleazy quid-pro-quo governs editorial content in these "respected" medical publications. With millions invested in research, the pharmaceutical companies have the clout to insist that the studies supporting their drugs are what's published and get the big play. That's how advertisers are reimbursed for their support. Clearly, the journals that flood doctors' offices are unlikely to include pro-chelation reviews, when none of their advertisers make a dime on EDTA.

There is always the possibility, of course, that doctors who have snubbed chelation just don't know any better. Most physicians, poorly informed about the intricacies of analytical biochemistry, physiobiology, molecular biology, bioinorganic chemistry, nutrition and cybernetics, don't have the knowledge or background to evaluate health and disease on a molecular or cellular level. As diligent readers have found out, free radical theory and the science of EDTA is complex and formidable. It's not apt to rival Johnny Carson for late-night entertainment.

Even if doctors were to read the chelation research, many probably would not understand it.

Perhaps the problem with medicine is not too little science, but too much. Today's physicians are notably devoted to the pursuit of single organ specialties - ("I do right thumbs, take your left knee to someone else".) In the quest for high-tech progress, many have lost touch with the rightful business of doctoring - the patient. A recent *Washington Post* headline suggests that is a real possibility.

LET'S ASK CONGRESS?

"Congress asked to study what does and does not work in medicine . . ." the news article began, reporting that a group of prominent doctors and medical scientists were urging passage of an "Effectiveness Initiative," to help them figure out which treatments make patients better, which make them worse.

That's as scary a story and sure to trigger a nightmare as any Stephen King thriller. Imagine going to a doctor so lacking in confidence and so out of touch with patients, he must ask Congress if he's helping people or not. That couldn't be *our* Congress - the one that can't balance its checkbooks - these docs want to consult, could it?

Bad joke. As we noted at the beginning of this chapter, chelationists don't have that problem. As they've long said: "People come in sick; they leave well. What else do you need to know?"

A story circulating at a medical meeting told of a man who had decided to give up everything scientists have linked to cancer.

The first week, he cut out smoked fish and
charcoal broiled steaks.
The second week, he cut out smoking.
The third week, he cut out having relations with women.
The fourth week, he cut out drinking.
The fifth week, he cut out paper dolls.

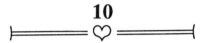

10

WHAT ELSE DOES CHELATION 'CURE'? DON'T ASK: IT'S A SECRET

A case could be made that it's easier to name an ailment chelation does NOT correct than to list those conditions it is known to relieve. From the first human trials almost forty years ago - (with the lead poisoned battery workers and the ship-painting sailors) - chelation specialists have observed an astounding array of seemingly unrelated health improvements.

Unanticipated benefits in place of toxic side-effects is so refreshingly different from what happens with other drugs, you'd expect chelation doctors to celebrate the distinction. Why don't they? Why do most of them cautiously avoid claims that chelation frequently reverses or reduces the symptoms of Alzheimer's Disease, senility, schizophrenia, rheumatoid arthritis, osteoarthritis, gout, arthritis, kidney stones, stroke-related coma, gall bladder stones, multiple sclerosis, lupus, Parkinson's Disease, Lou Gehrig's disease, osteoporosis, chronic fatigue syndrome, varicose veins, hypertension, memory loss, scleroderma, Raynaud's Disease, digitalis intoxication, intermittent claudication, diabetic ulcers, cold hands and feet, emphysema, leg ulcers, venomous snake bite, impotence, emotional difficulties, vision and hearing problems and many other signs of aging?

What else would chelation doctors prefer to keep to themselves? They shy away from saying chelation has a beneficial effect on almost every modern health disaster you can name, from AIDS to tension headaches, from colds to cancer, preferring to focus primarily on conditions stemming from inadequate blood flow due to atherosclerotic plaque.

Before delving into the reasons for their characteristic reluctance, here's a short list of benefits traceable to treatment with EDTA:

- **Reduction of liver-produced cholesterol;**
- **Lowered insulin requirements in diabetics;**
- **Lowered blood cholesterol levels;**
- **Reduced high blood pressure;**
- **Normalization of cardiac arrhythmias;**
- **Relief from leg muscle cramps;**
- **Reduction in allergic symptoms;**
- **Normalized weight;**
- **Improved psychological and emotional status;**
- **Enhanced sensory input: better sight, hearing, taste;**
- **Fewer excessive heart contractions;**
- **Lessened varicose vein pigmentation;**
- **Lightened age spots;**
- **Fewer aches and pains, arthritic and otherwise;**
- **Less reliance on pain medication;**
- **Hair loss stopped and reversed;**
- **Reversal of impotence;**
- **Alzheimer's Disease symptoms reversed;**

- **Reduced need for diuretics;**
- **Cold extremities warmed;**
- **Chronic fatigue syndrome overcome;**
- **Memory, and mental concentration improved;**
- **Post-cataract surgery vision loss is restored;**
- **Cosmetic changes, including more lustrous hair, added eye sparkle, stronger unsplit nails, better skin color, fewer visible wrinkles and a more youthful appearance.**

The longer the list grows, the more discomfort to those in the front lines of the effort to 'mainstream' chelation. Here's why. The current medical paradigm favors an aggressive approach to one disease at a time. Doctors are trained to approach ailments as though they were waging war on each sick organ separately - to conduct search and destroy missions on a target ailment. Throughout their careers, physicians are encouraged to seek out symptom-specific diagnoses and cures, as if it is possible to treat one biological system without affecting all others. Medication for a bladder infection, for example, is prescribed as though the urinary tract is not connected to the rest of the body.

Each year this trend away from generalism and towards specialization grows stronger. From medical school through internship, up and coming doctors have their eye on one goal: finding their niche in a profitable sub-specialty. The result is tunnel-vision medicine. As though they wore blinders, doctors see only 'their' chosen portion of the human anatomy - the smaller the area of concentration, the better.

Even if specialization were not in vogue, chelation's cure-a-lot reputation would be a detriment. An inevitable stigma dogs any remedy that does too much, making it vulnerable to 'snake oil' devaluation. One of the main reasons for the controversy surrounding EDTA, is the unavoidable evidence that it *is* so successful in a variety of serious conditions.

As one image-conscious doctor with a prestigious background confessed: "It's downright embarrassing to find myself endorsing a cure-all like a patent medicine side-show hawker."

THE MORE CHELATION CURES,
THE WORSE PRESS IT GETS

Why are the doctors with the most to gain so reticent? So restrained? So reluctant to speak out about their most dramatic results? Because valid or not, claims for such widely varied health benefits would, without doubt, further alienate or inflame anti-chelation critics.

Let's take a closer look at a few of the more common hush-hush healings. Ask the average American what disability he most fears, and nine out of ten will name "loss of sight." What does chelation have to offer?

There's good evidence that chelation improves vision in people suffering from diabetic retinopathy, and also decreases macular degeneration, dissolves small cataracts and aids other eye disorders, including intro-ocular hemorrhages and glaucoma. To be believable, such impressive claims need independent top notch verification. We've got it.

A BETTER LOOK AT LIFE

Consider the case of a 61-year old hospital administrator treated by Dr. Michael Schachter (Suffern, New York). The patient's peripheral vision, severely limited by diabetic retinopathy, improved more than 50% after four chelation treatments. Referring to his case notes, Dr. Schachter recalls: "The patient's ophthalmologist documented the change, and said he was 'astounded' when his patient, who was almost legally blind, could drive his car once again."

A similar case involves a lady whose vision problems grew so severe she could no longer read, knit, watch TV, paint or get around town unaided. The 82-year old became both angry and depressed.

"Not fair," she complained. "I'd rather be dead than blind."

With almost all vision in one eye gone, and the sight in the other rapidly failing, she began a course of chelation, more out of desperation than with real hope. The day following her fifth treatment, she was lying on her couch in front of a large picture window, and unexpectedly caught sight of a neighbor's terrier racing across her front lawn. She screamed! She cried! She thanked God!

"It was the most wonderful moment in my life," she recalls. "I jumped up and ran outdoors, relishing the sight of flowers, trees, birds, the blue sky. Let me tell you, I made so much noise, I stirred up the whole neighborhood."

Just before going to press we heard of new EDTA-related vision recoveries from an ophthalmologist turned chelationist, Dr. Harold Byer of Fountainville, Pennsylvania who discovered (by accident) that chelation undoes the damage to sight suffered by cataract victims. While many cataract preventives have been proposed - Vitamin E and Vitamin C supplementation among them - the statistics on cataracts are staggering, with more than twenty percent of Americans over the age of 65 currently requiring surgery.

Current theory has it that the most common form of cataracts is the direct result of oxidative damage caused by free radicals. EDTA and other preventive measures, begun early enough in life, may serve to protect eyes against damage. But what about those whose cataracts have already formed, and require cataract removal? The operation traditionally leaves tiny vision-impairing scars which have formerly been considered irreversible.

"Not so," says Dr. Byers, who is carefully documenting results in concert with a Harvard University eye specialist. "While it's too soon to predict what percentage of post-surgery cataract patients will enjoy fully restored sight, it's not premature to suggest chelation will prove an important therapy for many suffering from this common cause of impaired vision."

NEW HOPE FOR THE 'INCURABLES'

If the possibility of losing your sight doesn't terrify you, how about the prospect of losing your mind? Call it senility, or Alzheimer's Disease, mental impairment with the degrading dysfunction that goes with it, is the second most feared condition among the aging. Once past sixty-five, most seniors worry about the loss of memory, speaking and thinking abilities.

"Once my mind is gone, what's left?" is the way one fading senior citizen put it.

No one can comfortably face the time they can no longer write checks, handle everyday responsibilities, care for themselves or conduct their affairs. Nonetheless it happens to many an elder whose physical status may seem sound, but whose mental capacities have diminished so badly, they are nursing home candidates. What hope for help? Traditional medicine has nothing to offer.

Dr. William Irby Fox (Abilene, Texas) took on just such a case - an 86 year old cowboy, married for 61 years, so far gone, he could no longer recognize his wife.

"What a tragedy," people said.

"No problem," according to Dr. Fox, who chelated the senior citizen back to normal mental function and gave him a chance to celebrate his diamond wedding anniversary.

Equally inspiring is the case of Lucy Romano, who had to give up her home, pets and independence when advanced arteriosclerosis led to senility. Although only sixty-eight, this widowed lady had gradually found managing her husband's estate, the upkeep of her property, and tending daily affairs were just beyond her.

After going food shopping, she'd stand before the fridge,

not knowing whether to store items away or take them out; she'd go up and down stairs, not remembering whether she'd gone up for something, or come down to put it away; she once went to the mail box, and opened the letter she'd intended to mail. Her daughter and son-in-law, fearful she would do something foolish, started investigating the legal procedures for declaring Mother Lucy incompetent, when a neighbor suggested chelation.

"Let's give it a try, before we have to pack mom away," Lucy's daughter decided.

Week by week for the next three months, those who knew Lucy best noted small gradual changes - all for the better. "It was like watching someone come out of a fog," is the way her daughter put it. Day by day, mental acuity replaced mental confusion until suddenly, the old Lucy was back. She emerged full blown, laughing, telling jokes, her memory intact, and in every way the person her family knew and loved.

The same story can be told about James Schuler. With his memory so bad he couldn't remember his name or hold conversations with other patients, he was headed for 'veggie land' when he started chelation treatments. Six sessions later, with mental faculties fully restored, he began giving lectures on the benefits of EDTA treatments to his fellow retirement village residents.

CHELATION DOCTORS NEVER SAY "NEVER."

Unless you've known the heartache that goes with being a close relative of a stroke victim, you cannot imagine how distressing it is to see someone you knew as an intelligent, personable, well-functioning personality reduced to drooling incompetence. In the worst case scenario, the sufferer loses use of hands or arms, has facial paralysis, cannot control bodily functions, and is unable to communicate. With such severe disability, the stroke patient is shuffled off to a nursing home, comatose, bedridden or confined to a wheel chair. In time, the more fortunate may be able to limp along with the painful help of crutches, canes and four-legged walkers.

It's a grim picture, with no known treatment - except chelation. Take sixty-two year old Gregory Trenton. He had several of the disturbing symptoms of an impending stroke - memory lapses, occasional mental confusion, uncharacteristic personality changes such as temper outbursts and extreme irritability - when the disaster happened. He suffered a stroke following total occlusion of a carotid artery.

Physicians learn that the prognosis for persons like Gregory is not good. Even when the individual survives the stroke and rehabilitation starts immediately, chances are he will never again be normal. Physiotherapy, gait training exercises and speech therapy are some of the more ambitious therapies frequently prescribed, but they have limited value. Many stroke victims find talking nearly impossible, cannot move about without help, have depressed immune function, are incontinent, and face a sorry future. As a result, they normally grow so withdrawn, hopeless and depressed, they give up and die.

Getting back to Gregory, he rates to be as seriously damaged and hopeless a stroke victim as doctors have seen. After his episode, he was comatose, curled into a fetal position. He could neither feed himself or swallow properly. Pureed food poured into him through a rubber tube kept him alive. He had no control over his bladder or bowels, and could make no intelligible sound other than an occasional groan or mumble. Imagine anyone suggesting his condition could be reversed. Imagine a doctor willing to tackle such a challenge. Luckily for Gregory and his family, a chelationist agreed to take him on, and he was trundled off for treatments.

As soon as treatments began, there were signs of change. First he could utter a few words; then he started speaking in sentences. As he became more articulate, he regained physical competency and progressed from walker to crutches. Finally, he could walk without assistance, care for himself, and return to his pre-stroke lifestyle. The renaissance from total incompetence to able-bodied wellness took less than a year. No doctor familiar with the case has dared suggest something other than EDTA is responsible for this remarkable recovery.

Chelation doctors handle such dramatic cures gingerly indeed. No matter how many stroke patients are similarly restored thanks to EDTA, they don't publicize it. Clearly they fear repercussions should tales of near-miraculous recoveries get out. Only the naive expect applause. Most are savvy enough to realize bragging about their 'biggies' will only further discredit them with close-minded colleagues.

AN X-RATED RECOVERY

Sexual impotence may not seem as serious a health problem as those already discussed, but to the man who can no longer make love when he wants to, it's psychologically devastating and has life-shortening implications. While we know of no patients who have undergone chelation specifically to cure impotence, there are many whose sex life was unexpectedly restored.

Dr. John Olwin, former clinical professor of surgery at Rush Medical College at the University of Illinois, recognized this phenomenon many years ago, when he reported patients experiencing a startling variety of unanticipated chelation-related benefits.

"Patients note increased nail and hair growth, many saying they've been getting more frequent hair cuts and manicures. There's been a decided increase in libido among many others, who tell me they're more interested in sex than they have been for fifteen or more years. One woman, married to an eighty-year old lawyer who'd been chelated because of senility, called to ask why her mate had suddenly 'become horny' after so many years of disinterest. 'Not that I'm complaining,' she was quick to add. 'It's exhilarating to have a mate who's been sexually 'dead' for decades, suddenly exhibiting sexual desires.'"

Were these results more generally known, it could revolutionize treatment for this sexual disorder. Contrary to what sex therapists would have you believe, impotence is more likely to have a physiological origin than to be a sign of psychological dysfunction. It's not surprising that psychologically-oriented treatments are generally unsuccessful. No cure is possible while the healer maintains the fiction that a man experiencing erectile failure has a mental hangup, when he is probably suffering severely restricted blood flow to the lower limbs and pelvic area.

That's not pure speculation. More than a decade ago, photographs taken by a penis-linked camera established restricted blood flow as the underlying cause of both male impotence and female frigidity. Those studies, conducted by the Danish psychologist and human sexuality specialist Dr. Gorm Wagner, go a long way to explain why impotence is so common among male diabetics and middle-aged men showing other signs of vascular problems and symptoms of arteriosclerosis.

Chelation therapy's potential as a cure for impotence is finally going to be put to the test by chelation expert Conrad Maulfair, M.D., who is currently conducting rigorous clinical studies.

NOT OLD ENOUGH TO BE CHELATED? THINK AGAIN.

In recent years, surprisingly large numbers of symptom-free young people in their 20's and 30's have turned up in chelation clinics. Why? Mindful of the potential harm from environmental pollution, the health-conscious twenty and thirty year olds are showing up for preventive treatments.

This much younger and healthier population of patients is adding new and exciting awareness of chelation's potential, as these essentially well young adults report that after chelation they think more clearly, are less sluggish, concentrate better, have fewer headaches, more energy. Dr. James Julian of Hollywood, California, has chelated his fair share of 'thirty-somethings', many of them well-known celebrities, and reports, "Chelation is proving to be a real solution to the 'yuppie' disease of the 1990's: chronic fatigue syndrome."

Philadelphia's Dr. Alan Magaziner has made the same observation, noting he has "chelated young professionals - both men and women - suffering from recurring tension and migraine headaches, and other stress-related symptoms, all of which vanish after a few treatments."

Dr. John Ettl (El Paso, Texas) risks alienating psychiatrists, psychologists and the whole mental health community when he states "chelation is a potent answer to 'executive burnout'.

"Call it what you will," Dr. Ettl states, "emotional wipeout, workaholic fatigue, professional disenchantment, the stress of success, or some similar career-related complaint, in many instances these subtle psychological symptoms are not the result of psychological dysfunction, but the adverse physical effects of a toxic environment."

PLEASE DON'T TALK ABOUT C-A-N-C-E-R!

"While there are several chronic diseases more destructive to life than cancer, none is more feared." That was true when Charles H. Mayo said it in 1926; it is much truer today. Cancerphobia is rampant in the U.S. - and with good reason. Despite the billions of dollars spent, the government's all-out war on cancer has been all but lost.

While the National Cancer Institute claims conventional treatments - surgery, radiation and chemotherapy - now cure half U.S. cancer patients, non-government biostatisticians disagree, and find the NCI's assertion as optimistically self-serving. In fact, studies published in reputable medical journals conclude that mortality rates have not improved since the 50's: two of three cancer patients still die of the disease or related therapy within five years of diagnosis.

Even more dismal is the medical establishment's record when it comes to cancer prevention. Widely publicized advice to seek early diagnosis and treatment, has not been productive. Nor has routine 'screening' made a difference. Breast cancer has become so prevalent, and the cure rate so poor, oncologists now recommend women with a family history of breast cancer undergo a mastectomy prophylactically - (that means they think your best shot at avoiding breast cancer is to remove your breast!)

Admonitions to quit smoking, fatty foods, eat more fiber, avoid carcinogenic preservatives and toxic environments while certainly valid, have not made a dent. Several decades back, one in ten was expected to develop cancer; current projections are for *one in three!* No wonder people dread the Big C, it's our leading growth industry.

What if the incidence of cancer could be cut back to ten percent of current rates? Or, better still, prevented? Imagine how that news would be treated - with news bulletins, banner headlines, prime-time documentaries, Congressional honors and a Nobel Prize, for sure.

The fact is, such a discovery has been made, and announced and caused hardly a ripple. Published research suggests chelation may well be the simple, easily available and effective countermeasure to developing cancer.

Who's been keeping this news under wraps? Everyone, including the chelation doctors themselves, who are as guilty as their more orthodox brethren in keeping the lid on what may one day prove to be medicine's best-kept secret.

"We've whispered about this among ourselves for years," one chelation doctor said after swearing us to secrecy.

"Don't use my name," he begged, "but every physician who chelates people must notice our patients just don't get cancer."

"A privately acknowledged phenomena," is the way another chelating doctor put it. We sit around and talk about this when we get together. Chelation doctors find it hard to name even one patient who has had EDTA chelation therapy who later comes down with cancer."

JIG'S UP - THE STORY'S OUT

Dr. E. W. McDonagh, the well respected Kansas City, Missouri physician and a founding member of the International Academy of Preventive Medicine, has broken ranks with his chelating colleagues, investigated what others whisper about, and then gone public with his findings.

This is what got Dr. McDonagh's attention and what he did about it. During the past 27 years. this highly respected Kansas City, Missouri physician, has chelated approximately 25,000 patients. He noted that contrary to national stats, which show the incidence of cancer is fast approaching one in three - (suggesting that at least 7,500 - perhaps more - of his patients should have contracted cancer) - but among those who did not have cancer before visiting his clinic, only *one* has ever later been diagnosed with the ailment.

Dr. McDonagh decided to investigate further. He identified 65 Vietnam veterans severely poisoned by Agent Orange, later treated with EDTA infusions, and studied their files.

"Every patient returned to normal function," states his yet-to-be-published report. Any cancer in the group? "Not a one," asserts Dr. McDonagh.

Unsubstantiated observation or documented fact? Is it

possible that cancer can be prevented and the news has been buried? Possibly. Sadder still, this cannot be rightly called 'new' news.

Chapter Seven of the first edition of *Bypassing Bypass* includes a detailed account of a 1980 study undertaken by Swiss scientists from the Institute for Radiation Therapy and Nuclear Medicine at the University of Zurich. It was originally published in the scientific journal *Environmental International* and comes to a dramatic conclusion: chelation with EDTA **cuts the incidence of cancer by 90%.**

Despite obvious extraordinary implications if the study were replicated and the finding found reliable - or even only half true - the report was ignored in 1980, ignored in 1984, ignored when republished by an ACAM physician, and is still ignored today.

What's going on? Why haven't chelation doctors pestered every science writer? Why has this potentially life-saving revelation been kept under wraps?

"Oh, my God - you're not going to suggest chelation can stop cancer!" one ACAM member exploded when I asked for his comments. "Don't we have enough trouble without getting the NCI (National Cancer Institute) on our backs? If you go to press with this, it'll sound as though we've joined the laetrile camp. Do you want to see chelation outlawed?" he fumed. "Keep it quiet or you'll do us all in."

HOW CAN A SIMPLE STUDY CAUSE SO MUCH CONCERN?

The study that started the furor began innocently enough. The researchers, not in any way part of the chelating community, set out to investigate the link between lead-based gas fumes and cancer incidence, with the hypothesis that exposure to automobile exhaust was carcinogenic. To test their theory,

Drs. W. Blumer and T. Reich examined the health records of 231 Swiss citizens living adjacent to a heavily trafficked highway. They determined that cancer mortality among this group was indeed significantly higher than among persons living in a traffic-free section of the same town. In both groups, the subjects studied were life-long inhabitants of their respective areas, adding validity to the comparison. The original hypothesis proven, the study should have ended right there.

As it happened, one group of the fume-exposed population, had developed such severe symptoms of lead poisoning, they'd been detoxified with the usual treatment for lead poisoning: EDTA. This serendipitous event resulted in Blumer and Reich being the only researchers to date who could compare long-term death rates in a matched population of chelated and non-chelated patients.

Again, that's not what they set out to do. When the researchers examined the data kept on the two groups for the following 18 years, they unexpectedly uncovered so significant a mortality difference between the studied populations, they found it hard to believe their stats. Of the 231 people living close to the highway, 59 adults had chelation; 172 matched controls did not. Only *ONE* (1.7 percent of the chelated persons) died of cancer, as compared with *THIRTY* (17 percent) of the non-treated.

After exploring all possible explanations for this vast statistical disparity in cancer mortality, the authors concluded: chelation was solely responsible for the 90% decrease in cancer deaths!

Still nervous over their conclusion, the researchers subsequently submitted their data to several independent Swiss epidemiologists for review. Only when these acknowledged experts confirmed and validated their findings and determination, was the study published.

If this is the first you've heard of that research, it's because everyone has looked away: the chelation doctors, the scientific community, and the news media that so loves a cancer story, they rush to print any time an oncologist gets good results with a lab rat.

WHAT WILL IT TAKE TO TAKE ANOTHER LOOK?

Why no attempt to replicate the study? Why, with all the billions the government spends on exotic approaches to cancer prevention and cure, no funds to check out the odd chance that there's something to this? If there's even a remote possibility that chelation reduces cancer mortality, why not check it out?

One of the most authoritative spokespersons among chelationists is Dr. Jonathan Collins, editor-in-chief of the prestigious *Townsend Letter*. His reaction to the Swiss research was a published warning to the chelation community not to inflame their powerful enemies by publicizing, or circulating copies of the study. He cautioned against taking any action that might suggest a link between chelation and cancer prevention.

Dr. Collins' admonition was based on, but not limited to, the valid observation that the Blumer study could be scientifically flawed. There were no double-blind controls; a placebo response could have skewed results; the researchers did not spell out their criteria for including subjects; and the findings might be compromised by the lack of carefully defined parameters. All perfectly true, but we've seen shoddier studies taken seriously.

Faulty or not, this research rates a follow-up investigation. While findings have never been confirmed, they've never been challenged, either. As Dr. Collins points out, the study might have merit, and if so, millions of people have a stake in the results. It would not be difficult or costly to replicate the survey with a more carefully designed protocol. Given an appropriate forum, chelation doctors could contribute more than sufficient numbers of case histories to assemble a massive epidemiological study. How sad to note these doctors are so fearful of a backlash, they'd rather not pursue the truth.

What about getting the story out in the popular press? *Sixty Minutes* isn't interested; neither is the *Washington Post*, the *Larry King Show*, or Phil Donahue. We never tried *Nightline*, but each time we proposed a segment based on the published report, it was turned down, occasionally with the forthright objection, "You know we can't do a pro-chelation piece."

Once we tried to sneak the story by - with the attention-grabbing headline, "Getting the lead out cuts your cancer risk!"

"Great story," commented the editor, until he came to the part that credited chelation by name.

"What are you trying to pull?" he snarled and crumpled the file in the trash.

Possibly, the trouble with chelation is not that it's *too* controversial, but that it's not controversial enough!

11

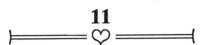

EVERYTHING ENQUIRING MINDS NEED TO KNOW ABOUT CHELATION

Much of the science behind the EDTA phenomenon, be it postulated or proven, is of questionable value to someone in pain or facing an uncertain future. Some theories are so esoteric, few patients have anything to gain speculating whether they're sound or not.

If you're in the grips of angina, unable to walk across the room without stopping for breath, have cold hands or toes turning black from circulatory disease, do you care whether chelation decalcifies arteries, or establishes cellular homeostasis, inactivates coenzyme inhibitors, reverses biochemical lesions, or neutralizes free radical activity? Will you recover from cardiac arrhythmias more quickly knowing EDTA is proven to stimulate parathormone production, reduce platelet aggregation, increase blood flow ala Poiseuille's Law relating to fluid dynamics and some complex interaction of these and other not yet discovered mechanisms?

WHEN PEOPLE NEED HELP, THEY WANT TO KNOW *IF*-NOT *HOW* - CHELATION THERAPY WORKS.

Where do you turn to find out if chelation is for you?

If you question the cardiologist who recommended some form of surgery, he'll advise against chelation and mumble something like, "It's unproven, untested, dangerous, worthless."

If you question a chelation doctor, he'll discourage surgery and probably assure you EDTA is successful with better than 85% of his patients.

If you phone the American Heart Association, they'll endorse your cardiologist's advice, and offer pro-surgery literature.

If you contact ACAM, the medical association that supervises training and certification of chelation doctors, they'll endorse EDTA and offer pro-chelation literature.

If you go to the library, you can read any number of pro-chelation books written by doctors, any number of pro-surgery books written by doctors, any number of "Try my magic formula" books written by doctors.

Confused? Cynical? No doubt. Where can you find objective counsel when every source you contact has something to sell or an axe to grind?

There's a simple solution. You don't have to take any authority's word for anything. You can check it out for yourself.

BE AN EDUCATED CONSUMER

Approach the medical marketplace thinking like a consumer, not a patient. Be prepared to be as critically inquisitive as you are when considering any major purchase. When you're in the market for a new car, a washing machine, a video recorder, what do you do? If you're like most people we know, you probably seek a more reliable source than the dealer who wants to make a sale.

Perhaps you check out product ratings in your library's advertisement-free *Consumer's Guide*. What happens when a major appliance needs fixing? You probably ask someone you trust for the name of a repairman they found reliable.

You can apply the same measures to health care. Medical treatments **are** competing products. Collect the data and shop around. If sifting through reams of published reports is daunting, you can enlist the aid of the pros at World Research Foundation (15300 Ventura Blvd., Suite 405, Sherman Oaks, California) a non-profit organization with access to 400 databases of traditional and alternative medicine.

WRF computers scan more than 5,000 medical journals from 100 countries, including the Soviet Union and China, and their information center contains more than 10,000 books, periodicals and research reports. There is no charge for using the library yourself. A staff member will conduct a search for you for a nominal fee. If you're in a rush, you can call them at (818) 907-5483, or FAX them at (818) 907-6044.

Another place to do research is the National Library of Medicine in Bethesda, Maryland, the world's largest single-discipline library. NLM is a resource used by other libraries and researchers nationwide through interlibrary loan and computer data bases. Individuals can obtain citations and abstracts electronically with their personal computer using Grateful Med software which can be ordered from the National Technical Information Service, (703) 487-4650.

THE MOST RELIABLE INPUT COMES FROM PEOPLE WHO HAVE BEEN TREATED

Do you consider yourself a good judge of character? Do you think you know when people are lying and when they're not? In sportscaster lingo, "let's go to the tape." Examine the evidence for or against a close call by checking it out first hand.

If surgery versus chelation is the issue, ask your vascular

surgeon to put you in contact with patients treated two or more years ago. Call them to find out how they're doing. People love to talk about their operations. Listen carefully. Take notes. Many communities have regular meetings of the local "zipper club" self-help groups of 'bypassed' and 'angioplastied' survivors. Check it out. Compare people's first hand reports with what you've heard and read.

If you're considering chelation, but are nervous as to what to expect, it's understandable. No medical procedure is "simple" or "minor" to the person about to undergo it. Glib assurances - "there's nothing to it" or the bakery-shop standard, "it's a piece of cake" - leave most people feeling worse, not better. We can think of no more desirable way to relieve natural anxieties than to talk things over with chelation patients.

Fortunately, that's easy to do. You can phone the nearest chelation doctor (see *Physician Directory*) and ask for people willing to share their experience. Better still, you could request an opportunity to visit the clinic and talk to people while they're taking treatments. That's what we did. Here's what we found out.

MEET THE PEOPLE

Contrary to what some skeptics maintain, chelation patients are not naive, trusting, poorly educated or highly suggestible. Quite the reverse. Surveys show they have above-average intellect, are well-read, and not easily duped. For the most part, they're tough-minded realists. On a typical day, treatment rooms nationwide are full of informed, articulate men and women. They are trustworthy information sources, eager to share what they know.

On our first visit to a chelation clinic, we met an impressive group: a 62-year old retired college professor, the 72-year old chief executive of an automobile dealership, a couple wealthy enough to seek treatment anywhere in the world, an 80-year old lady whose middle-aged children - one a lawyer, the other a computer specialist - were paying for her treatments, a farmer and land-owner who was a community leader and church elder, an IBM mid-level administrator on extended sick leave, the 47-year old comptroller of a large insurance underwriting firm and several self-employed businessmen forced by health problems to close up shop.

They were people you'd be happy to invite to your next dinner party - forthright, clear-minded, individualists with one striking characteristic in common: they were indignant at the suggestion they could be 'fooled' into believing they were getting well.

"How could I 'think' my toes pink?" asked one man whose gangrenous foot was gradually healing despite earlier warnings that only amputation would save his life

"Eight months ago I could hardly get out of bed. Now, I'm well enough to fend for myself," said the elderly lady, planning a birthday party for one of her seventeen grandchildren.

"I'm going back to work the day the doc says it's okay," laughed the financial expert who'd been pensioned off with a full disability after two heart attacks.

You better not tell the man whose brothers carried him in for his first EDTA infusion that he's experiencing a placebo effect or been taken for a fool. You'll have a fight on your hands. Within two weeks of his initial session, he was driving himself to the doctor's office, walking in under his own steam. After 30 treatments, he could go fishing, chop wood, and dance. What next? He was about to reopen his auto repair shop.

"I'm embarrassed to say I didn't think it would work," he confessed. "I thought if it did, all doctors would be doing it."

"The local Rotary club was preparing my memorial service," reported the auto dealer. "That was six months ago. The first time I bounced back into a breakfast meeting, the guys looked as though they were seeing a ghost. Now they're saying they'll have to look into this chelation thing."

And this from the once bed-ridden farmer. "Imagination? That's a laugh. If my imagination was good enough to get me walking again, maybe I should package it and make a mint."

The most humorous rebuttal came from the academician who had researched the chelation literature and found that, according to an outstanding expert in veterinary medicine, Dr. Lloyd S. McKibbon, chelated race horses turn into track superstars. The 'Professor' as his fellow patients called him, chuckled at the idea that the 'placebo effect' would work with horses.

"If chelation doctors are so good at mesmerizing patients, I say, 'More power to them'. What we need is more such wizards!"

A TREAT OF A TREATMENT

If you're beginning to suspect that the chelation experience is different than all other encounters with the medical community, you're right. For starters, chelation clinics, unlike most treatment facilities for the seriously sick, reek optimism.

Any one who's 'spooked' by a visit to the dentist or doctor, or whose blood pressure soars at the thought of needles, x-rays, tongue depressors, cavity probes and other diagnostic indignities, will be soothed by the sight of a room full of people, hooked up to intravenous equipment, behaving as though they're at a family picnic.

Chelation newcomers, almost without exception, express surprise when they find the clinic a place of fellowship and good cheer. There's none of the grim-faced, stiff-upper-lip false jocularity so prevalent in other medical facilities. Why do these people look so happy? Why are they smiling and joking? Have they lost their marbles, or has the doctor slipped some 'feel good' juice into their IV drip?

The answer. It's the 'Lazarus Syndrome' - the great joy experienced by those returned to life after facing certain death.

Almost every patient you meet, at one time thought himself a 'gonner', and relishes the reprieve. Even those who've only begun treatment - still painfully ill - are buoyed by the expectation they will recover as well as those whose progress they observe.

"Why don't the TV cameras come in here and record what goes on?" asked one lady, exhilarated to have witnessed patients who discarded crutches, walkers and wheelchairs.

Patients encourage each other. "Remember Joanne? The lady from Vermont who couldn't recall her name? When she left, she could rattle off her social security, Medicare, checking account and credit card numbers. We heard her do it."

Someone else tells about John, a stroke victim who made the transition from a speech-impaired, fuzzy-minded, near-cripple to an alert, talkative, personable fellow - and it happened right before their eyes.

The individual just starting treatment may not see, hear, breathe, or walk well; he may have leg aches, chest pains, breathing difficulties and other symptoms of serious disease; he may feel older, less energetic, weaker and more tired than he'd like, but the anticipation of eventual recovery will keep a smile on his face.

♥ ♥ ♥

Assuming you've decided to look into chelation, where do you find a trained physician? Since that's proven a problem for so many people (you won't find chelation specialists conveniently listed in the yellow pages) we've included a *Physician Directory* (Appendix B).

One word of caution: all doctors, even those we've included, are not equally competent or experienced. If you are uncomfortable, for any reason, with the first physician you visit, don't hesitate to seek out another.

To help readers know more about the doctors available to them, we've instituted the Chelation Oversight Project

(C.O.P.) and urge all to write us to report their treatment-related satisfactions and dissatisfactions. The information you provide will be passed along to future inquirers. Working together, we can all make a good therapy even better. There's more about C.O.P. following the *Physician Directory*.

❤ ❤ ❤

Now to the rest of your questions.

12

MORE QUESTIONS -
MORE ANSWERS

"What does it feel like to be chelated?"

"Does it hurt?"

"How long does it take?"

"What if I get sick? Nauseous? Panic? Faint?"

"I've had a bypass. Is it too late for me?"

"Am I too old to be chelated?"

"Do I need someone to drive me home?"

"How long before I see results?"

"What does it cost?"

"Where do I find a doctor?"

"How will I know it works?"

"What if I have to quit half-way? Or, get started and don't like it? Or, move and can't find a chelationist?"

"What do I do about my other medical treatments? The drugs I'm taking for arthritis? Diabetes? Ulcers? Whatever?"

"What do I tell my 'real' doctor? How do I go back if I need him?"

If you're considering chelation, chances are you're wrestling with all the above questions - and perhaps dozens more.

Most people facing this decision are filled with doubts. Defying conventional wisdom by selecting a frowned-upon treatment, imposes special burdens. Since your physician, family and friends are all likely to support some form of drugs or surgery - the 'accepted' treatments - it may seem somewhat easier to be 'bypassed' or 'angioplastied' than 'chelated'.

No matter how poorly an orthodox therapy turns out, you're off the hook. You'll receive unqualified sympathy. On the other hand, if you opt for chelation and fail to recover, you'll have to shoulder the blame. You'll be judged guilty of having made an unwise choice.

CONSIDERING CHELATION? TAKE THIS TEST FIRST

Are you a candidate for chelation? Only an experienced physician can tell you.

Are you psychologically fit for chelation? Only you know whether you're equipped to buck social, cultural and professional pressures.

To help you decide your mental readiness for chelation, take this test. In each statement, choose the response that comes closest to your own, then check the scoring and analysis that follows:

1: When my doctor prescribes medication, I: **(A)** Take it without question; **(B)** Ask about side effects; or **(C)** Check it out in the *Physician's Desk Reference?*

2: When dissatisfied with the service at a restaurant, I: **(A)** Complain to the manager; **(B)** Complain to the server; or **(C)** Leave a smaller than usual tip.

3: When a doctor advises surgery, the smart thing to do is: **(A)** Request a second opinion; **(B)** Investigate non-surgical alternatives; or **(C)** Check into the hospital at once.

4: When disappointed by a play, movie or concert, I: **(A)** Sit through the entire performance; **(B)** Leave during an intermission; or **(C)** Walk out as soon as possible.

5: I've **(A)** Never; **(B)** Rarely; or **(C)** Occasionally - questioned a doctor or hospital about a medical bill.

6: When family members argue, I become: **(A)** Uneasy; **(B)** Shaken; or **(C)** An objective arbiter.

7: When I have a medical checkup, I find it: **(A)** Difficult, **(B)** Easy or **(C)** Somewhat uncomfortable - to ask for an explanation of the tests, findings and their significance.

8: I **(A)** Rarely; **(B)** Sometimes; or **(C)** Always - return faulty merchandise.

9: I find it **(A)** Easy, **(B)** Difficult, or **(C)** Impossible - to disagree with my doctor on a health issue.

10: I have **(A)** Never; **(B)** Rarely, or **(C)** Frequently - been talked into a purchase by a high-pressure salesman.

11: If I were to opt for an unconventional medical treatment, I would have: **(A)** A great deal, **(B)** Some, or **(C)** No - difficulty sticking by my decision over the objections of family and friends.

12: When faced with a major decision, I rely most heavily on: **(A)** My mate's advice; **(B)** The advice of many friends, or **(C)** My own judgment.

SCORING: Give yourself points for your answers as follows:

1: (A) 0 (B) 1 (C) 2	7: (A) 0 (B) 2 (C) 1
2: (A) 2 (B) 1 (C) 0	8: (A) 0 (B) 1 (C) 2
3: (A) 1 (B) 2 (C) 0	9: (A) 2 (B) 1 (C) 0
4: (A) 0 (B) 1 (C) 2	10: (A) 2 (B) 1 (C) 0
5: (A) 0 (B) 1 (C) 2	11: (A) 0 (B) 1 (C) 2
6: (A) 1 (B) 0 (C) 2	12: (A) 0 (B) 1 (C) 2

ANALYSIS:

If you scored from **0 through 6 points,** you are pained by the possibility of being thought an 'oddball', and thus tend to avoid doing things others might consider unusual or controversial. To find the social support and reassurance you need to be chelated, talk to people who have undergone treatment. Pick their brains.

If you scored from **7 through 12 points,** you are somewhat uncomfortable in unfamiliar situations, and tend to shy away from new experiences. Read up on chelation; familiarize yourself with details of the treatment's procedures and you'll gain the self-confidence necessary to make a non-main stream medical decision.

If you scored from **13 through 18 points,** you are a strong-minded outspoken individual who has little trouble standing by your convictions. You have what it takes to evaluate chelation objectively and unemotionally.

If you scored from **19 through 24 points,** you couldn't care less what other people think and are gung-ho to try anything new. Your enthusiasm and impatience might work against you, causing you to quit before chelation can prove itself out. While 85% of those who submit to treatment DO experience health benefits, there are no guarantees. Sometimes positive results don't materialize as rapidly as you expect. Those most likely to start and *stick with* treatments, have one extra quality working for them: patience.

Those most likely to opt for chelation therapy score between 13 and 24 points. They're self-confident, curious, and can stand up to criticism.

THE TIME FACTOR

Psychological hurdles to one side, time pressure is the second most frequently cited reason for refusing chelation.

Case in point: strong-willed George R., advised that he

required balloon angioplasty to restore adequate blood flow to his heart, knew all about the advantages of chelation, yet he chose surgery. Why?

After losing his job in the hard-hit computer industry, he spent six months in the unemployment lines before deciding to go into business for himself. He bought a 'quick print' franchise, put in seven days a week, and was just beginning to cover expenses, when he got the bad health news.

"My doctor, who's a good friend of mine, insisted on the angioplasty. I knew the drawbacks. Cecil (his wife) didn't make things easy. She kept insisting that *real* doctors who work at *big* hospitals and advise treatments covered by medical insurance were the way to go, but I stood my ground.

"Then, I started thinking. This chelation business was going to cost money - and time. Ten to twenty treatments at three hours a pop adds up to 30 to 60 hours, not counting travel back and forth, and hours spent in the waiting room. I just couldn't afford it, time-wise.

George opted for angioplasty and almost three months to the day after his operation, suffered a massive stroke.

Americans suffer as much from the 'hurry up' disease as from anything else. Moreover, our TV-controlled educational environment which conditions us to getting the news in 30 second sound bites, leads us to expect solutions to the most pressing problems in 24 minutes (the length of the average sit-com sans commercials.) When we fall sick, we want to be cured - 'fast'.

What works on TV is not good medicine in real life. Quick-fix cures are okay for a trauma-created health problem: a broken leg, burn, sports mishap, accident, wrenched back, accidental poisoning. But when dealing with a degenerative disease - atherosclerosis, for example - or any condition that's been developing for years, chances are it cannot be reversed overnight.

And now for the questions.

What does it feel like to be chelated? Does it hurt?"

Trust us. You'll hardly feel a thing. One of the nicest things about chelation treatment is how easy it is to take - comforting news for anyone who is doctor-phobic.

The most discomfort you're apt to experience will be the IV needle's pin-prick that starts the infusion (not even close to a novacaine injection.) A tiny needle is used, and most technicians are skilled at inserting it painlessly into a vein in the back of your hand or forearm. Super-sensitive patients can have a mild local anesthetic such as procaine or lidocaine added to the solution.

Once the EDTA drip begins, you won't detect anything strange or unusual. You may feel a bit restricted tied to the IV equipment, but to enhance your comfort most chelation technicians will tape your arm to a padded arm rest propped on a pillow, permitting you to move your arm without dislodging the needle.

Since your IV bottle hangs from a wheelable stand, you can go to the bathroom, take telephone calls, move around and stretch your legs, change seats - you are not immobilized.

How long does it take?

You'll have to learn to be a *patient* patient. Each treatment session should take from 3 to 3 1/2 hours. Properly administered, chelation is no 'quick fix' remedy. To begin with, before each session, your doctor (or doctor's assistant) will weigh you, and take blood and urine samples. Since cardiac patients have a tendency to retain fluids, renal function must be closely monitored. Pre-treatment testing is an important precaution, assuring appropriate adjustment of medication dosage, rate of dosage and the safe interval between infusions.

Once the IV infusion is in place, the clock starts running. Settle down for a pleasant respite. What you make of the time is up to you. Knit, read the latest best-seller, do a crossword puzzle, watch TV, catch up on your correspondence, update your shopping list, balance your checkbook, petition your Congressman, sleep, listen to a self-improvement tape, play a computer game, gossip with other patients, work on your laptop computer. Trade recipes, shopping tips, pictures of the grandchildren. It's not too bad once you make up your mind to use the time productively.

One and a half hour infusions (using a comparably smaller dose of EDTA) have now been shown to be as effective in a just completed, as yet unpublished study by Drs. Grant Born and Tammy Geurkink. Their finding - no reduction in benefits and no ill effects - duplicates results of an earlier Brazilian study which also showed EDTA to be just as effective at the lower dose. The 'half bag' treatment, easier to tolerate and schedule, now appears to be an acceptable - even preferable - option.

What kind of tests must I take?

Before your first chelation treatment, the doctor will do a complete workup - a physical examination that will include your medical history, blood chemistry profile, cholesterol levels, kidney function, arterial circulation, mental status, weight and blood pressure readings, heavy metal toxicity, nutrient deficiencies, metabolic abnormalities. Your doctor also will ask about your drinking, eating and smoking habits.

No need to worry that tests will be painful, or dangerous. Holistically-oriented chelation doctors DO NOT submit patients to the coronary catheterizations (angiograms) and thallium scans routinely ordered by cardiologists. Chelationists generally base diagnosis on harmless, non-invasive tests, and can spot circulatory disorders with the aid of thermograms, ultra-sound Doppler analysis, echocardiograms and plethysmograms. Once the doctor has determined your physical status, chelation treatment, if found advisable, will be tailored to your individual requirements.

The basic EDTA treatment, as established by the accepted protocol, consists of 500 to 1,000 ml of solution in an infusion bottle, with an EDTA dose based on your weight and kidney function condition. The intravenous solution might contain, among other substances, magnesium, a sodium bicarbonate buffer, a local anesthetic, heparin (to reduce the incidence of localized phlebitis), Vitamin C (a free radical scavenger), and miscellaneous nutrients such as the B-complex vitamins.

What if I get sick? Nauseous? Panic? Faint?

What better place to have an anxiety attack than in a doctor's office? Since the EDTA solution normally contains no preservatives, allergic reactions are extremely rare. Should you experience any adverse reaction, chances are it'll be psychological - not physiological. To our best knowledge, NO ONE has ever died while being chelated!

Most chelationists are alert to the possibility of an exceptionally sensitive patient having a bad reaction and are ready to deal with such a happening. Reputable physicians monitor their patients frequently, and their assistants are on the lookout for anyone requiring special assistance. The larger, better organized chelation clinics have an easily accessible "crash cart" that contains the medical supplies and equipment needed for emergency pulmonary resuscitation.

Can I be chelated if I've had a Bypass?

Absolutely, and often the sooner the better. One of the least publicized studies of the bypass procedure shows that fifteen to thirty percent of vein grafts (used in the bypass) become obstructed within one year. Chances are that within five years of surgery, your cardiologist will either advise another bypass - or tell you your condition has deteriorated to the point where "you're not a good candidate."

The same holds true if you've undergone angioplasty or any similar procedure. The odds are you will need remedial treatment sooner than not.

An informal survey of people taking chelation treatments revealed nearly half are bypass 'rejects' - or, previously bypassed or angioplastied people whose treatment did not cure their underlying disease or prevent it from recurring.

Am I too old to be chelated?

Never too old. Chelation has proved safe and effective with people well into their nineties, with a history of tuberculosis, liver disease, congestive heart failure, severe renal insufficiency, Alzheimer's, Parkinson's Disease, and other age-related ailments. There are probably NO absolute contraindications to the use of EDTA, other than for extremely allergic persons.

Should someone accompany me?

That's strictly a matter of personal preference. Usually, if you were well enough to get to the doctor's office on your own, you'll be able to see yourself safely home. Occasionally, a patient will feel a bit weak, tremulous, or have a mild stomach upset - and in such circumstances, it can be comforting to have a friend on hand. In any event, your doctor will not allow you to travel if you're unable to do so.

How long before I see results?

There's no pat answer to this question. Every individual is different. A 63-year old California stockbroker, diagnosed as having 90% blockage in four arteries and advised to have a quadruple bypass, chose chelation instead and was playing tennis with his wife in three weeks after just six treatments! Most patients, of course, are not 'instant winners'. The average course of treatment may take from one to three months, or require ten to thirty treatments. You'll probably experience small health improvements almost immediately - more energy, less pain, less difficulty breathing and walking.

Once the therapy takes hold, you'll have no difficulty recognizing results. You'll not only feel better, friends will begin commenting on how well you look - or asking whether you've had a face lift or found romance. Your complexion will take on a healthy glow. Wrinkles might become less visible, age spots may fade away or vanish, if your hair has turned gray, it might regain some of its color. What else? You'll enjoy a renewed vigor, interest in life and eagerness for productive activity. Best of all, you'll feel sexy again.

What if I have to quit in the middle? Or, Have to move and can't find a chelationist?

No problem. Chelation is not like a roller coaster - once on, no getting off. With chelation, you can begin - and stop - any time. Every treatment produces some benefit. When you stop, you retain benefits up to that point. Benefits accrue when you continue treatments, provided you begin again within one year of your last treatment.

Relocating should not prove an insurmountable problem. There are practitioners in almost every part of the country, and new ones opening offices every month. Physicians who have taken courses offered by ACAM (American College of Advancement in Medicine), GLACM (Great Lakes Association of Clinical Medicine) or through the "Howw Tooo" seminars run by Dr. Charles Farr (800-235-4788) follow pretty much the same protocol. Treatments from one doctor to another might vary, but they shouldn't differ significantly.

What do I do about the drugs I'm now taking?

Your chelation doctor will carefully monitor the drugs you've been prescribed. Chances are you'll require fewer - and much lower doses. Often, people can discard drugs entirely, particularly those that control blood sugar levels and angina pains.

What do I tell my 'Real' doctor?

Tough question. Doctors tend to become offended when a patient disregards their advice, and your fear of alienating your doctor is understandable.

Usually, honesty is the best policy. Tell your doctor what you're doing and why. Offer to keep him informed of your progress. Ask if he would like copies of your medical records as treatment progresses.

If you're not up to an open and above-board approach, do what one patient did. When his physician questioned his remarkable improvement, he smiled and said, "I've changed my diet."

It sounds too good to be true. No side effects?

Unpleasant side effects are always a possibility with any medical treatment, but the odds overwhelmingly favor your not being discomfited. Any problem you encounter will probably be minor. Any one of the annoyances might crop up on rare occasion:

- **Puncture site problems.**

Having a needle stuck in your arm is probably not your favorite pastime, but for most people the momentary pin prick is over and quickly forgotten. Occasionally, however, the IV infusion produces a burning or stinging sensation, a rash, some slight swelling, perhaps a black and blue bruise in a thin-veined or super-sensitive person. If setting up the IV proves to be a problem, injection sites can be rotated, from one arm to another, from the back of the hand to a foot or leg.

- **Anxiety reactions.**

Fainting spells, dizziness attacks, feelings of weakness, light-headedness, or extreme lethargy are all possibilities. While most such symptoms have an emotional origin, sometimes it's a lowered blood pressure treatment response. Resting for an hour or more with feet elevated until pressure normalizes will usually do away with this problem.

- **Stomach upsets, nauseous feelings and/or headaches.**

Aspirin and other pain relievers will usually eliminate tension headaches; upset stomach, with accompanying nausea, is extremely rare and can be readily treated.

- **Unexplained fever.**

Occasionally a patient experiences a sudden, temporary fever spike within 24 hours of starting treatment. The specialists do not consider this occurrence serious, and it usually vanishes as quickly and unexplainably as it arrives, but should be reported at once to the doctor.

- **Blood sugar instability.**

If your blood sugar levels are somewhat erratic, or you're subject to hypoglycemic reactions, chelation treatments may trigger a 'woozy' or weak feeling. Drinking a glass of fruit juice before treatment, and enjoying a healthy snack during treatment should ward off such problems.

Diabetics must have their blood sugar levels monitored diligently. Insulin requirements may change drastically during treatment, and every precaution must be taken against the possibility of hyperinsulinism.

- **Nocturnal leg cramps.**

Approximately 5% of patients voice this complaint, which may result from the chelation-induced changes in your body's calcium-magnesium balance. If this happens to you, additional magnesium can be added to the IV solution, and should relieve the problem.

- **The 'trots' and the 'runs'.**

"I've been living in the bathroom. What goes?" Loose-stools, diarrhea, and having to wake up to urinate several times a night are the most common difficulties. EDTA is a mild diuretic. One proof that it is restoring cellular integrity in all body organs is the evidence that it is ridding the body of accumulated fluids. Should you have to 'pee' a lot, be happy. You're not only getting healthier, you'll be several pounds lighter.

I'm still confused. Why does the American Heart Association 'bad mouth' chelation?

Let's look at some of the reasons they give (in their pamphlet, *Questions and Answers About Chelation Therapy*) for turning thumbs down.

For rebuttal to the extensive disinformation rampant throughout the pamphlet the AHA sends in response to inquiries, we turned to E. Cheraskin, M.D., Ph.D, a learned researcher who does not treat patients, but is one of the world's leading authorities on chelation therapy. It would be great fun, and quite enlightening, if we could bring an AHA spokesperson and Dr. Cheraskin face-to-face for a debate. But since that's not possible, we've done the next best thing: quoted what the AHA claims in their pamphlet and reported Dr. Cheraskin's verbatim response:

AHA: " . . . the benefits claimed for this form of treatment aren't scientifically proven."

DR. C: "Yes and no. It all depends on what you mean by scientific proof. If over half a million people benefiting from chelation is not scientific proof, I don't know what better proof there is. By the way, less than twenty percent of treatments used today, including bypass and balloon angioplasty haven't been scientifically proven to be beneficial - that is, they've not been tested in a double blind trial with a large number of subjects."

AHA: " . . . insurance companies and Medicare won't reimburse patients who undergo the treatments."

DR. C: "So what! Historically, the American Medical Association has at one time or another been against every progressive medical idea. They were against Social Security, Medicare and Medicaid. And to suggest that a profit-motivated organization like an insurance company being against chelation is proof it's no good, is just plain nonsense."

AHA: "It's possible that patients feel better not because of chelation therapy but because of something else (life style changes or the placebo effect)."

DR. C: "That's possible. Anything is *possible*. It's also *possible* the same holds true for many accepted procedures.

AHA: "The danger of kidney failure is very real. EDTA is also known to cause bone marrow depression, shock, low blood pressure, convulsions, disturbances of regular heart rhythm, allergic type reactions and respiratory arrest. In fact, a number of deaths around the country have been linked with chelation therapy. Also, a number of people are now on dialysis because of kidney failure caused, at least in part, by chelation therapy."

DR. C: "Going up. Second floor - ladies underwear, shoes, Halloween costumes and dirty tricks. The answer to that absurd laundry list of made-up slurs is that I've either been personally involved in research or know of research that shows that: (1) EDTA does not tear up kidney function. It actually improves it; (2) EDTA increases blood serum calcium and increases bone density in individuals with osteoporosis; (3) EDTA restores regular heart beats in patients with irregular heart beats; (4) as far as deaths are concerned, they're minimal compared with bypass (about 30 over the past three decades as against 4,000 with bypass); (5) blood pressure is in fact reduced in people with hypertension. I know of no case where a patient has become hypotensive after chelation; (6) when it comes to shock, convulsion, allergic-type reactions and respiratory arrest, I've never heard or seen such reactions. But I suppose it *can* happen. The question is *has* it happened or is the AHA just using scare tactics to cloud the issue?"

AHA: " . . . people who begin relying on chelation therapy may delay undergoing proven therapies like drugs or surgery until it's too late."

DR. C: "Again, that's possible. On the other hand, more than half the people who go for chelation have had the drugs and surgery and weren't helped. That's precisely why they're there."

AHA:(edited) "The idea that removing calcium from plaque will reverse or prevent atherosclerosis hasn't been proven."

DR. C: "Of course it hasn't. Back in the 70's, it was speculated that EDTA worked by removing calcium from plaque, but the amount removed was so infinitesimal, that theory didn't hold up. From the 80's to the present, the prevailing explanation is that by removing toxic metals, EDTA increases enzyme function and reduces free radical activity. By the way, the AHA knows that EDTA infusions remove toxic metals. They seem to be caught in a time warp, faulting an old explanation that was discarded by knowledgeable scientists more than a decade ago. Either the AHA hasn't done its homework, or this organization is so eager to 'get' chelation, it resorts to questionable tactics."

HOW WRONG CAN THE AHA BE? LET'S FIND OUT.

AHA: "In the first month, patients usually receive from five to 30 treatments ... Often the patient is then advised to continue preventive treatment once a month."

DR. C: "That's nuts. Five to ten treatments *a month* is par for the course. When the series of treatments are over, the patient is advised to return for an annual check-up (anything strange about that?) at which time a booster series of five infusions may be appropriate. The AHA seems to be making this stuff up whole hog."

AHA: "The truth of the matter is that physicians who treat cardiovascular diseases could significantly increase their income if chelation therapy was a scientifically proven treatment procedure ... Surgery, after all, can be performed on only one patient at a time ..."

DR. C: "The truth is, cardiovascular surgeons are not hurting for income. Every survey shows they earn more than all other specialists. Surely even the AHA can't pretend surgeons are nobly sacrificing potential profits when they reject chelation! 'One surgical patient at a time' is a quick $40,000 clip - quite a bit more than the $2,000 or so a chelation doctor receives from treating one patient over a three month or longer time period."

We decided to give Dr. Cheraskin the last word in this 'mock' debate. Here's what he said.

"All in all, this supposedly consumer-oriented folder is full of distortions, misrepresentations, and falsifications. I'd like to challenge the AHA to provide the scientific studies to back up their contention that EDTA chelation therapy is a dangerous, non-effective treatment. I'd like to see what they come up with."

Good idea, Dr. C. We did as you suggested and sent a registered letter to Phil Kibak at AHA headquarters in Dallas, Texas requesting full documentation of their anti-chelation charges. Three weeks later, came a response in the form of one obscure 28-year old study accompanied by the following note: "Enclosed is a 1963 study of chelation therapy (published in the _American Journal of Cardiology._) This is the _only study on the subject in our files_ (emphasis ours). The poor quality is due to its being a copy from a microfilm reader. - PK"

We called Dr. Cheraskin back.

He laughed. "That's the old Kitchell-Meltzer research chestnut - the one they called a 'reappraisal of EDTA'. It's bad science married to smelly politics. And if you read through it, you'll note, not one of the dangers attributed to chelation in the twelve-page AHA pamphlet is touched on in the Kitchell-Meltzer work. Their study involved 38 patients, and after three months of EDTA treatments, concluded that '66 percent of these 38 patients exhibited _improved_ anginal patterns, and 40 percent showed _improved_ electrocardiographic patterns, and none of these effects was long lasting.

"What that means," Dr. Cheraskin explained, "is that despite documenting _positive_ benefits from a sizable percentage of the EDTA-treated patients, the study is nevertheless quoted by the AHA as the _only_ scientific rationale for condemning the treatment! The AHA couldn't come up with anything more damning for a simple reason: I don't know of any such studies and neither does the AHA."

THE REST OF THE STORY

We are not alone in viewing this revisionist report with suspicion. After all, it's common knowledge among those familiar with pre-1963 chelation research that this superficiously negative study was in direct contradiction to all the rave reviews (twenty or more) these very same researchers had previously published. What had happened? How to explain the 180 degree turn-about? Dr. Garry Gordon, an astute physician, knowledgeable about the scientific shenanigans so prominent in chelation's long history, shed some light.

"First of all, know this," Dr. Gordon explained: "the researchers were paid some $1,500,000 to complete this study, an amount far above the going rate in 1963 for a 3 month project involving less than 50 patients. Second: Kitchell and Meltzer virtually disappeared from the research scene after this study was published. Third: I followed up on my hunch that something was seriously amiss, and thirteen years later, in 1976, I succeeded in getting Dr. Meltzer to admit that he had been 'pressured' - some would say 'paid off' - by National Blue Cross and Blue Shield to take a stance *against* chelation."

Shocking? Yes. Unusual? No. When science and profits clash, no contest as to which wins out. Just a few months back, science fraud investigator Walter Stewart concluded, after years of studious review, that as much as 25 percent of all research papers may be intentionally fudged.

SO HOW MUCH DOES CHELATION COST?

Chelation costs vary from doctor to doctor, but in most cases run about $1,000 to $3,000 for a full course of treatments. Some of these costs - initial medical workup, diagnostic tests, supportive therapy - may be covered by your health insurer. The treatments themselves, probably will not. Let's talk a bit about money - and why you'll have to foot the larger part of the bills when choosing to recover with the help of EDTA infusions.

"Skyrocketing" is the adjective most frequently used to describe the cost of health care in America. The numbers have zoomed from about $50 billion to $550 billion in a dozen years, and are rapidly approaching 12% of the gross national product. To make matters worse, every study suggests costs will continue to explode in the years ahead, as the population ages and sickens.

Pushed to the limit, health insurers work overtime searching for reasons to refuse reimbursement to policy holders. Documents presented in a 1989 legal action against Aetna Life and Casualty Company showed just how far insurance companies will go to deny benefits. According to court testimony, Aetna set overall dollar amounts it wanted its offices and individual employees to save on payouts; they evaluated employees and recommended bonuses on their ability to cut policyholder claims; they targeted claims just over the $500 statutory threshold that claimants must cross to file suit for other damages; they conspired to make the treating physician a party to suits over contested health claims thereby encouraging the doctor to settle the case rather than spend time away from his office.

As one witness testified in open court: "Aetna officials were telling their workers, 'We want you to save $10,000. We don't care how you do it - just do it. Cut people off.'"

THE 'UNINSURANCE' SCAM

With growing frequency, the patient's freedom to choose whatever medical care he deems best is restricted by the claim adjuster's power to wield the "denied" stamp. When a treatment not blessed by the AMA crosses the desk, the insurance company has its best excuse to turn it down, irrespective of potential benefit. Once the establishment labels a procedure "experimental," "unproven," or "not usual or customary," insurance carriers can easily justify withholding payment. To complete the vicious circle, critics of a "controversial" test or treatment, point to the insurance companies' reimbursement refusals as evidence of unacceptability.

Talk about "Catch 22," this is it. Chelation is twice-damned, by the way the medical industry's big guns work hand in hand to shoot down anything they don't like. Logical thinkers find it hard to understand why health insurers don't make an exception and pay for chelation.

"It's so much less expensive," people point out. "If they're so cost-conscious, why don't insurers encourage people to get well without spending big bucks?"

On the surface, that argument presents a legitimate point of confusion. Dig deeper and you'll realize, as we have, that chelation therapy is potentially so costly to the insurance industry they cannot afford to have it approved!

Why? Because not just the currently ill, but most men and women over the age of twenty-one - (and some kids still below voting age) - probably can establish a valid basis for needing and demanding chelation therapy.

Autopsies done by the U.S. Army Department of Technology revealed that 70% of 3,000 soldiers killed in Vietnam exhibited "significant" occlusion of the arteries. If 70% of the U.S. adult population were to be chelated at $2,000 to $3,000 for each treatment series, cost to health insurers would total a whopping $300 BILLION to $500 BILLION, a sum that would undoubtedly break the bank and leave their stockholders howling. Medicare and Medicaid also stonewall payments for chelation, and for the same reason. It's no secret the government is hard-pressed to find funds for currently approved treatments, and like private insurers, seeks ways to cut benefits, not expand them.

The large medical centers are co-conspirators. High-tech in-hospital procedures (bypass and angioplasty, to name two) have grown to a $6 billion bonanza, and administrators are not about to share this cash cow with chelation, a competitive out-patient procedure.

We certainly agree the health insurers are not only callous, but short-sighted as well. At the very least, they might grant people who opt for chelation a reduced rate on their insurance premiums - the same as they do under other "Healthy American" plans - that reward low-risk non-smokers, non-drinkers, and people who carefully fasten their seat belts, stay out of gay bars and practice safe sex.

HERE COMES THE JUDGE

All may not be lost. In 1988, the Aetna Insurance Company got a swift kick in the wallet when a Ohio court ordered them to pay for chelation. The judge in the case, George H. Ferguson stated, "Although chelation therapy may not be the *treatment of choice* for atherosclerosis, it appears to be a broadly accepted professional treatment since 300,000 patients have received intravenous EDTA chelation therapy over the past 30 years with fewer than 20 deaths compared to more than 4,000 deaths caused by coronary artery bypass surgery in approximately an equal number of patients."

In another section of the judgment, the judge also spoke to the matter of costs, saying the policy holder had "saved the insurance company the expensive cost of a coronary bypass surgical operation."

True. But this one case is not apt to change things. The bottom line is this: unless you're willing to spend years - and big bucks - fighting for your rights, you'll probably have to dig into your pocket to pay for EDTA infusions. Chances are, when you look back, you'll call it a bargain. You'll cut future drug and medical bills and enjoy added years of pleasurable and productive activity. What a deal.

I've read there's an FDA study on chelation therapy. How is it coming along?

It's not. The FDA-approved study begun with such high hopes in 1985 never really got off the ground. In his final accounting to the FDA late in 1991, Dr. Richard Guardino (the study's Medical Director) reported progress on 32 of the 120 patients on the original agenda. Of those recruited during the six years of active funding, only 23 completed treatment. Four patients dropped out and five were in post-treatment phase when the project came to a halt with no conclusions drawn.

Later that same year, Wyeth-Aherst, a subsidiary of pharmaceutical giant American Home Products, agreed to allocate some $6.3 million to complete the aborted EDTA project. Less than six months later, in February of 1992, they unexplainedly withdrew. So much for eight years of great expectations.

How realistic were those great expectations? What chance that a successfully completed FDA-approved study would lead to insurance coverage? Take the heat off chelating physicians? Since hundreds of confirming studies have been ignored by the medical establishment, we cannot envision any study so definitive and persuasive, it would compel anti-chelation forces to do a 180 degree turnabout. It's easier to believe in the tooth fairy than to expect an overnight conversion by those dedicated to denying decades of accumulated published data.

What are the prospects for future acceptance? Ironically, the worse the economy gets, the better the chances. Chelation and other non-surgical, non-pharmaceutical approaches to chronic degenerative disease offer the cost-effective options health care reformers claim to be seeking.

One study that makes the case is "A White Paper on Cost Effectiveness of Alternative Medicine in the Workplace", prepared for the Great Lakes Association of Clinical Medicine by Dr. Chappell and a host of GLACM associates. Specifying chelation therapy, the researchers note: "In the United States for 1991, $10,000,000,000 (that's ten billion!) was spent on a medical procedure, bypass surgery, that in most cases was not indicated, according to the best medical literature available."

Work out the numbers for yourself. If 230,000 surgeries costing on average $44,000 each were replaced with an equal number of chelation therapies at an average cost of $3,000, we're talking about a $9.43 billion saving! When you add the costs of failed angioplasties, unnecessary amputations, catastrophic strokes that could have been avoided .... well, you get the picture. If the economic crunch worsens, both private and government insurers may eventually be forced to offer the chelation option. When that happens, it's apt to be a 'good news/bad news' story. On the downside, we anticipate one or all of the following scenarios:

1. Insurance coverage may be limited to the most serious cases of arterial blockages. It won't extend to sub-clinical peripheral circulation problems, cases of infrequent TIA's, or preventive treatments.

2. Chelation may be covered by insurance *only* if performed in a facility that meets insurance company requirements - i.e. limited to hospitals and practitioners with access to expensive diagnostic and resuscitation equipment. That may prove a real wallop in the wallet for the consumer who ultimately foots the bills;

3. Hospitals may require extensive (expensive and dangerous) testing as a prerequisite for treatment. Hospitals have been aggressive promoters of such 'services' in recent years. In the fall of 1990, Reston, Virginia's Hospital Cardiology Center ran full page ads with the tempting headline "You ought to Be in Pictures", inviting the unwary to "drop in" for a cardiac catheterization as though they were offering as simple and innocuous a procedure as donning a blood pressure cuff. Only

after we threatened the *Washington Post* with a class action suit charging false advertising and a Congressional hearing, did the ads cease. Obviously, cardiovascular departments have a huge investment in diagnostic equipment they are not about to sling on the scrap heap.

4. With hospital doctors 'in charge', patients requesting chelation may well be coerced into surgical procedures by staffs more familiar with bypass, angioplasty and the like. Every survey proves doctors, like automobile mechanics, continue to perform those procedures for which they're trained and have experience: surgeons operate. That's the way of the world.

Whether any or all of these concerns prove valid, only time will tell. Meanwhile, with national health insurance a looming prospect, the window is closing. There is little time left for those interested in having chelation therapy available to all when and how they want it, to pressure local, state and federal legislators to include chelation in all health care plans.

The outlook is not all grim. There's a good chance chelation will be mainstreamed sometime in the forseeable future. There are signs this is already happening. Encouraging numbers of eager-to-learn physicians are signing up for chelation training at seminars offered four times a year by ACAM and GLACM, and weekly by Skoshi and Charles Farr, M.D., of Oklahoma City. OK.

In any event, more people everyday are learning about the chelation alternative. That's good news, indeed.

How do I convince my stubborn father (spouse, in-law, friend, close relative) he or she should be chelated?

Don't try too hard. There's probably no more painfully frustrating experience as failing to persuade someone you care for to do what you're convinced is best for them. We know; we've been there.

When you find yourself in such a predicament, your best

bet is to locate someone who has been chelated to talk to your loved one. If that's not possible, try to get him or her to read this book. If he does not have the patience to read, or has poor eyesight, you can send for the audio version of this text, a one hour taped adaptation. (See ad in back of book.)

If despite your best efforts, the person opts for bypass or angioplasty - or nothing - take it in stride, and hope for the best. Take comfort from Winston Churchill who once remarked: "Americans can always be relied upon to do the right thing after they've exhausted all other possibilities."

Where do I find a good chelation doctor?

You'll find a directory of doctors at the back of this book. If you don't find one listed at a convenient location, call ACAM 1-800-532-3688 or GLACM (Great Lakes Association of Clinical Medicine) 1-800-286-6013. If you want to find out whether a particular doctor has taken the advanced training which qualifies for certification by the American Board of Chelation Therapy, contact ABCT 1-800-356-ABCT. If you want to know more about any one doctor, call us and we'll tell you what patient reports are on file.

I've heard chelation doctors are Quacks. Are they?

Glad you asked. The next chapter speaks to that issue.

Doctors are whippersnappers in ironed white coats
Who spy up your rectums and look down your throats
And press you and poke you with sterilized tools
And stab at solutions that pacify fools.
I used to revere them and do what they said
Till I learned what they learned on was already dead.

Gilda Radner on Doctors

13

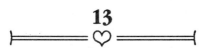

DUCK! HERE COME THE 'QUACKS'

"Quackery," a disreputable part of the American heritage, has a distinguished history both in our country and abroad.

Dr. Elisha Perkins of Plainfield, Connecticut, obtained the nation's first medical patent in 1796 on a device he called "tractors" - two metal rods with which he would stroke patients to relieve their pain. He sold tractors to such notables as the Chief Justice of the U.S. Supreme Court and, as legend has it, George Washington. Not until Dr. Perkins took his tractors to New York City to fight the yellow fever epidemic, and died of the disease, did anyone suspect he was a bona fide 'quack'.

In the early 1800's, Samuel Thompson, an unschooled New Hampshire farmer's son, shook the medical establishment with his "self-healing system." He published claims that every man could be his own doctor with steam baths and herbs. Thompson was eventually discredited, but his anti-professional crusade triggered such an outpouring of public outrage, his 'quackery' inadvertently helped abolish other questionable medical practices such as bleeding and massive mineral doses.

Not all innovative medicine is later found fraudulent. Ignaz Semmelweiss, for example, was a Vienna physician who bucked the medical establishment with the idea that handwashing prevented puerpural infection among hospitalized pregnant women. Even after he proved himself right by almost eradicating obstetric ward mortality, his peers remained unimpressed, and ultimately drove him out of the country.

Dr. Edward Jenner, a country doctor, experienced his share of difficulties establishing a vaccine for smallpox. Imagine how much worse the outcry, had he revealed that the procedure he favored was a female contrivance. Unbeknownst to his critics, he adopted work introduced in England 81 years earlier by Lady Mary Wortley Montagu, a radical writer, feminist, and medical pioneer.

History is replete with examples of innovators, initially labeled charlatans, only to be posthumously recognized as geniuses. But not until chelation pioneers banded together more than twenty years ago, has the medical establishment libeled so large and well-credentialed a group.

WHO ARE THESE "QUACKS"?
WHERE DO THEY COME FROM?

Would you believe Harvard University? Case-Western Reserve? University of California? Indiana University? Duke, Georgetown, Texas A&M, Michigan State? Almost any prestigious medical school you might name is the alma mater of one or more chelating doctors.

What were these doctors doing before adding EDTA to their black bag of tricks? Were they defrocked elsewhere? Deported refugees from third-world countries? Health-providers with failing practices? The record shows otherwise.

Check the professional credentials of the more than five hundred ACAM members and you'll find a surprising number are board certified cardiovascular surgeons - (which means they could be performing bypass surgery and similar operations if they so chose). Others are Fellows and/or passed the Boards of AMA-affiliated medical specialties, hold hospital staff appointments, and are elected officers in local, state and national medical societies. An impressive number have had their research published in mainstream medical journals and/or received honors and awards from their colleagues.

DO THEY GET RICH QUICK?

What makes conventionally trained doctors defect? Are they greedy opportunists hungry for easy money?

Not likely. You won't see a lineup of chauffeur-driven BMW's parked in front of an ACAM meeting. The latest survey of physician incomes reveals chelation doctors rank way down the list compared to cardiovascular surgeons, cardiologists, neurosurgeons, obstetricians, dermatologists - even pediatricians.

Heart surgeons get top dollar. A recent report revealed that they earned an average $383,520 in 1989. Other medical specialties earned between $250,000 and $300,000, and since many doctors benefit from such unreported financial 'perks' as 'kickbacks' from pacemaker manufacturers, referral dividends from investments in million-dollar CAT scan and MRI imaging centers, and profits from doctor-owned pharmacies, those lofty incomes may in fact be significantly higher.

Chelation specialists, by contrast, not only earn less ($150,000 on average), they get to *keep* less. The legal costs of defending an unpopular medical practice has bankrupted more than one chelation doctor. It can be expensive - financially and emotionally - to continue chelating. Dr. Warren Levin of New York City claims to have shelled out more than $100,000 over a two year period, battling a licensing board that has ruthlessly persecuted him for almost a decade. Ironically, no patient has ever filed a complaint against him, but that hasn't helped Dr. L's bank balance a bit.

"Every time I attend my medical school reunion, I'm reminded that I'm the poorest guy on the block," chelation specialist Dr. Jonathan Collins, editor of the prestigious *Townsend Letter* remarked. "I estimate my earnings fall in the bottom fifth percentile of my graduating class."

"Chelation a big money maker? Don't make me laugh," explodes Dr. Milton Fried. "I can make more suturing a simple laceration than doing a whole chelation treatment and it takes a hell of a lot less time. If it were really profitable, you'd find ten times as many doctors doing it."

"My practice is for sale - any day, at any price," exclaimed one physician who asked to be anonymous. "Income is down, pressure is up. At some point, you've got to call it quits!"

If not money, what? Surely not prestige.

You get no 'brownie' points and little public acclaim for practicing chelation. Chelationists are routinely and maliciously attacked by organized medicine, licensing boards, government agencies, and health insurers. The tactics used against chelating physicians include smear campaigns, entrapment, illegal wiretaps, politically inspired IRS audits. Some chelation doctors spend almost as much time defending their right to practice as treating patients - an obviously costly, time-consuming and ego-bashing undertaking.

THE NIFTY FIFTY FESS UP

So, why do they do it? We asked more than fifty chelation doctors that very question, and discovered the vast majority converted in response to a personal health problem. Either they or someone they loved got sick, and they could find no other cure! Having discovered chelation, they would rather fight the medicrats than revert to conventional medicine, despite professional costs.

When doctors face life or death decisions for themselves - or their loved ones - they frequently investigate unfamiliar therapies. When they find an unorthodox treatment that offers some promise, it doesn't matter if their colleagues approve or not. They're not influenced by the lack of double-blind studies or prestigious backup. Conventional guidelines are shoved aside when the life of someone they love hangs in the balance.

One prime example is Dr. Dan Roehm, of Pompano Beach, Florida, Chief of the Department of Medicine at Broward General Hospital, certified as a Diplomate of the American Board of Internal Medicine and a Fellow of the American College of Physicians.

Dr. R. was a main-stream cardiologist until his wife began exhibiting symptoms characteristic of subclinical mini-strokes, any one of which might one day escalate into a full-blown fatal attack or disabilitating episode.

"I had nothing to offer; there was nothing I could do to ward off what I saw on the horizon," Roehm realized, and so began his urgent search for some way to forestall the looming calamity. Once he discovered EDTA, he tried it. When it restored his wife's health, Dr. Roehm added chelation and other alternative treatments to his practice - and says it's "more satisfying than the drug-and-surgery oriented medicine I was practicing before."

THE DOCTOR SAVES HIMSELF

When the doctor becomes a patient, he's *in* the bed instead of standing next to it, and everything looks different. Medical decisions are no longer simple when instead of operating, you're going to be operated on.

Dr. Grant Born of Grand Rapids, Michigan, became involved with chelation to save himself from that trauma. He was just forty-three, with no previous history of heart disease, when he went into cardiac arrest while attending a football game.

"My heart just stopped," he recalls. "They revived me, got me to the Mayo Clinic, where the doctors agreed I needed bypass surgery - perhaps a heart transplant. While I was wrestling with this news, a guy walks into my room with a book about chelation therapy and asks, 'Do you know anything about this?' It was like somebody sent him.

"What I read convinced me. I went for treatments. After chelation saved my life, I really got interested."

Dr. Born speaks from experience when he admits there are social as well as professional pressures NOT to practice chelation.

"My first wife was dead-set against my getting mixed up with a controversial therapy. Even though EDTA helped me survive, she argued against it when I wanted to do it. She worried her reputation with the country club set would be wrecked if word got out that I was practicing 'quack-style' medicine."

Dr. Born resolved his problem. He changed specialties and wives. The new Mrs. Born (Dr. Tammy Guerkink) has no hangups about chelation - she works at his side.

Dr. Jack R. Vinson, of Dallas, Texas was a 'young' forty-two years of age, when he was told he only had two or three years to live, perhaps five on the outside.

"I had a serious heart condition - arrhythmia, angina, posterior infarction and had gone into congestive failure. Conventional medicine didn't have much to offer, except the common symptom-relieving drugs.

"I couldn't work. It was bad. There I was, with a wife and two teenagers, forced to retire to a quiet backwater community in the Arizona desert and prepare for the end. While I was waiting for the coroner to call, I did a lot of reading, and an article headlined 'Doctors in California Using Chelation Therapy for Heart Disease' caught my attention.

"I was on the next plane to find out what it was all about - and one week later, back in Arizona with enough EDTA to treat myself, began therapy. Two months, and thirty treatments after that, I was well enough to discard all my drugs, get back on my feet, and return to work."

That was in 1970. Dr. Vinson is still in practice, still chelating himself, and all others for whom he deems it to be a suitable treatment.

John Ettl, M.D. an El Paso, Texas chelationist, was also his own first EDTA patient. A rock hobbyist, he discovered he was suffering near-fatal levels of lead toxicity thanks to his hobby of casting unusual specimens.

"I had all the usual symptoms - irritability, anxiety, bad temper, sleeplessness, forgetfulness, mental disorientation, blurred vision and poor hearing but thought they were age-related problems, though I was only in my mid-50's.

"Fortunately for me, Dr. Harold Harper, a pioneer doctor in this field, convinced me it was lead poisoning - not mid-life crisis - and told me to read up on the treatment of choice, chelation. As a pathologist, I was extremely wary of the potential dangers, and went about it very cautiously.

"I began slowly, but eventually gave myself over 200 treatments before I got my lead levels down to normal. By that time, I was symptom-free, and a chelation expert."

THEY DID IT FOR DAD

Dr. John Parks Trowbridge in Humble, Texas, learned about chelation therapy from his 70-year old father who'd read about it in a health magazine. The elder Trowbridge wanted his son to look into EDTA because he'd suffered an aortic aneurysm and had other serious circulatory problems.

Young John, just emerging from a surgical residency in urology, responded predictably. "Forget it. It's quackery. If it was any good, wouldn't I have heard of it? Wouldn't the medical journals publish reports on a marvelous way to reverse atherosclerosis? Wouldn't doctors be using it?"

It wasn't until several years later that Dr. Trowbridge, a bit older - a lot wiser - was embarrassed to remember those hasty, cocky words. His parents had grown older, too - and sicker when a chance meeting with physician/nutritionist/chelationist Robert Haskell, M.D. encouraged him to take a second look. What Dr. Haskell showed Dr. Trowbridge amazed him - medical records of recovered patients whose test readings and clinical exams proved beyond doubt how much they'd benefited from chelation treatments.

Still only partially convinced, Dr. Trowbridge flew from one chelation clinic to another to check things out - to Alabama, Pennsylvania, Oklahoma, California. He made dozens of stops in as many cities, as he criss-crossed the country in search of more data.

"Every chelation doctor I visited was so enthusiastic about what he was doing, and so eager to open his patient files, I could no longer question effectiveness. Cabinets full of case histories clearly showed chelation therapy was a revolutionary method for overcoming degenerative disease. It blew my mind!"

No question as to Dr. Trowbridge's motives when he changed from critic to advocate. The first patients he chelated were Claire and Jack Trowbridge, his mom and dad.

Dr. Harold Huffman of Hinton, Virginia is another doctor whose first chelation patient was good old dad.

"It was 1982, and my father, 70 years old at the time, was a diabetic, suffering from diabetic retinopathy, and had already lost one foot because of gangrene and was facing the loss of the other. A physician himself, he knew the prognosis was not good. I called a nurse in Indiana who knew a lot about alternative medicine, and asked her what we could do. She recommended chelation and I said 'what's that?'

"She filled me in on the fine details. I learned how to do it, and while I wasn't convinced it was any good, knew it was dad's only hope of avoiding a second amputation.

"Talk about reluctant - I don't remember which one of us had more qualms, him or me. But we sure went into it with our fingers crossed - and were more surprised than anyone when the treatments worked. It saved his remaining leg - even restored his eyesight - and he continued practicing medicine for five more years."

THE 'NAGGED' AND THE 'NUDGED'

Dr. Michael Schachter's infant daughter inadvertently changed the course of his professional career. The two and a half year old had cerebral palsy, and despite intensive therapy at a prestigious rehabilitation center, was still unable to get up on all fours or to crawl.

"My office nurse suggested I try Vitamin E. I read up on it, found it had been used with some success on brain-damaged children, and thought 'what the heck.' Within three days of giving Amy 100 units of Vitamin E daily, she was noticeably more alert, more responsive, even started rocking back and forth.

"That shook me up. How was it possible my nurse knew more about restoring health than I did? I began investigating alternative medical treatments and have been proud to offer chelation and other forms of homeopathic treatments to the people of Nyack, New York ever since. What's more important - I'm still learning."

Seventy-eight year old Dr. James D. Schuler of Smith River, California, had a chelation practice unceremoniously 'thrust upon him' when a colleague and good buddy had a stroke.

"His wife turned his sixty chelation patients over to me and said, 'You take care of them.' I said, 'What good is chelation if it didn't prevent John's stroke?'

"She had a ready answer. 'He didn't take his own good

advice. He smoked, drank, ate lots of meat and fatty foods. Even chelation won't save you if you're determined to do yourself in.'

"I was stuck. I was an orthodox practitioner, general surgeon, and knew almost nothing about this chelation business - never practiced it, never referred anyone. But with sixty new patients, I was motivated to become educated - fast. Once I read up, and started treating these people, I discovered how great chelation is, and I've been doing it ever since. Lucky for the patients. Lucky for me."

Dr. Ronald Hoffman of New York City, an outspoken advocate of holistic medicine, looked into chelation after having dinner with a talkative nurse.

"Throughout the meal, this lady regaled me with tales of miracle cures: patients who'd been brought back from the brink of death and were now symptom-free. and one hard-to-believe story after another about people whose legs had been saved from amputation. I couldn't get her to talk about anything else.

"I thought, either this dame's a nut - or chelation is worth a closer look. I decided to investigate and discovered everything this lady said was the absolute truth. That was nine years ago, and I've been practicing chelation ever since."

Skeptical at the outset, Dr. Terry Chappell of Blufton, Ohio, latched on to chelation after listening carefully to what people told him.

"I was nagged into it (chelation) by a patient," he admits, telling about "an important local honcho. This executive of a very large corporation had been traveling more than 11 hours each way to get chelation treatments from the nearest doctor he could find. Since he didn't want to spend all that time on the road, he kept after me, pestering me every other day to insist I check it out.

"I wasn't terribly interested, but I wasn't hopelessly doctrinaire, either. I was mildly curious about nutrition, meditation, hypnosis - things like that. This guy was so persistent, I gave in, and visited several chelation doctors. Once I checked things out, I had no choice. Chelation works and here I am."

David Freeman, M.D. of North Hollywood, California is yet another non-believer who was dragged into chelation, protesting all the way that he would *NOT* get involved with quackery.

"A dozen years ago, I'd have sworn this chelation was a bunch of garbage. I was well up on the conventional medical literature, and believed what I read: 'no proven value', 'fraudulent claims', 'anecdotal evidence from unreliable sources'. Who needed it!

"As it turned out, many of my patients thought *THEY* needed it - a lot. One after another, they began bugging me to look into it. I turned thumbs down.

"Then, as luck would have it, an old medical school chum visited me. I knew this guy was a solid scholar, totally reliable with a sterling intellect and unquestionably ethical. We'd interned together, and I'd trust this doc with my life. When *he* started praising chelation, spinning astonishing tales of miracle cures, I just had to listen. Since then, I've learned a lot - About chelation, and what it means to be labeled a 'quack'."

When we asked Dr. Irby Fox of Abilene, Texas how he came to join the quack squad, he said, "It was an accident. A patient who had a bypass that failed, was in pretty bad shape, and begged me to chelate him.

"I hedged a lot. I don't know anything about this, I told him. But I'll check it out, and if that's what you want, I'll do it, provided you sign an agreement that if your wife, kids or their relatives sue, I can use your estate to defend myself.

"I was being pretty cautious, but once I got started, I couldn't stop. This first guy got well; the next chelated patient did also. It's incredible. I really didn't want to get interested in anything so controversial - I'm no hero. The real heroes are the patients who insist on being chelated despite all the bad things their doctors say about it."

Dr. John Schwent of Festus, Missouri was a conservative main-stream physician until he lost several young patients only a short time after undergoing bypass surgery.

"It was frustrating," he recalls, "to send thirty- and forty year-olds off for bypasses only to have them die in a couple of years."

Then Mrs. Schwent's best friend, an attorney, began having angina attacks and instead of bypass surgery, opted for chelation treatments - "and results were fantastic. He got well!

"I got a book about chelation and sat up all night reading it. One of my classmates, a Chuck Curtis, was mentioned in the book, so I called him. 'Are you practicing this voodoo medicine?' He laughed and said, 'For eight years now' and when I asked, 'Killed anyone yet?' he got serious and replied, 'No, but if you've got two weeks to spare, I can use every minute telling you great stories about the lives I've saved.'

"I wound up spending an entire year visiting chelation clinics all over the United States. Then I took the ACAM course and still didn't give the first treatment. I was very reluctant to get into it. I knew that introducing chelation into my practice would jeopardize my professional standing, and perhaps lead to my being ostracized. In spite of it all, I had to go ahead. It wouldn't be honest to know how to cure people and refuse to do it."

A PATIENT MADE THEM DO IT

Dr. James Swann of Independence is a "show me, I'm from Missouri" sort of physician.

"I first heard about chelation in 1973 at a Jackson County Medical Society meeting when a Dr. Paul Williams, the author of two medical textbooks, tried to educate us on its usefulness for atherosclerosis. Nobody in the room knew anything about it - we couldn't even spell it.

"The lecture over, I hung around to chat with Paul, and it surprised me to learn that the *American Journal of Cardiology* had published favorable reports on this treatment. It bothered me that almost no one was following up, investigating, or using it."

Dr. Swann's moment of decision came when a close friend whose triple bypass had failed (all three grafts had closed) only four months after surgery, came to visit. She'd been sent home to die, but had heard of chelation and there she and her husband sat, in Dr. Swann's living room, begging for the treatment.

"'Lill', I said, 'I sure would like a better case than you to practice on. You're going to die on me, and we'll all look bad.'

"She was a spunky rascal. When she said, 'I'd rather die trying, than die doing nothing,' she got to me. I said 'OK. If you're willing, I am.'

"We started her out on three chelation treatments a week. That was twenty years ago, and she's alive today and still going strong. That's the case that brought me around."

It would be hard to find a more conservative physician than Dr. Conrad ("Connie") Maulfair, Jr. of Mertztown, Pennsylvania. A farm boy and Pennsylvania Dutchman, reared in the land of the Amish, you can imagine his reaction when a patient brought him an article about chelation in a holistic-type magazine published - where else? - in California. He snorted. He sneered. He said, "What can you expect from those west coast loonies?" He dismissed the idea without a second thought. But then came a second, third, fourth patient - all asking questions about chelation, all bringing books and articles, or as Connie puts it, "telling tall tales".

True to his heritage, Dr. M. refused to be "pushed". For six years, he shrugged the subject off, before coming around to investigate for himself. That was ten years ago, and now he not only treats patients, he trains other doctors how to administer EDTA infusions properly.

Dr. Milton Fried of Atlanta, Georgia, insists that he never set out to be a rebel.

"I'm very thin-skinned and hate doing anything that exposes me to criticism - BUT - on the other hand, I'd feel worse not doing what I know to be best for patients.

"I was a resident in a New York hospital when a patient with a blue leg and gangrene of the toes and foot, was scheduled for amputation. When he told us he was going to get chelated instead, we warned him that it was bunk, and advised against it. He got chelated anyhow, and weeks later came back with the leg healed, and just lorded it over us.

"The other docs ignored the whole thing, but I thought, 'Hey wait a minute. There's something to this.' I started studying chelation. That was the easy part. Working up the chutzpah to do it was tough. I knew it meant parting company with the 'respectable' docs, taking a lot of flack, jeopardizing my reputation and income. It was a hard decision - but I had to do it.

"I've never been sorry. I get a lot of 'nachis' - that's Yiddish for 'pride and satisfaction'. I'll tell you what makes me mad - all the doctors who come to me for chelation when they get sick - or send their wives, friends, relatives - and never let it be known. They tell me, 'I wish I had your nerve'. I tell them they're gutless wonders."

Dr. Gerald Parker of Amarillo, Texas, says Dr. Fried is the perfect example of chelation doctors who should be proud to be called 'quacks'.

"There's a fine breed of 'Quacks' - they're the rare medical birds who are not satisfied with what they're taught in medical school and are willing to explore new approaches. These 'quacks' become frustrated when they can't help a patient recover, and they look for a better way."

TO SAVE A 'GOLDEN GIRL'

That definition fits Dr. Harold Sparks of Evansville, Indiana, who got into chelation because his 85-year old widowed mother-in-law's mental faculties were fading due to advanced arteriosclerosis.

"The local hospital docs checked her out and said, 'Nothing to be done. Put her in a nursing home.' My wife said, 'No way. You're a doctor. Fix her.'

"What was I to do? I'd heard about chelation, but didn't want any part of it. Why get into something that's going to bring you nothing but grief - that every doctor will fight you on? My wife nagged and nagged. I decided to do chelation - just once, for my mother-in-law. After seeing her recover - her mind cleared and she went back home to care for herself - my conscience got me. I couldn't deny my other patients. That was 1976, and I've been chelating ever since."

Dr. Harold Walmer of Elizabethtown, Pennsylvania is the Lancaster County version of TV's Dr. Welby - an old-fashioned country doctor perfectly content with "being a pillpusher and collecting my fees," as he puts it.

The least likely M.D. to stray from the fold, Dr. Walmer's chelation involvement is a fluke.

"I had some extra room, and when a few patients started asking for chelation, I investigated and thought 'It can't hurt'. I studied up, took the ACAM course, and decided I'd chelate very selectively - just a few close friends, and people I knew real well.

"Before I knew it, I was getting patients from all over. I have no idea how those out-of-towners heard about me, but they started coming in droves. Then the local paper ran a story about how I'd cured a real basket case. Who needed that! My phone started ringing off the hook.

"I've been in practice forty years, minding my manners and getting along with my colleagues, and now look what's happened. I'm a small town doctor and am not at all interested in being a lone wolf fighting the establishment."

Dr. Walmer is not as ornery as he pretends.

"Let's put it this way. I'm not out selling chelation," he says. "If you come and demand it, OK. Otherwise, forget it. I wouldn't mess with it at all, if I hadn't seen the results and know it works."

PUT THE BLAME ON MAMA

What red-blooded American mother doesn't hope her son will grow up to be president - or, next best, a doctor?

A doctor "Yes'; a 'quack', "No."

"It's my mother's fault I got into this 'quack' medicine," says Dr. Robert S. Waters of Glen Ellyn, Illinois.

"All through med school and internship, my health got worse and worse - while my mother was getting stronger and healthier. She kept nagging me to pay closer attention to my diet, to take vitamins, and all that stuff - and I thought, 'What does she know? She's only a high school graduate and I'm a doctor."

Mom kept nagging, and Waters gave in. He began to read up on nutrition and nutritional supplements, and other frowned-on self-helps.

"Then came the day one of my mother's close friends came to me after suffering a minor stroke, that resulted in temporary loss of his facial muscles and the use of one arm. I knew it was just a matter of time before he had another stroke, and ended up totally paralyzed. A neurosurgeon had examined him and determined he was not strong enough to undergo bypass surgery. The arteries in his legs were so badly blocked, he could only walk a block at a time. On top of all that, he had emphysema and arthritis.

"While I was trying to decide what to do, a patient who'd read about chelation brought me a book on the subject and asked for my advice. I stayed up all night reading and told myself, 'Either this is quackery or something important'. I talked to my mom, and she said, 'Give it a try'. I talked to our friend, and he agreed to be my guinea pig.

"I found a doctor who did chelation and kept tabs on the man's progress. After 27 treatments he was walking two miles at a clip, leg pains gone, no more angina. A Doppler test on his carotid artery revealed it was open and clear. The pulse in his feet was normal. It was amazing. When I reported the dramatic results to my mother, she told me to start calling all my near-dead patients who'd been given up by their cardiologists and get with it - start chelating them. That's what I did - and I've been doing it ever since. Thanks, mom."

FROM DROP-OUT TO NOBEL PRIZE NOMINEE

Charles Farr, M.D. made headlines as the first doctor in Oklahoma City to perform open heart surgery, but his fame and fortune soured when he realized the bypass was more sizzle than science.

As Dr. Farr put it, "It was exciting for a short time, until I noted post-bypass patient outcomes weren't living up to advance notices.

"I was one of the medical society's better paid performers," he laughs, "but wasn't the least bit unhappy to drop out of surgery to plow into a more humane and sensible approach to heart disease."

Dr. Farr's rise in his newly adopted field of natural medicine has been meteoric. A few years after leaving the surgical arena he became Founding Chairman of the American Board of Chelation Therapy. ABCT sets the protocol for administering EDTA and oversees the training and certification of new chelation doctors.

An avid researcher, Dr. Farr has gained international recognition for his research in free-radical biochemistry and bio-oxidative medicine - and in 1993, his name was submitted for nomination as candidate for the Nobel prize in Medicine.

"It's worked out well," Dr. Farr chuckles, remembering that one of his early victories involved an aging bypass candidate whose family was aghast that their ailing dad was rejecting surgery in favor of chelation therapy.

"The man's wife, two daughters and a slew of relatives, certain chelation was a fraud and I was a 'quack', were determined to 'rescue' him. They were tough, but he and I stood firm. I chelated him and he got well."

Why does this case stand out after so many years?

"That's easy," he smiles. "Once Skoshi, his daughter, witnessed her dad's complete recovery, she couldn't say 'No' when I asked her to marry me."

A PSYCHIATRIST GIVES UP THE COUCH

Many doctors we questioned switched to chelation out of frustration with accepted, but ineffective therapies. That's the case with Dr. Serafina Corsello of New York City.

A board certified psychiatrist, Dr. Corsello once had a psychoanalytically-oriented psychiatric practice - "lots of couch-talk, but few good results. No matter how hard I tried, people were just not getting better. I didn't like the side effects of mood-changing drugs.

"People must be physically well before dysfunctional behavior patterns can be modified. I understood the impact of exercise, sleep, nutrition on health - you don't have to convince an Italian of the importance of food!"

Dr. Corsello's quest for effective treatments led her to orthomolecular therapies, biochemical modalities, nutrition-oriented programs, and finally, to chelation.

"Now, I do it all - whatever works! It's very rewarding to be part of a medical community where doctors are truly excited about what they're doing. And I like it that we don't have to send many sympathy cards to our colleagues' widows."

IS RUSSIA FREER THAN AMERICA?

Dr. Vladmir Rizov of Austin, Texas, first learned about chelation in his native Russia, where it's the recognized therapy for atherosclerotic disease.

"When I came to this country, I thought I'd have the freedom to practice whatever medicine suits the patient. I prescribed chelation where indicated, and it surprised me to find that medical doctors who came to me for treatment, didn't refer any of their patients.

"'What's going on?' I asked. 'How can doctors separate themselves? Do one thing for themselves, another for their patients?'

"Finally, one patient/doctor said, 'Don't you know the AMA doesn't approve of chelation and has a lot of influence in this country?' I told him: 'So does the Mafia. Who cares?'"

Dr. James Carter of New Orleans, Louisiana, describes the 'real' quacks as "the doctors who sneak in for chelation, or send their relatives to out-of-town chelationists so they won't be found out."

That's a common complaint. Thousands of doctors are secretly chelated, both in the U.S. and abroad. The conspiracy of silence includes some high-placed physicians, according to Dr. Garry Gordon of North Highlands, California, who threatens to start naming names.

"One government doctor, when told he needed a bypass, knew enough to realize the overall mortality rate was bad, and since he didn't want to add to the stats, came to me for chelation. I did it at his request but am really angry that he's refused to let anyone, not even his heart specialist, know what cured him."

Dr. Ronald M. Davis of Webster, Texas, first learned about chelation from a doctor on his hospital staff who confided he was chelating 'secretly' and getting fantastic results, but insisted on doing it on the Q.T.

"I spent six months with this fellow, to see how it worked, and then decided to use it in my practice. Then, somehow the hospital found out what we were doing. They told us to give it up or get out. My friend quit chelating. I didn't and was kicked off the staff. It wasn't even a tough call."

CHELATORS ANONYMOUS EXPOSED

We estimate that for every doctor who has 'gone public', there are two or more "closet chelators," who limit EDTA treatments to themselves, family members and close friends.

How do we know? Easy. We have a list of doctors who are regular purchasers of EDTA - the chelating drug - and less than one-third are on any list of physicians who accept chelation patients or referrals.

THE LAND OF THE BRAVE

Talk about putting your money where your mouth is, nobody outperforms Dr. David Steenblock of El Toro, California, who practices "naked" - sans medical malpractice insurance. In these litigatious times, when patients sue doctors at the drop of a suture, how has Dr. Steenblock found the courage to chelate without coverage?

"That's easy," he says. "Chelation works. What have I got to worry about?"

Dr. Albert Scarchilli, with offices in Farmington Hills, Michigan, is so confident of positive results, he permits patients to "put chelation treatments on the cuff." When insurance won't cover costs, and patients are strapped for dough. Dr. Scarchilli carries the account.

Risky?

"Not at all. I've never had a patient miss a monthly payment. How could they? Chelation is keeping them alive."

TARNISHED HALOS

So what's the bottom line? Are chelation doctors more ethical, noble, moral, self-sacrificing than their more orthodox colleagues?

No. Within their ranks are doctors with hidden agendas: money-hungry egoists seeking fame or power; self-promoters hoping to profit from pet theories; vitamin 'pushers'; proponents of questionable exotic products; 'bad' doctors running chelation mills; ambitious physicians who'd rather be interviewed by Johnny, Geraldo, Oprah, or by-line a best-seller than treat patients. There is the same political in-fighting within ACAM circles that makes one wince when AMA doctors harrass each other.

And if the God-complex is a failing common to many physicians, more than a few chelation doctors who share that fault come easily to mind. Not surprising. It's a heady experience to be blessed day after day by patients who swear, "You saved my life." Some physicians 'forget' it's the EDTA that deserves most of the credit.

Taken as a group, however, chelationists are unique in one important regard: they are more consistent than doctors in other specialties when it comes to practicing what they preach. Unlike the cardio-vascular surgeons who panic and scream "No bypass for me" when it's their turn at bat, chelationists routinely take the treatments they've given hundreds of thousands of patients.

CHELATORS GET CHELATED

Dr. James Julian of Hollywood, California chelated himself first - "next came members of my immediate family, then friends, and last of all, patients." He's typical.

"How many treatments have you had?" is the most popular question ACAM members ask each other when they meet semi-annually. It's an ongoing competition. I doubt there's a patient anywhere who has had as many EDTA infusions as last year's 'winning' doc, who claims to have chelated himself 437 times.

More impressive yet are the results of clinging to conviction. When 46 chelating physicians were compared with 36 who do not use chelation therapy in their practice, the chelating group was found to be generally healthier (despite being on the average older) and to suffer significantly fewer symptoms related to heart disease: fewer dizzy spells, morning head-aches, indigestion that could be angina, tachycardia and abnormal heart rhythm.

YES, VIRIGNIA - THERE *ARE* QUACKS

Most chelationists have learned to laugh off the term 'quack', which originated in Germany during the last century and described doctors who administered 'quak silber' (quick silver, or mercury). Patients so treated would often get violently ill and doctors who prescribed this treatment were called 'quacks'.

"Now doctors who want to chelate mercury - and other toxic metals - out of people's bodies, are called 'quacks'," Dr. Evers pointed out when interviewed in 1989. Dr. Evers , who has since died claimed: "I'm the oldest living doctor doing chelation in America - that means I must be the biggest 'quack' of all. It makes me proud."

Dr. Annette Stoesser of Roswell, New Mexico brags she's a "certified quack" - and she is. She's been inducted into the American Quack Association, shows off the framed membership certificate on her office walls and proudly explains what her brand of quack stands: "quality care with kindness."

Who then, are the 'real' quacks? You be the judge.

We have some candidates:

- Doctors who practice 'fad' medicine, promoting popular operations (bypass surgery, for one) that don't help patients but do produce hefty fees;
- Doctors who knowingly (or unknowingly) prescribe medications that worsen the conditions they're supposed to cure. A good example: anti-arrhythmia drugs, hailed as preventing heart attacks, which actually increase the mortality rate among heart patients by 7%;
- Doctors who underplay the hazards and overplay the benefits of profitable procedures. As illustrated: angiograms advertised as a simple diagnostic procedure, when in truth cardiac catheterization is dangerous and inconclusive, its main purpose an excuse to rush patients into the surgical suite;
- Doctors who pretend modern medicine's handmaidens, drugs and surgery, are the answer to improved health and well being. Fifteen years ago, about 40% of Americans polled reported not feeling well. Today, despite all the advances in diagnosis and treatment, that figure has climbed to 60%. More people feel sick more of the time than at any time in our history.
- Last but not least, the doctors who would rather you die of your disease than be cured by a 'quack'. Funny? Not really. There are indeed self-serving "quackbusters" determined to protect their cookie jar. If you find this difficult to swallow, read Dr. James Carter's well-documented expose, "Racketeering in Medicine".

STAND BY YOUR DOC!

Each time a chelating physician's medical license is threatened, "people power" saves the day. Ordinary citizens are chelation's unsung heroes. In Texas, Evia Hobbs, now in her eighties, has led a 12-year struggle to foil the state medical society's stated goal of "getting those chelation docs one at a time." In Virginia, 150 patients got up at dawn to squash the medical society's intent to 'regulate' chelation out of business. Alaska was the first state to guarantee citizens the right to the medical treatment of their choice, thanks to activists who sprang to Dr. Robert Rowen's defense when the medical society attempted to defrock him for practicing chelation.

Chelation was unavailable in Canada until Ted Dickson began organizing chelation clubs. Now, six years and hundreds of meetings, rallies, protests, circulars, newsletters, and petitions later, there are a dozen chelators in British Columbia, and more on the way in Alberta and the eastern provinces.

A two year effort in South Dakota resulted in the first state law protecting chelation therapists from trumped up attack. In North Carolina, Carolinians for Health Care Access (CHCA) won a monumental battle against a vicious AMA-inspired campaign to outlaw chelation and other alternatives.

According to CHCA director, Dudley Wilson: "...what we did was alert people ... (and) ... thousands got a hold of their legislators and educated them. When we started, most legislators had no idea what "alternative" medicine was. Now, we've got legislators seeking out alternatives for their own medical problems!"

What can you do to help?
- Spread the word about the benefits of chelation;
- Encourage your physician to investigate chelation;
- Organize a SUFYCD (Stand Up For Your Chelation Doc) group;
- Solicit legislators to suppport freedom of choice in medicine.
- Urge your Senators and Congressmen to increase funding of NIH's newly organized Office of Alternative Medicine.

*It is our duty, my young friends, to resist old age; to compensate
for its defects by a watchful care; to fight against it as we would fight
against disease; to adopt a regimen of health;
to practice moderate exercise;
and to take just enough food and drink to restore our strength
and not to overburden it.*

Cicero, On Old Age (106-43 B.C.)

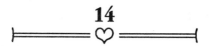

14

THE POST-CHELATION LIFESTYLE

The time has come, as the Walrus might have said, to speak
of many things… of smog-filled skies and fat-filled foods… and
a bunch of other nasty challenges Alice never had to deal with
on her trip through Wonderland.

How best to fend off internal and external pollution? What
can you do to retain the health benefits of a completed course
of EDTA infusions? What comes next?

On the upside: Chances are you breathe easier, walk
further, have more energy, look younger and feel sexier than
you have in years. On the downside: You're not home free.
You can't rely on any one treatment to do it all. Not even EDTA
comes with an American Express-style money-back guarantee
that will keep you from getting 'broke' again.

The truth is, being chelated is the easy part. Now comes the
real challenge - making the switch from the doctor's 'patient'
to 'partner'. To remain detoxified, prevent new plaque accu-

mulations from clogging your arteries, maintain an efficient immune system, and protect your cells from further free radical damage, will take some doing on your part. You must do more than show up periodically for some 'booster' shots.

BE HAPPY YOU'VE BEEN GIVEN A WAKE UP CALL

We doubt that you welcomed whatever health problems propelled you to action. You probably moaned "Who needs this?" when you got the bad news some serious ailment was about to disrupt your life. Consider yourself lucky. The wheel of misfortune dealt you a timely warning to get on the fitness bandwagon - quick!

Not too many years ago, any diagnosis of serious degenerative disease was equivalent to a death sentence. At best, it condemned the sufferer to a never-ending round of doctors and drugs. Similarly, people who'd reached a 'certain' age assumed it was 'all downhill' from then on. Once past fifty, they expected progressive decline and few felt there was much they could do to slow the ravages of time.

LIVING TO A HEALTHY 100 IS WITHIN REACH

In case you've not noticed, your chances of becoming an OAP (old age person) are rising dramatically. America is in the midst of a boom of centenarians, with over 10,000 new members joining the 100+ club in just the last five years. Now that you know you might live that long, doesn't it make sense to take better care of yourself?

Census Bureau demographers expect the trend to continue and accelerate. They predict four times as many hundred-year olds by the year 2000 and that by 2050, over a million Americans will celebrate more than 100 birthdays. Such optimistic forecasts are based on the recognition that the human body has an inherent ability to endure and function reasonably well for a century or longer. How close you come to realizing that potential, given your genetic inheritance, is up to you.

Equally encouraging, longevity is 'in'. Today's oldsters are living longer and loving it. And it's not only for celebrities like George Burns, Bob Hope and the ageless Zsa Zsa that the clock and calendar seem to have come to an accomodating halt. Ordinary citizens, Beatrice L. Cole for one, who appeared on national TV in 1981 to extoll the "joys of being eighty," fit the pattern. Now ninety, Beatrice states "I can truthfully say that the last ten years have been the most satisfying to date." Meeting Beatrice dispells the notion that living past eighty means vegetating in a nursing home.

What's life like for today's active ninety-year olds? For Beatrice, the day starts at 8 o'clock when, no matter the weather, she walks her dog. It ends some fourteen hours later with a game of Scrabble or bridge. In the hours between, she shops, cleans house, entertains, does volunteer work, attends concerts, reads, watches TV and does crossword puzzles. Weekends, she visits her daughter and son-in-law at the country house they all share. Not a bad agenda at any age.

Is Beatrice, vigorously romping through her ninth decade unique? Not any longer. Just the other day, the *Donahue Show* featured a bevy of professional strip-teasers, all of them grandmothers, all of them still working at their craft! The 'baby' of the lot was past fifty-five; the oldest had been eligible for Social Security for some fifteen years!

What's going on here? No doubt there are many explanations, but the one given the most credence is that as people learn to take better care of themselves, they see results. The odds of your living longer and healthier improve when you have accurate information and act upon it. The more you know, the better your opportunity to make health-promoting lifestyle choices.

The opening stages of the longevity revolution began in the late seventies when the concept of preventive medicine first took hold. When people began to accept the idea they could no longer entrust their long-term health status to doctors, public awareness sparked fundamental change.

As new scientific knowledge evolves, it spurs further upheaval in attitudes toward medical care and promotes the 'health yourself' movement. The willingness to assume personal responsibility for how you look and feel is buttressed by the considerable publicity given the payoffs.

For example, there are the stories telling what happened to the fifty heart patients recruited by internist Dean Ornish of the University of California at San Francisco. Half the group entered a special self-help health improvement training program in which they practiced yoga, meditation, and visualization techniques, had psychological counseling, did moderate aerobic exercise, and went on a low-fat vegetarian diet. The other twenty-five - the controls - relied on conventional medical treatments.

After a year, health professionals examined both groups using such high-tech tools as PET scans and quantitative coronary angiograms, and 80% of the self-help group showed significant improvement, while most of the medically-treated got worse.

FIT OR FAT? IT'S UP TO YOU

Every survey of American health habits reveals startling contradictions between what people *know* and what people *do*. For example: 45 million avid exercisers sweat it out at the gym, then 'pig out' at the table. Another 68 million, are conscientious dieters but are equally perverse. They know the calorie and cholesterol count of everything they eat, but when it comes to exercise, let their fingers do the walking.

Prolonging good health and sustaining an active life style is within reach, but primarily YOUR responsiblity. If you want to spring out of bed each day raring to go, follow an active and energetic schedule, and continue to function in an able-bodied manner well into your eighties and beyond, you can. It's up to you.

EDTA: A JUMP START TO GOOD HEALTH

Most chelating physicians are completely up-front with their patients. Few pretend that EDTA infusions are the total answer to complete and lasting recovery. Fewer still neglect to offer sound advice on the lifestyle changes they consider most vital. Like non-professionals, however, they all have their pet theories.

Some of the doctors are exercise buffs, and sincerly believe some form of regular workout - calisthenics, aeorobics, jazzercise, rebounding, swimming, the essential component in any back-to-health program.

Others prefer dietary control, and recommend some adaptation of the low-fat regimen first proposed by a non-doctor, Nathan Pritikin (an engineer). It was Pritikin, by the way, who produced the first clinical evidence that a drugless, non-surgical appoach could reverse atherosclerosis, and he did it in the face of virulent AMA and AHA objections. Both organizations, of course, have since "borrowed" his ideas, and now gratuitously present a similar dietary program, pretending it's their own.

Still other doctors are convinced that boosting immune fuction by whatever means - vitamins, antioxidants, mineral supplementation - is the key: Not to leave out the doctors who stress 'stress' - and emphasize the importance of developing psychological defenses to the biological damage suffered by those whose lives are out of control.

The true holistic approach, of course, is the one recommended by those who understand no one methodology works best for everyone, especially since no serious health problem can be traced to a single cause. Most people need to patch together bits and pieces of this and that into an individualized plan that fits like a tailor-made suit.

How well you fare on any health-improvement program depends on three factors: **1:** whether you base your life-style changes on valid information; **2:** how responsive your body is to the chosen regimen; **3:** how well you follow through on your good intentions.

Taking these issues one at a time, beginning with the first factor, the chapters that follow are aimed at providing you with many things you need to know to design a personalized healthy-for-life routine.

The second factor has to do with heredity. As some wag put it long ago, "The best health insurance comes from choosing the right parents." You may have inherited bad genes. If so, you will probably have to work harder to overcome inborn weaknesses. Think of it this way: you can always fall back on drugs and surgery if more benign approaches fail.

The third factor is the 'toughie' - developing the determination to stick with it. It's tricky to resist all the advertised bad-for-you temptations designed to lure us astray.

When you lunch out do you order a double cheeseburger with everything, a side dish of fries, a chocolate shake and some lemon pie, while your conscience nags you to settle for a spinach salad and grapefruit juice?

One thing for sure - as you might suspect - most of us cheat. Even when we know for sure it's bad to smoke, drink, eat rich desserts, agonize over 'small things' and slump into an overstuffed chair to watch TV for hours on end, we do it - perhaps only occasionally, but usually much too often.

EVEN HEALTH NUTS 'SIN' OCCASIONALLY

Many years ago, we were friends with a North Carolina couple who most surely deserve recognition as pioneer 'health nuts'. They preached, on radio and TV shows, on college campuses, to friends and relatives and to all who would listen, about the dangers of processed foods, hormone-treated meats, chemical preservatives, nitrosamine-laden smoked delicacies, fat-laden pastries and breads, additives and artificial colors and decried the health-destroying potential of the typical teen 'hamburger, french fries and coke' diet long before others. And underscoring their warnings - they lived by their beliefs.

This pair of foresighted mavericks were growing sprouts, serving tasty nutrient-rich backwoods weeds in salads, concocting yogurt-based oil-free homemade dressings, purifying their water, and shopping for organically grown fruits and vegetables twenty years prior to the advent of the health food movement.

Visitors who smoked were barred from their home. Dinner guests learned to expect spartan fare - fresh baked whole wheat muffins, bowlfulls of unfamiliar greens, 'meatless' meat loaf, steamed, lightly seasoned fresh vegetables from the farmer's market, herb tea and whatever fresh fruit was in season.

Then came the night we happened upon this couple devouring a pizza and guzzling cokes at a local pizzeria. What a shock. We could have been tactful and pretended not to see them. No way. We sallied over to their table and demanded, "What are you two doing here?"

"Well, it's only human to cut loose and enjoy yourself once in a while," was the shame-faced excuse. Don't sneer. Do you do better? Does anyone?

It's easy to slip from a health program. Especially after being chelated, feeling better than you have in years, and thinking you've got your problem beat.

THE SHAPE-UP PIG-OUT SYNDROME

If you're like most people, you can stand to be 'good' just so long. After a few days - or weeks - of munching on rice cakes, drowning your sorrows with mineral water, sticking to a lean cuisine and bypassing the fix-your-own dessert bar, chances are you suddenly switch gears and dig into chocolate cake heaped with Haagen-Dazs ice cream, and try to forget what you've done with a stiff drink.

Psychologist Ray Browne, chairman of the popular culture department at Bowling Green State University, says this is a very familiar eating pattern. "Once a dieter strays from the straight and narrow, he goes nuts."

Dr. Barry Popkin, professor of Nutrition at UNC, calls this recurring syndrome the 'Yuppie Diet': exercise like crazy, cut back to 700 calories a day, then splurge on a whipped cream dessert and a bag of candy bars.

Why do we do it?

"People who have been virtuous feel they've earned the right to be self-indulgent," he says.

If you've asked yourself: "What does it matter if I cheat a little?", know this. Every holistic doctor agrees: It's absolutely vital for you to *PERMANENTLY* change your life style. But no doctor can do it for you. The best they can do is offer informed advice, but after that, you're on your own. To put it simply: everyone is responsible for fastening their own seat belt.

WILL POWER ALONE WON'T DO IT

If you've ever tried to diet, quit smoking, cut down on sweets, stop nail biting, or rid yourself of any annoying habit, you already know that subconscious yearnings can undermine your determination to do what's good for you. The conflict between reason and desire can sandbag your best efforts to withstand temptation.

Why don't we all take better care of ourselves? For starters, even when we know enough to realize which pastries, cream sauces, luscious grilled steaks and other wonderful-tasting foods are deadly, we optimistically hope that indulging - just once in a while - won't do us in. Dieting vacationers, for example, pretend calories don't 'count' while they're on holiday; party-goers play the same game - "I've held myself in check all week - I can afford to enjoy the weekend."

And to varying degrees, we're all 'deniers'. Ironically, the more fearful we are of the consequences of our actions, the more apt we are to pretend that 'the rules' don't apply - that we are 'above it all'. To deny our morality, we defy the gods, take irrational chances and succumb to health-endangering indulgences.

Even people who've had a close brush with death often exhibit paradoxical bravado. Lung cancer patients frequently continue smoking; so do emphysema sufferers. There's a published case of a seventy-four year old gentleman who developed cancer of the throat, was successfully operated on and survived, and went right back to smoking! His cancer reappeared. A second operation again restored his speech and swallowing ability.

After two close calls, you'd think he'd give up smoking. Wrong. When doctors asked him why he still smoked and drank, he responded: "What difference can it make at my age?"

Such a response is not unusual. People at great risk are wont to say, "We're all going to die sometime, why worry about it?"

Supporting that sentiment: we all know people who've lived happily into their eighties despite breaking all the rules. There's 'Uncle Charlie' dining on steak and french fries seven times a week, and healthy as a horse. There's George Burns, still puffing ten cigars a day at age 96. We forget that some people can get away with all sorts of bodily abuse because they've been genetically blessed with a phenomenal immune system. Unfortunately, few of us are that lucky. Even those with long-lived ancestors have no assurance they'll survive in like fashion because of the damaging effect of a multitude of modern-day assaults which can defeat the sturdiest genes.

Psychologists agree: we all harbor a natural reluctance to accept unpalatable truths. People rarely believe ominous statistics apply to them. Disguised optimism - "It can happen to *HIM* but it can't happen to me" - and an irrational retreat from reality underlies much self-destructive behavior.

TAKING THE PAIN OUT OF DOING WHAT'S BEST FOR YOU

Are you really serious about maintaining the health benefits you've enjoyed? Are you intent on switching gears to healthier habits? Are you ready to sign up for long term changes? What can you do to get going and keep going?

- **Want it.** Once you're certain there are real benefits to a changed lifestyle, you must decide if better health, improved quality of life and longevity are really important to you. Unless you are convinced that in some way your life depends on your behavior, you're apt to drop out of your self-improvement program before it's done you much good. Desire is the fuel that sustains effort.

- **Believe it.** Do you trust health advice? Do you think it works as well as advertised? Or do you secretly believe you're too old or too far gone for lifestyle changes to make a difference for you. Lose faith and you'll waver. To reinforce conviction, buddy-up with other health-conscious people. Develop a strong social network of folks dedicated to growing younger and healthier.

- **Expect it.** See yourself as a more energetic, creative, active, lively, healthier individual. Be positive. Tell yourself good things: "I'm full of energy"; "I enjoy doing what's good for me"; "I'm not geting older, I'm getting better." Upbeat self-talk is an effective motivator. Tell yourself good things and it will help them happen.

One more secret of success: have a longevity goal - or several. The more reasons you develop to keep living, the better. What are you looking forward to next year, the year after, ten, twenty, fifty years down the line? Grandchildren? Great-grandchildren? A second career? Around-the-world travel? A Florida retirement home? Becoming a Life Master at bridge? Do what we've done: buy a parrot and try to outlive it.

Whatever your incentives, focus forward. Live *FOR* the future, not *IN* the past.

> *By Chance our long-liv'd Fathers earn'd their Food;*
> *Toil strung the Nerves, and purified the Blood:*
> *But we, their Sons, a pamper'd Race of Men,*
> *Are dwindl'd down to threescore Years and ten.*
> *Better to hunt in the Fields, for Health unbought,*
> *Than fee the Doctor for a nauseous Draught.*
> *The Wise, for Cure, on Exercise depend;*
> *God never made his Work, for Man to mend.*

John Dryden (1631-1700) Fables Ancient and Modern

15
══ ♡ ══

EXERCISING YOUR RIGHT TO GOOD HEALTH

"The toughest thing about exercise," said George Allen, former Washington Redskins football coach, "is getting started. Even for a fitness nut like me, getting up in the morning when it's chilly and dark is tough. I consider a day without exercise a day that's been wasted, but I still have to force myself to do it."

If Mr. Allen who was chairman of the National Fitness Foundation found exercise tough going, what about the rest of us? Many studies show that nearly fifty percent of 'new' exercisers drop out before they're six months into an exercise program. More than half of them don't sweat it out more than three weeks. Fully twenty-five percent who enroll in a program, fail to show up for the first session.

If you've bought a rowing machine, stationary bicycle, treadmill, trampoline or similar gadget that's turned into a dust-collector, you're not alone. Most home-style exercise equipment for sale in the classified ads at flea markets, garage sales and on radio swap shows, is indeed 'practically new' as advertised.

UNFASHIONABLY UNFIT - AND LIKING IT

Just as you might suspect, the fitness boom is a mirage. Despite all the health club ballyhoo, and Cher's urging to join her in the body-building craze, most Americans still exercise their minds more than their bodies. One survey showed that 87% of all running shoe buyers *never* - you guessed it - *run!* Thinking about exercise is obviously a lot easier than doing it. That's especially true if you're financially comfortable. Statistics confirm the more money you make, the less physically active you are. Upward mobility expands the waistline as well as the bank balance, it seems.

TV star Susan St. James, now well into her forty-somethings, confesses she's resorted to hiring a seventy-five dollar an hour personal trainer to come to her home daily. "If the doorbell doesn't ring, I hardly move," she tells.

In this respect, she's kin to the not-so-famous - especially those middle-aged and older who consider it real exertion when they get up out of their easy chairs to switch TV channels instead of using their remote tuners.

PRIME TIME PUDGIES

Warning: Television may be harmful to your health. It's not what you watch, but how much that distinguishes fat from thin and fit from flabby, research now shows.

Americans devote more time to watching television than they do on any activity beyond working or sleeping, surveys find, and as the time spent sitting in front of the TV screen increases, - now about four hours a day - fitness fades away.

In a study of more than 6,000 men conducted at Alabama's Auburn University, TV watching proved to be the determining difference in their level of obesity. Those who watched television more than three hours a day were twice as likely to be obese as men who watched only one hour a day.

The connection between television and tubbiness is confirmed by newer studies. The Harvard School of Public Health in cooperation with Tufts found the more kids watch TV, the more likely they were to be obese. The *American Journal of Public Health* reported similar findings early in 1991 when a study of 5,000 working women, (average age of 35) revealed obesity doubles as TV-viewership escalates from one hour daily to three or four.

The outlook is the same for teens, the *Tufts Diet and Nutrition Letter* warns. In a study of nearly 400 teen-age boys, researchers found that those who watched four hours of TV daily were significantly less fit and could do far fewer push-ups, pull-ups and sit-ups than their counterparts who spent half as much time in front of the tube.

The next question of course, is why? Tufts suggests two theories:

- People already overweight may be more sluggish or self-conscious about their bodies and therefore choose to avoid physical exertion in the first place;
- Watching TV may actually contribute to weight problems because (a) the stillness required can limit the number of calories burned, and (b) the number of calories consumed while watching is high. Research has shown that people consume more calorie-laden foods during their favorite programs, Tufts says.

So if the most exercise you've gotten lately is jumping at the chance to avoid any activity that might cause you to perspire, you're part of the sluggish majority. About 80 percent of the American population has the same problem.

SO, CAN WE ALL SIT DOWN NOW AND TAKE IT EASY?

Not so fast.

According to health experts, once people begin to exercise regularly, they tend to take better care of themselves in other ways as well - including improving their diet. The typical 40 year old man who doesn't exercise, also doesn't wear a seat belt, smokes two packs a day, and is 30% overweight. As noted experts in sports medicine have observed, 'exercisers' become more health-conscious and are more likely to make health-promoting changes in all aspects of their lives.

Ironically, it doesn't always work the other way around. People who DO take rather good care of themselves in other ways, often neglect exercise. Many fitness buffs who don't smoke, drink, eat a sensible diet and stick to their vitamin regimens, fail to appreciate the importance of exercise.

One of America's best known nutritionists, Carlton Fredericks, whose books, syndicated newspaper columns, radio and television programs brought health education to millions, was fond of quoting a 1930's era wit who said: "The secret of my abundant health is that whenever the impulse to exercise comes over me, I lie down until it passes away."

After which Fredericks would add: "I get all the exercise I need acting as pallbearers for my friends who exercise."

Funny - but hardly supported by the facts that provide powerful ammunition for the pro-exercise camp. Prominent among the exercise drop-outs are those who believe - or hope - they've stored up enough exercise 'credits' in their youth to last them a lifetime. High school and college 'jocks' are the prime culprits. They gaze fondly at mementos of their school day exploits and figure they've done enough running, stretching and jumping to insure a healthful future.

They're kidding themselves. Unless you keep on exercising, you're no better off than the guy who sat on the sidelines and cheered. Studies show that middle-aged men who were once very active in sports, have no fewer heart attacks than their sedentary counterparts - UNLESS they continued keeping in shape.

The older you are, the more benefit from exercise. It doesn't matter how fit you once were. After you stop exercising you lose almost all measurable benefits. If you want to live longer, it's more important to exercise when you're old than when you're young.

We'll wager this is not the first time you've read that health authorities make a big deal of exercise. Sports medicine expert Dr. Gabe Mirkin reports, "The research data shows that the more fit you are, the less likely you are to suffer a heart attack. High intensity exercise prevents heart attacks.

"A study published in the *New England Journal of Medicine* showed that a high level of physical fitness is associated with a markedly reduced susceptibility to developing heart attacks."

How come? Exercisers have high HDL levels - and the more HDL (the 'good' cholesterol) you have in your blood stream, the less likely you'll have a heart attack. At least, that's the current opinion.

Dr. Paul Thompson of Brown University has looked into this phenomena and feels that HDL may not prevent heart attacks directly, but may be a marker signifying a person's increased ability to clear fat from the bloodstream.

As Dr. Thompson explains: "Lipoproteins are large balls that float in your bloodstream, that contain cholesterol, a fat called triglyceride and are covered with a protein coat.

"When you exercise, LDL lipoproteins bring triglycerides to muscle cells to supply them with fuel. Simultaneously, they release cholesterol to HDL lipoproteins and increase blood levels of HDL."

Dr. Thompson's message is clear: "You can raise HDL levels by exercising."

The latest research on cardiovascular disease suggests that raising HDL levels is far more protective than lowering overall serum cholesterol levels.

If the prospect of keeping your heart healthy is not sufficiently motivating, how about this? A Harvard University study shows that a regular exercise program can keep you young sexually. Other studies show that people who compete in sports in later life exhibit fewer signs of aging, such as high blood pressure, rapid heart rates and weak muscles.

Two more good reasons to exercise: it stabilizes blood sugar levels - (important for diabetics) - and can normalize eye pressure - (a possible preventive for glaucoma).

Harvard University researchers believe there is a link between exercising and a lowered risk of specific cancers: breast, colon and cancers of the reproductive system.

For women, exercise can be crucial in preventing osteoporosis - a common health threat that results in progressive bone loss that in time can cause fractures and hip problems. It also can alleviate this ailment once it occurs, since bone, like muscle responds favorably to stress.

Most know what exercise can do for your heart and body. You may even have discovered it can boost your spirits and self-esteem, but you may not be aware it can be a genuine therapy for common emotional problems. Psychologist Keith Johnsgard, a professor of psychology at San Jose State University in California, prescribes exercise for the emotionally disturbed.

According to the newest psychological theory, moving the body mends the mind. Hostility is reduced by exercise; so is depression, anxiety, and guilt. The evidence is accumulating - exercise does all this and more. It relieves mental stress, beefs up the immune system, is a brain energizer, and adds years to your life.

What good is all this pro-exercise info, if you can't bring yourself to get with it?

"NO PAIN, NO GAIN"? - WHAT BUNK!

It's really much easier than you suspect to become a lifelong exerciser. First, you must find an activity you like; second, you must start slowly and gradually integrate it into your daily life; third, you must keep yourself motivated.

Let's start at the beginning. Since people normally do things they enjoy, it's a mistake to work out simply because you 'should' or with a sense of martyrdom. Subjecting yourself to discomfort or displeasure is self-defeating. Before very long, you'll find excuses to legitimatize quitting - 'I don't have enough time', 'It costs too much', 'I'm bored' - are the more common excuses.

It doesn't take a huge investment of time or money to reap the benefits of exercise. When it comes to exercising, especially for those in the older age brackets who have allowed themselves to get all out of shape, less is best. Even very minimal exercise can be of tremendous medical benefit.

You might not think a weekend of gardening, playing with the grandkids, or doing home repairs would amount to much of a work-out, but this may be all you need to live many more years.

That's what a major study of Harvard alumni showed. It linked a 20 percent reduction in the death rate with very mild work-outs. Tack on a few more recreational activities such as sailing, badminton and biking, and death rates nose-dived by another 10 to 20 percent.

Here's something easy for starters: give up your *Lazy-Boy* recliner and substitute a rocking chair. That's how chelation patients at the Farmington Medical Center in Michigan are introduced to exercise. Dr. A. J. Scarchilli tells us, "I get people moving, even while they're in treatment. I've furnished my facility with rocking chairs. At least once during each EDTA infusion session, we encourage each patient to take a turn on a stationary bicycle. Though it is somewhat inconvenient, we keep patients up and walking, even while connected to the IV apparatus. Circulation is restored more quickly when people are active and move around."

Dr. Scarchilli gives every patient an 'exercise prescription' that includes the following recommendations:

- Exercise must be daily and of constant duration.
- Exercise at an invigorating, but not exhausting pace - one you can maintain without strain.
- Exercise at least 20 minutes a day. Ease into the exercise, then maintain a constant heartbeat for a minimum of 15 minutes.
- Recommended forms of exercise, all of roughly equal value, are swimming, stationary cycling, rebounding (on a home-size trampoline) and walking.

WALKING IS A WINNER

What's your idea of the perfect exercise? How about an activity that's free, doesn't require lessons, advance planning, special equipment, training or skill, can be done anywhere, in all climes at every time of the year, is suitable for all ages, that you can start right now. It's walking, called "man's best exercise" by Hippocrates, that makes for a "long life" according to an ancient Hindu proverb.

"I have two doctors - my left leg and my right ," said an ancient philosopher.

Contrary to what you may think, walking is not too "lightweight" an activity to produce fitness results. The research shows that a regular walking program (at least 30 minutes a day, five days a week) can produce dramatic pay-offs: brain stimulation, mood elevation, pumped up lung power, lowered resting pulse rate, reduced blood pressure, decreased levels of artery-clogging blood fats, stepped up bodily metabolism, slimmed down legs, hips and bodies.

Good enough? There's more. For every hour you walk,

promises a Harvard expert, you add that hour - and one or two more to your life span. Still not convinced?

"Walking is a case of benefit without risk," says so eminent an authority as Dr. Barry Franklin, Director of the Cardiac Rehabilitation and Exercise Laboratories at William Beaumont Hospital. He's convinced that walking may be the "best method for the average person to become fit."

A physician's belief in the life-saving benefits of walking might have changed the course of history. According to published reports, Harry S. Truman's personal doctor, Dr. George S. Carter, pulled no punches when the then-Senator Truman, distressed at seeing so many of his Congressional colleagues dying prematurely, asked him, "Will I be next?"

A plain-spoken man, Dr. Carter responded: "I don't know how you've lived this long, abusing your body with inactivity and smoke-filled rooms. You're in worse shape right now than some men whose funerals you've attended. Walk or die."

We all know how Truman benefited from this straight talk. He lived to take his place in history as our thirty-third president, and his early morning walks, with reporters half his age struggling to keep pace, became his legendary trademark.

Mr. Truman proved that no one can claim to be too busy or too burdened with work or personal responsibilities to establish a daily routine of walking as though your life depended on it. Probably it does. Get up an hour earlier, if necessary. Walk part way to work, traveling a bit more distance on foot each day. Park further and further away from your destination when you drive. When you travel by bus, train or cab, get off a stop or two sooner than necessary.

To derive the utmost in health benefits, however, slow walking won't do it. 'Power' walking, 'fitness' walking, 'health' walking, 'aerobic' walking, 'race' walking - whatever you call it, the key is to walk vigorously enough to huff and puff.

To build up walking speed, take longer strides and quicken your pace. Here's what Dr. Mirkin recommends:

"Every time you move your left leg forward, swing your left arm backward. Bend your arms at the elbow as you coordinate arm swings with leg movements. The faster you move your arms, the faster your legs will move.

"To take the longest strides possible, waddle from side to side. Swivel your hips one hundred eighty degrees as you stride forward, swinging your arms and bending your elbows as much as you can.

"Don't overdo it. When your legs feel tired, or heavy, slow your pace until they recover and then gradually pick up the pace again. No need to do this every day. Three thirty minute fast-walking sessions a week will keep you fit."

If 'walking' sounds dull, there are lots of new twists to this old standby. Here are some novel ways to spice up this plain vanilla activity, and turn it into an enjoyable 'fun' experience:

- **TRY BIRD-TREKKING.**

Add purpose to your walk. Buy an inexpensive bird-watcher's guide, and keep on the lookout, giving yourself points for every bird you can name, extra points for exotic varieties or rare species. See if you can spot hawks, owls, and household-pet escapees such as canaries, parakeets and parrots. Keep a daily tally and try to beat yesterday's score.

- **BECOME A 'WALKING ENCYCLOPEDIA'.**

There's an unlimited number and variety of educational books on tape for mind improving-walking. Everything from foreign languages to skill training is yours for the listening. So is self-help for whatever ails you. Inexpensive - ($20.00 for the cheapest) - portable 'Walkman-type' tape players are available. Check out your local library. Most branches offer a good assortment. You could amuse yourself by listening to the latest fictional best-seller' - or turn your walk into a real learning experience. You could indulge your love of music, poetry readings, 'pop' psychology or get your fill of self-help advice,

• TRY 'MALL-WALKING'.

An estimated half million early risers arrive at the nation's shopping centers each morning, long before the stores open for business. Dressed in sweat suits and jogging shoes, throngs of 'mall-walkers' stride past the shuttered storefronts, whipping their way around kiosks and potted palms, working out in the weather-insulated, security patrolled safety of the Great American Shopping Center.

These indoor arcades - mild in winter, cool in summer, free of bugs, bikes, beggars or muggers - have become so popular, many astute shopping center managers are making their premises even more inviting, by laying out a prescribed measured course for their walkers. The Garden State Plaza in Paramus, New Jersey, one of the largest malls in the country, sponsors a "Club Tread" and offers the 300-plus members a prize for every fifty miles logged.

'Mall-walking' earns high praise from one New Jersey lady who reports: "It's good for me physically - I've made a major comeback from open heart surgery; it's good for me spiritually - my mall-walking group includes my best friends; it's good for my pocket-book, too - I get first look at what's going on sale."

• BUDDY-UP FOR YOUR WALKS.

Sign on a walking companion and you'll feel free to stroll around unfamiliar neighborhoods without fear. Teaming up with another walker has many social and psychological benefits. Married people will be encouraged to learn that couples who walk together, stay together. They have better marriages, says Ira Glick, Professor of Psychiatry at Cornell University Medical School, who has found walking is not only good exercise, it affords a relaxed forum for communication, providing time to share thoughts and feelings.

• WORK UP TO 'WOGGING'.

As the name suggests, 'wogging' is the happy compromise between walking (not strenuous enough for some) and jogging (too much bone-jarring exertion for many). Dr. Thomas W. Patrick, Jr., of Fort Lee, New Jersey, who coined the term, defines 'wogging' as "walking fast for pleasure, exercise and fitness at different rates from brisk to rapid."

Dr. Patrick recommends that beginning 'woggers' start easy, about a block or two at first, working up gradually to about twenty minutes a day. Check with your physician to get his advice on what's safe for you.

- **THE ULTIMATE: RACE-WALKING.**

For those who are able, race-walking provides all the aerobic benefits of running without the injury-inducing jarring. Competition is keen at regularly scheduled meets; there is a chance for good fellowship with the exercise. One dedicated race-walker is Georgetown University Professor of Medicine and Director of Preventive Cardiology Program, Dr. Samuel Fox, III. He believes race-walking will give your heart the best workout with the greatest margin of safety, lower your blood pressure and triglyceride level, reduce stress, and help develop your mind and body.

THE SAFE WAY TO GET FIT

If you hanker to be a Jane Fonda look-alike, but resemble Roseanne Barr instead, don't even consider trying to make yourself over with an all-out effort. With most beginners, less is more. Informal, nonstructured exercise may be all you need to keep your muscles loose, your joints flexible and improve cardiovascular function. If you have any serious disease, or have been habitually sedentary for years, you must NOT go at it vigorously.

Equally inappropriate at any age, in any condition, is to become a 'weekend jock' - deskbound five days a week, then packing in tennis, handball and volleyball on Saturdays and Sundays. Irregular bursts of vigorous activity not only won't do you much good - they can be very dangerous.

MARRIED TO YOUR EASY CHAIR? GET A DIVORCE!

Just as important as establishing a seven-day-a-week exercise routine is avoiding inactivity. Try not to sit in one spot for longer than twenty minutes at a time - at home or in the office. Break up your TV-watching with a short walk around the room; get up from your desk periodically; attach an extension cord to your phone and pace while you talk.

Give up step-saving devices and strategies - take the stairs instead of the elevator, disconnect telephone extensions, throw away remote tuners, push a lawn mower, wash dishes by hand, park as far from the supermarket as you can. Better still - walk to the store, and carry your groceries home.

Find fun things to do to keep active: get a dog, baby-sit a toddler, make love. The importance of LTPA (leisure time physical activity) cannot be overrated.

A recent study of 3,000 white, male, middle-aged railroad workers, followed over a period of 17 to 20 years, showed that those who were sedentary in their leisure time (couch potatoes) had a 30% to 40% greater risk of dying from coronary heart disease and all other causes than those who expended just 1,000 to 2,000 calories a week in LTPA.

The biggest surprise was the men didn't have to be doing anything really strenuous to enjoy tremendous life-saving benefits. Moderate activities such as gardening, strolling, bowling, sailing, fishing, golf and ballroom dancing was action enough to keep them hale and hearty.

Of prime importance is to routinely include more physical activity in the everyday things you do, and you'll find many pleasurable ways to get more physical and improve your health.

Raring to get going? Good! Here's how to keep yourself motivated:

- **Make a commitment.**

Remind yourself that exercising regularly can be a life or death decision - once you believe that your life depends on sticking with it, chances are you will.

- **Have fun.**

Enjoying yourself is critical. Find ways to keep exercise as entertaining as possible - perhaps by rewarding yourself periodically with new walking shoes or sports gear - for going a whole month without missing a workout.

- **Fight boredom by adding variety.**

Walk with different friends; invite family members along; investigate new routes; join a hiking club; try a competition.

- **Visualize yourself a younger, slimmer, more energetic person.**

Seeing yourself brimming with vitality will beef up your expectations and fuel your resolve to stick with it. What it all adds up to is this: As the sense of work fades and a feeling of playful enjoyment begins, exercising regularly will become easier and easier.

*All samples of the fossil record suggest that some death-dealing
enemy, swift, merciless and irresistible, lurked in every corner of the
world. This enemy, we believe, was the medium in which the early
vertebrates were undergoing evolution; it was an enemy they could
not see but one that pursued them every minute of the day and night,
one from which there was no escape though they deployed from
Spitsbergen to Colorado - the physical-chemical danger inherent in
their new environment: their fresh-water home.*

Homer W. Smith (1895-1962)

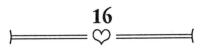

16

CLEANING UP YOUR ACT

WASHINGTON'S MOST POPULAR MONUMENTS IN LOSING BATTLE WITH TOXIC ENVIRONMENT
Washington Post, April 9, 1990

If the 68-year old Lincoln Memorial and the 47-year old
Jefferson Monument are crumbling because the capital's toxic
environment is mutilating the venerable cement and steel
structures, imagine what effect the area's foul air is having on
like-aged human bodies.

Is there something unusually noxious about Washington's
atmosphere? Except for the hot air discharged by resident
politicos, the region is relatively free of industrial pollution.
Think how much worse it must be in smoke-stack choked areas.

There is no question but intolerable levels of air-born
poisons are daily bombarding millions of Americans. One
documented result: environmental super-sensitivity, the so-

called "ecological illness" that Rachel Carson predicted in her book *Silent Spring* thirty years ago, has reached epidemic proportions. As our planet becomes increasingly polluted, individuals with weaker constitutions - those Dr. Alan Gaby has called the "human canaries" - fall ill, signaling grave danger ahead to the rest of us, just as the birds miners took with them into mines gave early warning of noxious gases or insufficient oxygen to sustain life. Infectious and allergic diseases, commonly associated with immunological breakdown, are now the fifth leading cause of death in the United States, accounting for thirty percent of visits to physicians' offices. A growing number of Americans react so badly to almost everything around them, they've had to abandon civilization to take up residence in the wilds.

The rest of us watch with horror as diseases unheard of - or exceedingly rare - a decade ago, escalate into modern plagues. Herpes, candida, chronic fatigue syndrome, lupus, and of course, AIDS, all appear to have one thing in common: they afflict the once hardy whose immune systems have crumbled under constant bombardment by environmental pollutants.

How essential to health is the air we breathe? None of the wants of the body are so constant and pressing. Fouled air is so destructive that confined to an air-sealed room, breathing nothing but our own exhaled air without any addition from without, we would die at the end of eight hours.

Think you're not at risk? **The U.S. Environmental Protection Agency (EPA) scientists report that the average American home is more of a toxic waste dump than a chemical plant.**

"The level of toxic fumes found in homes from paint to cleaning solvents is so high, indoor contaminants are three times more likely to cause cancer than outdoor airborne pollutants," states Harvard University's Dr. Lance Wallace, an EPA physicist and environmental specialist.

Before you say, "Not my home," check out this EPA list of common home-based free radical producers:

1: Carbon monoxide - from faulty furnaces, unvented gas stoves, exhaust fumes from attached garages;

2: Methylene chloride - from paint strippers and thinners;

3: Radon - from radioactive soil and rocks surrounding the home's foundation;

4: Formaldehyde - from furniture, fabric and pressed wood products;

5: Benzo-a-pyrene - from tobacco smoke and wood stoves;

6: Tetrachloroethylene - from fumes of dry-cleaned clothes;

7: Para-Dichlorobenzene - from air fresheners, moth crystals and mildew retardants;

8: 1,1,1,-Trichloroethane - from aerosol sprays. Old buildings are healthier to live in than new ones. Drafty corners let in fresh air. Army trainees housed in new energy-efficient (sealed up) barracks, had fifty percent more respiratory infections than those living in old style barracks.

TENNIS, ANYONE?

To illustrate how insidious these dangers have become, the chemicals in your 'tennies' may be courting trouble. Sport shoes made with certain kinds of sponge-rubber insoles can lead to itchy feet, says Purdue University pharmacology professor Jerry McLaughlin. The culprits are two chemicals, mercaptobenzothiazole (MBT) and dibenzothiazyl disulfide (DBTD).

"Many potential victims of tennis-shoe dermatitis could be spared distress if we can only persuade manufacturers to delete those harmful chemicals," McLaughlin says. Meanwhile, he proposes that toxic compounds should be listed on the shoe box.

Is there no safe place? Is every home a risk-ridden castle? What about on-the-job dangers? How secure are you at your office?

As you might have guessed, your nine-to-five world is also perilous. More than a dozen types of indoor pollutants have been found common in 'sick' office buildings. According to the World Health Organization, up to thirty percent of new and remodeled office buildings cause health problems.

For starters: carbon monoxide fumes seep in from underground parking garages; furniture, carpet, upholstery, insulation and other construction materials emit formaldehyde; filthy heating, ventilating and air-conditioning ducts often crust over with chemical pollutants and volatile organic compounds.

The unrelenting attack by toxic chemicals is cumulative. As the assault builds, it often buckles natural human defenses, laying the groundwork for free radical chain reactions. The result is health problems ranging from chronic fatigue to emotional distress, from allergies to asthma, from heart disease to cancer.

To make matters worse, environmental researchers report countless varieties of bacteria infect office building air ducts. To name but a few: stephyloccocus and streptococcus (common causes of skin, throat and eye infections), legionella (which can cause fatal pneumonia-like attack), aspergillus, cladoosporium, penicillium and phoma (implicated in hay fever and asthma).

COLOR THE AIR DIRTY

The air in the U.S. is getting dirtier and dirtier. The Environmental Protection Agency estimates 110 million Americans breathe air unfit for human lungs. Dismal as this report is, more alarming is the likelihood the stats are understated, since an estimated 200,000 'new' synthetic chemical agents (some 150 million tons) enter the environment each year. The toxicity of many newer compounds is completely unknown. All that is known is that our bodies can only tolerate just so much contamination before an overload triggers immunological dysfunction.

To lower the level of toxic fumes at home:

- Ventilate your house periodically. Open windows and doors and let fresh air circulate;
- Store leftover paints and paint thinners in an outdoor shed. If that's not possible, discard them;
- Have your wood stove, fire place, furnace inspected and cleaned annually;
- Vent stoves to the outside or use charcoal filters in units that throw fumes back into the kitchen. Install a window fan;
- Air dry-cleaned clothes outdoors for a day before wearing them or bringing them into the home;
- Replace aerosol spray cans with pump-activated products;
- Use disinfectants, chlorinated compounds, harsh cleaners, paints or thinners in well ventilated areas;
- Don't start or 'warm up' your car in an attached garage;
- Seal cracks in basement walls and floors;
- Install a fan in your basement to vent radon contamination outside;
- Decorate with spider plants. National Aeronautics and Space Administration scientists have found that the long tendrils on this species of house plant absorb formaldehyde and other toxic gases from the atmosphere.
- Invest in an air cleaner. Today's High Efficiency Particular Air filters (a huge advance over the old-style electronic air cleaners) is no luxury if you love your lungs enough to want to protect them against airborne assaults. A high quality HEPA can remove about 99.97 percent of the particles from the air, and works well against the many allergens: viruses, fungi, pollens, molds, yeast and bacteria, also dust and mites. It will keep your home environment as clean as you can get it for some two to

five years. A high quality air conditioner, equipped with an electronic filter, also will help clean the air and minimize allergies.

To protect yourself out of the home:

- When gassing up at a self-service station, set the nozzle latch on automatic and stand clear of the fumes;
- When possible, park in outdoor parking lots rather than underground facilities;
- Insist on the 'no-smoking' section when dining out;
- Travel on 'smoke free' airlines; reserve 'smokeless' hotel rooms.
- For on-the-road protection, install an air cleaner in your car.

THE HIDDEN HAZARD: LEAD

Conventional wisdom has it that lead in the home is primarily an inner city problem, with underprivileged children the main victims of lead-based paint flaking off walls.

That was until they found it in the White House when Millie, the First Family's dog, fell sick with lead poisoning. When Barbara, George and the dog all came down with some form of auto-immune disease, the White House physicians said the chances of that being a coincidence was less than one in 20 million.

"It's a terrible thing," President Bush said, noting the renowned English springer had gotten ill from licking flaking paint off her toes.

Less than one year later, a second shocker. High levels of lead were found in the Vice President's home. The testing was ordered after doctors remembered who the former residents of the century-old mansion were: the Bushes.

There's a world of difference between the ghetto and the White house, but not when the issue is lead contamination. Among the hidden hazards in the average home: lead in the water (from pipes), lead on the dinner plates (from ceramic glazed dishware), lead in the food (from cans), lead on the walls (from household dust and lead-based paints) - there's even lead in your wine (from the lead foil capsules that cover the bottle's rim and cork).

Discouraging? And how. There is no such thing as a 'safe' level of lead. Even very low levels, once thought to be harmless, are proving toxic. More discouraging still is the oft-repeated emphasis on lead being chiefly a growing child's health problem, blamed for all manner of problems from learning deficits to delinquency.

All probably true. But what about the post-puberty crowd? Why soft-pedal the news that as we grow older, lead does more, not less, harm. We've known about the poisonous effects of lead since the days of the Roman Empire. Since then, evidence is mounting that its effects are more subtle, wide-ranging and long-lasting than anyone suspected. Not only does lead decrease IQ by several points in the developing child, but in adults it affects reaction time, psychomotor performance, electrophysiological measures such as EEG patterns, potential and peripheral nerve conduction, all in a way that suggests a dose-response ratio. Heavy lead exposure is correlated with cardiovascular disease; modest exposure is linked to high blood pressure. What can you do about lead?

- Test your dishes for lead. A kit for this purpose is available from Frandon Enterprises Inc., 511 North 48th Street, Seattle, Washington 98103.
- Be wary of craft show pottery. Do not use lead-glazed ceramic products to store or serve food. Acidic foods like orange juice can release lead from the shiny glazes of ceramic products made in some foreign countries and those fired by amateurs.
- Have your water tested. If results are worrisome, replace the pipes or add filtration devices. Short of that, flush frequently when water has been sitting stagnant for

several hours; let the water run for about three minutes before using it for drinking or cooking.

- Don't use hot tap water to make coffee, tea or cocoa. Lead solder in pipes dissolves more readily in hot water.

WATER, WATER EVERYWHERE AND NOT A DROP SAFE TO DRINK

There's trouble at the water tap. Turning on the faucet may be dangerous to your health.

Who says so? All those health-conscious consumers so alarmed they spent $2 billion last year on bottled water.

Are people spending money foolishly? Not when you consider the evidence that your tap water is probably contaminated. Every day brings new and worrisome reports of high lead levels in drinking water. Equally troubling - municipal water is also treated with chlorine to kill bacteria. While many experts considered chlorine safe in small quantities several decades ago, recent research suggests it tends to combine with the organic matter often present in water to form dangerous chemicals known as trihalomethanes (THM's). The most familiar THM is chloroform. If it's breathed or ingested, it triggers free radical activity.

The outlook is gloomy. The very EPA officials charged with insuring the safety of the nation's drinking water are the first to admit that water pollution is among the top four environmental threats to health. As if this weren't bad enough, no one knows for sure what's really in the water or which of the thousands of the contaminants spewed into the environment each year are turning the nation's water supply carcinogenic.

The scariest scenario to date is this: your water faucet might be dispensing a radioactive cocktail. People living in areas fraught with radon face this added threat, for the gas not only permeates their homes, but also seeps into their drinking water. Preliminary studies of households in Maryland, Virginia and other affected areas (the New England and Western mountain states) reveal that as many as 17 million people may be exposed to excessive levels of radon gas. The noxious fumes are released not only via tap water, but during bathing and dishwashing.

How important is clean water? It's vital to the workings of every organ, muscle, tissue and cell in the body. Water helps flush poisons from the blood stream, bathes and cushions the brain and gives lungs the moisture they need to breathe. Without water, arms couldn't flex, eyes couldn't see, and the heart couldn't beat.

BYPASS THE PURE WATER HOAX

When it comes to the expensive bottled waters, be cautious. You can't assume you are getting the safety you're willing to pay for. The filthiest water can look and taste pure (and cost like the devil) but it can easily be contaminated by bacteria, warns health expert Dr. Gabe Mirkin. One airline used purified water on its planes until they found many pilots and passengers getting sick and discontinued the disappointing advertised 'luxury'.

What don't the bottled water ads tell you? Everything you need to know. Commercial bottlers don't have to date their products, or list an expiration date, so you have no way of knowing how long the product has been sitting on the shelf, or how many bacteria may have grown in the bottles. The products can contain coliform bacteria, gasoline residues, high nitrate levels, algae, plastic residues, high arsenic levels, mold, insect larve, cesspool contaminants, protozoa . . .etc. Several studies have found bottled brands no less polluted than what flows from the tap for free.

The scandal that brought the facts to light was the Perrier recall, said to have cost the French bottled water company some $40 million (an indication of the popularity of 'upscale' water products in the U.S.) when tests by the FDA showed shipments contained high levels of benzene, a cancer-causing chemical. At first, company officials trying to downplay the incident, claimed a careless maintenance worker and a flawed bottling procedure had allowed the contaminant to seep in. Later they changed their story when the truth seeped out: that benzene is *always* in the water, and then must be carefully filtered out to achieve advertised purity. Usually it is; this one time it wasn't.

A healthful water supply is of special importance to heart patients. Toxic metals such as lead and cadmium that are often present in old iron pipes, dissolve easily into the water supply and are known to be harmful to the heart. In such a circumstance, a water filter - or bottled water - can be a critical advantage.

Finally, find out if you live in a soft- or hard-water area. The World Health Organization and the National Academy of Sciences have both concluded there is a relationship between the hardness of our water supply and the incidence of heart disease. Specifically, harder water has been linked to decreased heart disease mortality. If you reside in a soft water area, up your intake of mineral supplements.

BUILDING A BRIDGE OVER TROUBLED WATERS

There are several things you can try before spending twenty to thirty dollars a month for a bottled substitute. Homeowners who don't like the taste of their water, worry about what's coming out of their faucets, or have quality concerns, should find out what impurities lurk in their water supply. If served by a public system, call the water department to get a copy of the latest analysis report. If you're supplied by a well on your property, get an independent laboratory analysis.

Consumer Reports advises boiling your tap water for twenty minutes to get rid of bacteria. Since chlorine is a gas that dissipates, letting water sit out for a time in an open container sometimes helps. When it comes to chemicals, filters that attach to the end of your faucet are not a good buy for they may give you a false sense of security. Most experts consider those devices ineffective.

A more sophisticated reverse osmosis purifier runs between four and six hundred dollars. Before investing in any costly filtration systems, request information from the Environmental Protection Agency, Washington, D.C. 20460. Check out *Consumer Reports'* magazine rating of available brands. If you're on a tight budget, you can build a system with a supply of granulated activated carbon, a large funnel, some coffee filter papers and a container to collect the filtered water. For complete directions, check out Carol Keough's book, *Water Fit to Drink*.

WHERE THERE'S SMOKE ...
THERE ARE FREE RADICALS

Dr. Joseph Giordano, best known as the surgeon who saved Ronald Reagan's life after the 1981 assassination attempt, says, "There is no one who comes into my office with peripheral vascular disease who doesn't smoke or have a history of smoking."

Smoking contributes to vascular disease in various ways, he points out. It causes plaque formation in the arteries producing blockages, causes leg arteries to constrict decreasing their ability to supply blood to muscles, reduces the ability of red cells to supply oxygen to the tissues, and increases clot formation. No matter your age, your arteries are subject to damage if you smoke.

At a 1990 meeting for science writers, researchers revealed they had for the first time linked smoking and blood cholesterol levels to hardening of the arteries in men under 35 years of age.

Dr. Henry McGill, one of the study's directors, said findings were based on autopsies of about 3,900 15 to 34 year old men who died violent deaths by age 34. Raised arterial lesions (the beginning of atherosclerosis) were prevalent in the most persistent smokers.

"In this age group, smoking and cholesterol are about equally bad," Dr. McGill told us. Given the wide play the subject's had, itemizing the health risks of smoking seems like overkill. However, here are some late-breaking bulletins you might have missed:

- **Even a few puffs hurt women's hearts.**
  So says a new study from Harvard University's School of Medicine that found females smoking as few as one to four cigarettes a day doubled their risk of heart attack.
- **Women who smoke are nearly 3 1/2 times more likely to develop cervical cancer as non-smokers,** and the risk is almost as great for women living with smokers. Dr. Martha Slattery of the University of Utah Medical School, whose study turned up the unexpected finding, pointed out they had previously thought that it was the number of sex partners and early onset of sexual activity that was the link with cervical cancer. Said the researcher: "Now we know it's smoking, not sex, that is the real deadly sin."
- **Smoking interferes with breast-feeding,** according to a new study. Norwegian researchers have found that 40 percent of babies breast-fed by smoking mothers had colic - they cried for more than two hours a day for no apparent reason. Smoking mothers were also more likely to give up breast-feeding because of 'too little milk'.
- **Smokers risk Crohn's disease** - an ulcerative colitis. Again, women are more at risk than male smokers.
- **Smokers suffer aching muscles.** A Scandinavian study supported earlier findings in the U.S. that linked smoking

with lower back pain and other musculo-skeletal problems as well.

- **Smokers take more sick leave.** Researchers in Missouri uncovered a 23% higher absenteeism from smoking employees, with male smokers, older than 40 or unmarried, the most likely to call in sick.

- **Smoking can stunt your career.** Your chance of becoming a company bigwig can go up in a puff of smoke, according to a survey by Robert Half International that found non-smokers are more apt to hold the top jobs in any company. Only 22 percent of the top guns at 100 of the largest corporations in America are smokers against 71 percent of their lower echelon employees.

Need a new reason to quit smoking? You've got it. Take pity on your pooch. Please don't light up around Lassie. Dogs whose owners smoke are at a 50 percent greater risk of getting lung cancer, according to a professor at Colorado State University's College of Veterinary Medicine.

"Dogs don't smoke," the researcher noted, "and lung cancer is extremely rare in dogs."

Okay, so you'd like to quit. But how?

The decisive first step, the research shows, is a matter of mind-set. Once you're convinced that continued smoking will do you in, you're more apt to give up this destructive habit. One survey of successful former smokers revealed:

- 90 percent quit on their own;
- 39 percent quit because a health care provider told them they must;
- The two most common reasons for quitting were "to maintain health" and "to take control";
- The most popular quitting techniques were "Throw away all cigarettes", "cut down on the number of cigarettes smoked", "set a quit date"; "use substitutes"; and "spend more time around nonsmokers."

You, too, can become an ex-smoker if you just put your mind to it. If you can't do it alone - only one in four can quit smoking by will power alone - get help. Join a Super Stoppers Club, or a Smokers Anonymous, or try hypnosis, or nicotine gum, or nicotine patches, or perhaps acupuncture will work, or ear pressure, or Smoke Enders, or what-have-you. Just do it!

One ex-smoker who finally quit after 20 failed attempts, told how she did it: "There was this little clipping I cut out of the newspaper. It read: 'You pay for cigarettes twice; once when you get them, and once again when they get you.'

"I stuck that clipping on the front of my refrigerator and read it every time I wanted a cigarette. And I finally made it - I joined the quitters club'.

The good news is, it doesn't matter if you're under 35 years old or over 70, whether you smoke five cigarettes a day or go through five packs, whether you smoke nonfilters or light - if you quit smoking *NOW*, you can cut your risk of a heart attack or premature death - whatever your present age or condition.

If you need more convincing, consider this fact: 1,000 people quit smoking each day - by dying!

LIVING WITH A SMOKER

What if the love of your life has resisted all your well-intentioned nudging and nagging and you are forced to live in a smoke-filled home? What can you do to protect your health?

If your spouse won't quit, and you don't want to quit the marriage, here are some ways to cope with second-hand smoke:

- Limit exposure. Try to get the smoker to smoke outside, or to confine smoking to one well-ventilated room of the house.
- Ask the smoker to put out all cigarettes completely immediately after smoking.

- Make it a rule that the bedroom is an off-limits smoke-free area.
- Protect yourself with extra Vitamin C. A recent study by four biochemical researchers at the University of California at Berkeley determined that ascorbate (vitamin C) is a potent antioxidant. It prevents body damage from external sources of free radicals such as cigarette smoke. Ditto Vitamin E. More on this in the next chapter.

TAKING THE BITE OUT OF INTERNAL POLLUTION

Most health professionals miss it: The Mad Hatter's Disease-mercury poisoning. That's because the most likely cause comes from a most unlikely source - the fillings in your teeth.

Take the case of Mark Peterson of Larkspur, Colorado. For ten years he suffered from devastating health problems no physician could pin down. Unexplained aches, pains, stomach upsets, muscle cramps, and continuous headaches defied explanation. Sleepy one day, he'd be hyper the next, on an emotional roller coaster, depressed without reason, on cloud nine without cause.

For twenty-five years, no one knew what was wrong with Jennifer Carter. She'd been suffering continuous, debilitating headaches, followed by dizziness, sick feelings and concentration difficulties since she was eight years old. At thirty-three, she felt old, sick and tired, complained of bad taste and smell, abdominal pain and diarrhea. When she also developed chronic bronchitis, and periodic arrhythmias, she grew tired of hearing "it's all in your head" and decided to get help.

YOUR DENTIST MAY BE YOUR BEST DOCTOR!

Luckily for both Mark and Jennifer, they happened upon a well-read specialist. He suspected the onset of their mysterious maladies could be traced to dental work done years back.

When tests confirmed high levels of mercury in their bodies, they consulted a dentist who removed the offending metals from their teeth, and their health improved.

The idea that many of your health problems could track back to the fillings in your teeth is undoubtedly news to many. Although largely ignored, many knowledgeable dentists consider undiagnosed chronic mercury toxicity the unrecognized cause of mysterious symptoms and baffling disease. If you're surprised to find dentists, rather than physicians, alert to this health threat, get out your history books. Dentists were the first to link diet with disease, since the gums, teeth and condition of the mouth provide first hand evidence of how quickly lifestyle effects health. One reason physicians find mercury-linked conditions so difficult to detect, is that until recently there was no good test, and symptoms are generally non-specific and confusing.

Swedish researchers are years ahead of American scientists on this issue. They've developed a 24-hour urine test that establishes the diagnosis of chronic mercury poisoning that formerly could only be made by post-mortem brain autopsy. This test is not yet available in the U.S. The Swedes have also taken the lead when it comes to banning mercury amalgam fillings. Sweden's foremost politicians, recognizing the documented health threat mercury poses, vowed "No more amalgam after 1991."

According to Sweden's Mats Hanson, Ph.D., a leader in the anti-amalgam movement, some people react so severely to mercury, they are almost totally incapacitated. Not long ago, Dr. Hanson reported the link between micromercuralism and multiple sclerosis.

As Dr. Hanson has stated: "The use of amalgam as a dental filling must cease. Amalgam contains mercury, which when dissolved into the human body, even in small amounts, precipitates such health problems as tiredness, lack of appetite, infections, joint and muscle pain, gastrointestinal and concentration disturbances. At higher levels of toxicity, there will be behavioral and personality changes. Also the immune system can be affected since certain white blood cells are reduced in number. There is also the potential for reduced kidney function."

In 1985, the Swedish Health and Welfare Board appointed a group of experts to examine the risk of low-level exposure to mercury. Their determination: mercury amalgam is an unsuitable dental filling from a toxicological point of view and should be discontinued - especially for pregnant women where there is a strong risk of fetal damage.

Other European investigators studying the problem have confirmed the long-lasting damage traceable to mercury. In one German study of 200 patients who had from one to twenty-two fillings, clear evidence of chronic poisoning started after six years. Patients with ten or more fillings suffered the most tormenting problems. Among other serious side-effects of amalgam-induced mercury poisoning is the likelihood of zinc deficiency, and that other poisonous metals like lead, cadmium and arsenic also will be retained in the body to a higher degree.

According to previously unpublished data, 98% of patients with amalgam fillings suffer some detrimental effect. Among case reports: a nine year old girl who had five amalgam fillings in one year, became extremely agitated, suffered seizures, and lost contact with her surroundings; a 30 year old female suffered continuous and debilitating headaches and low back and abdominal pain until removal of 11 amalgam fillings and chelation treatments; a 33 year old female with 14 amalgam fillings over a twenty-five year period, felt very tired, old, depressed, had constant vertigo, sick feelings, concentration difficulties and related problems. She complained about bad taste and smell, abdominal pain, diarrhea, and periodic arrhythmias and tachycardias, and developed a chronic bronchitis. Her health did not improve until removal of amalgam fillings and chelation.

Even after amalgam removal, health problems frequently persist. In certain treated cases, for instance, severe migraine headaches continued for four months. Worldwide there is increasing opposition to the use of silver/mercury amalgam dental fillings, as more and more research condemning amalgam appears in the scientific literature.

One third of West German dentists have signed a petition calling for government health insurance to cease paying for silvery/mercury amalgam fillings. Sweden has gone one step further State health insurance now pays for the exchange of amalgam fillings for a non-amalgam replacement at the patient's request. Canadian researchers led by Dr. Murray J. Vimy have published dramatic evidence of mercury-caused ailments. Australian TV has given wide coverage to anti-amalgam publicity.

In England, mercury-laden fillings received a really bad press when the British papers reported Princess Diana had her amalgam fillings replaced with composites several years back. How come? The Queen urged her to do so after she read of the harmful effects of mercury exposure.

Japan has just been host to a world congress featuring prominent amalgam biocompatability researchers. Chief among them, Dr. Kazuhiko Asai, who has pointed out that the combination of the mercury atoms and the free oxygen and hydrogen radicals from the amalgam fillings, constitute a free radical generator, right in your mouth.

WELCOME TO ROUND THREE
OF THE AMALGAM WARS

Despite all the scientific documentation of the seriousness of mercury vapor toxins released from fillings, and the very real potential for irreversible damage, the American Dental Association (ADA) has categorized the subject a 'frivolous concern', and persistently supports the continued use of mercury amalgam fillings with fanatical devotion.

This is not a new controversy, but one almost 150 years old. In 1845, the America Society of Dental Surgeons passed a resolution denouncing the use of amalgams as malpractice and further demanded that each member sign a pledge not to use amalgams. Expulsion from the society was automatic for any dentist not adhering to the restriction.

One and a half centuries later, the ADA has reversed itself and insists that the mercury in fillings is nothing to worry about. Really? At one time, this very same A.D.A. recommended that scrap amalgam, the material left over after filling a tooth, should be handled as gingerly as any toxic waste. No one was to touch it. It was to be stored under water in sealed containers, and disposed of only through local health departments. Many experts agree that if some dentist introduced mercury based fillings today, the FDA would not approve its use in repairing teeth.

Prominent among U.S. activists seeking a Sweden-style ban on silver/mercury amalgam is Dr. Michael Ziff who has called mercury amalgam fillings **"toxic time bombs."** Outraged citizen anti-amalgam groups, chartered as DAMS (Dental Amalgam Mercury Syndrome), are active in many states, and lobby for legislative action. Small bands of highly dedicated courageous U.S. dentists have devoted themselves to raising public awareness, risking the wrath and scorn of their see-no-evil colleagues.

Richard Fischer, D.D.S. of Annandale, Virginia, a practitioner of what's been called "biocompatible dentistry," has found, **"Eighty percent of patients experience some health benefits after amalgam replacement.**

"I haven't seen anyone get up out of a wheelchair, but have had some very astonishing recoveries nonetheless. One young lady with chronic migraines, which nothing had helped, now has only one or two per year - instead of one or two daily.

"I've talked to other dentists who've had patients recover from arthritis, diarrhea, lupus, digestive disorders, multiple sclerosis, and severe allergies once they had their amalgams replaced."

WHY ARE DENTISTS SO DOWN IN THE MOUTH?

For a long time, epidemiological researchers have puzzled over the unusually high incidence of suicide, divorce, alcohol and substance abuse among dentists. As a group, dentists have led all the professions in these unhappy statistics for many years.

Now at last, there may be an answer. Mercury toxicity does not end with the dental patient, but poses a serious occupational health threat to dentists as well. That became clear when in 1982, a research team from the University of Pennsylvania studied 300 dentists and found 10% with significant mercury levels in their body tissues. Of those, 70% suffered from mild neurological problems such as irritability, depression, anxiety and insomnia.

When University of Minnesota School of Dentistry researchers screened 1166 (1002 male and 163 female) dentists for undetected cardiac arrhythmias at the 1988 ADA/FDI World Dental Meeting, they found 14% of those dentists screened had an abnormal EKG showing one or more arrhythmias. Four percent were identified as having an arrhythmia that needed immediate medical follow-up. Two dentists were hospitalized with potentially life-threatening disorders that had not been previously identified.

Merely working in a building that houses dental offices can be hazardous. Polishing amalgams gives off considerable mercury vapors. If the building has sealed windows and central ventilation, employees and visitors may be exposed to toxic levels which far exceed OSHA limits, which are five times higher, by the way, than allowed by European standards.

What of the dangers to the environment at large? Dentists used 200,000 pounds of mercury in 1980; 400,000 pounds in 1990; estimated use in the year 2000 is 600,000 pounds annually. Data collected in Hamburg and Berlin has revealed at least 13% of the mercury in refuse water originates from dental clinics. The 100 dental clinics in Hamburg dump 0.4 tons of mercury into local waters each year - an alarming report that should alert American environmentalists to a possible explanation for the ever-increasing contamination of U.S. rivers and lakes.

No wonder larger numbers of people every day are developing unspecified health crises. Mercury kills unrenewable cells. Nickel alloys (used routinely in removable partial dentures) are the customary means of inducing cancer in laboratory animals. Tin poisoning from canned foods is well known. Silver causes argyria, an irreversible gray discoloration of the skin. Dental amalgams aside, there is an increasing load of toxic substances in the environment, resulting in constant exposure to unhealthy material. We are poisoned by lead-laden air, smoker's carcinogenic fumes, harmful chemicals in food, cosmetics and medications, and damaged by electromagnetic assault by outdoor power lines and our home-based radioactive appliances. They all have a detrimental effect on the immune system and the body's natural defenses.

SURVIVING ON A POLLUTED PLANET

Short of abandoning civilization and taking up residence on some uninhabited island, what can you do to keep environmental toxins from doing you in?

If you've been fortunate enough to inherit good genes, or your natural defenses have proven strong enough to fight off pollution, you're lucky, but not home free. As you age, your in-built defenses will weaken, and eventually, those nasty free radicals are liable to 'getcha' - more sooner than later unless you beef up internal fortification.

If you've already buckled under free radical attack, or fallen victim to environmental toxins, it's not too late to regroup and recuperate. Your body's defenses can be revitalized. Medicinals such as EDTA put safeguards back on track. Once you've done that, anti-oxidant supplementation combined with dietary changes and lifestyle improvements will provide you with the most reliable protection.

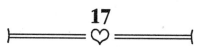

17

FIGHTING THE FREE-RADICAL FOE
POWER UP WITH VITAMINS

"If I had my way, I'd make health contagious, instead of disease," said Robert G. Ingersoll in the late 1800's.

The fact is: health *is* catching. When one member of the family commences on a self-health program, the life style modifications that follow inevitably affect everyone in the household. This is certain to be the case if the chief cook and bottle-washer (once called 'lady of the house') is the first to become health-conscious.

Dr. Cheraskin calls this the "spouse-likeness" syndrome and his research demonstrates that married couples - and even their pets - not only eat alike, they begin to look alike over time. The long married have remarkably similar cholesterol, vitamin and blood pressure levels; their blood chemistry profiles and clinical status are almost identical. If a husband and wife are fat, chances are the dog is also. If one of them starts to diet, both partners will lose weight.

We know how true this is from our own experience. Time was when we thought the Four Food Groups were "sandwiches, snacks, sweets and soda pop". Then, we met up with the preventive health movement (thanks to our happy association with Dr. E. Cheraskin with whom Arline co-authored *Psychodietetics*), and our home life changed. Journalists are quick to make the most of their insider's edge. Given access to newsworthy information, they not only broadcast it, but use it for personal gain. In our case, that translated into a cleaned-out pantry, rid of chemically-laden processed foods. We swore off Twinkies, fried chicken, Big Macs, Dunkin' Donuts, and ruled our favorite French-style gourmet restaurants off limit.

Being in the communication business, we didn't stop there. We nagged the kids, our parents, in-laws, friends, neighbors - everyone who would listen - to do the same. "No more potato kugel," we warned mama, and carefully refused dinner invitations from couples apt to serve food we wouldn't eat at home.

With that as background, let it be clearly understood that we've based what follows on what we've gleaned over the years. We are not in the 'advice' business; we are not doctors; we do not presume to know what's good for anyone except ourselves. We are willing to share the strategies we've adopted to preserve our loved ones' health. Keep it in mind, that what's worked for us may be all wrong for someone else.

Heading up our "How To Live a Long Time" list: we've been chelated. Our original intent was to experience at first-hand the therapy we were writing about, considering it dishonest to introduce readers to a procedure we had not tested.

Did we enjoy it? No. It was boring and swiped time from our super-busy work schedules. Did we benefit? Not having suffered any diagnosable symptoms, it's hard to document positive results. We were healthy pre-chelation; healthy post-chelation. It certainly did us no harm, and probably did us much good, since we continue (almost two decades into current careers) to follow as active, energetic and productive an agenda as people half our age. Most days we're up at 5:30, still hard at work at midnight. We're sufficiently pro-chelation to continue with periodic 'booster' shots of EDTA, convinced it's the best established defense against environmental-imposed toxicity and the normal ravages of aging.

Do we encourage others to do the same? We urge everyone to investigate the appropriateness of chelation for themselves.

What else? Here are some other strategies we consider important in our quest for robust longevity.

THE VITAMIN QUEST

Early in our training as medical journalists, we recognized the unmistakable truth that the 'balanced diet' was a myth - for all practical purposes, nonexistent. Guidelines for establishing optimal nutritional guidelines - individual requirements for carbohydrates, fats, protein, vitamins and minerals - are ill-defined. Even if it was possible to scientifically determine the ingredients of a balanced diet, the odds are poor - a thousand to one shot at best - that anyone could select foods to fit the formula.

In the best of all worlds, vitamin pills might not be necessary. Our food would be locally grown on the best quality soils, pesticide-free. In the real world, things are much different. Today's edibles grow on mineral-depleted soil, are manufactured with consideration to appearance, and processed to last on store shelves. They have lost nutritional value every step of the way.

Nutritionally 'enriched' foods are a very bad joke. This is how Dr. Joe Nichols, a founding director of the International Academy of Preventive Medicine, once described the "enrichment" process:

> *"Suppose a mugger ordered you at gun point to strip down to your birthday suit, giving up clothing, shoes, underwear, wallet, credit cards, jewelry - everything you possess. Then, should the thief take pity on you and return your wedding band, socks and perhaps your topcoat to cover your nakedness so you could go home, would you feel 'enriched'? We doubt it. That's the equivalent of what's taking place in the food industry. First they strip away everything of value; then they put back a token selection of necessities and convince the consumer they've been 'enriched' by the process. Don't you believe it."*

The problem doesn't stop there. Because of business, social or other concerns, we often eat in a hurry and rely on convenience foods. Compounding the problem, there are those irresistible urges that defy our best intentions to adhere to a clean-Jean diet. Add up all the obstacles, and you reach an obvious conclusion: it's close to impossible to secure your daily requirements of all the proper quantities of vitamins and minerals from foods.

Finally, there is the question of drug/nutrient interaction. As you might suspect, drugs have an unfortunate impact on nutrition. The most frequently prescribed heart drugs interfere with enzyme systems; some compete with drugs for the sites of action; some decrease nutrient synthesis. Many drugs, even those seemingly benign, compromise the taker's nutritional status by interfering with vitamin homeostasis. The most common offenders are the estrogen-containing oral contraceptives that put women using them at risk of a clinical folate deficiency. As people age, they tend to take many more drugs, depleting nutritional status at the very time of life that the immune system needs boosting. One seemingly innocuous example is mineral oil, used freely by the elderly, which causes malabsorption of Vitamin D.

Once we realized the desirability of obtaining an excess of each essential nutrient as a hedge against dietary deficiency, we thought we had the problem licked. All we needed was to assemble a medicine chest full of nutritional supplements.

In the beginning, there was Vitamin C. Persuaded by Dr. Cheraskin's extensive research, added to what we learned from Linus Pauling and gleaned from Dr. Fred Klenner, we were for a time convinced "C" was the sure-cure for everything from colds to cancer. Fortunately, we had few of the one and none of the other.

Next, we latched onto Vitamin E. Our working relationship with Dr. Wilfrid E. Shute (author of *Vitamin E for Ailing and Healthy Hearts*) convinced us he was 'right on' when it came to a nutritional antidote to ischemic heart disease and related circulatory disorders. Then when we became acquainted with Dr. Roger Williams, we were schooled on biochemical individuality, and the difficulties of satisfying personal needs with mass merchandised products.

Attending meetings featuring orthomolecular specialists - Drs. Abra n Hoffer, Alan Cott, Bernard Rimland - switched our focus to the B vitamins. We wrote at length about the likelihood that megadoses of many essential nutrients could be an appropriate strategy for those seeking drugless alternatives for common emotional disturbances, especially those normally considered to be of primarily psychological origin: schizophrenia, anxiety neurosis, depression.

As we gained a more sophisticated view, we realized the need to beef up with vitamins and minerals from A to zinc, and so began investigating a variety of shelf products. The treasure hunt was on - for a multi-vitamin preparation that would include all the essential vitamins and minerals plus the many so-called nonessentials as well. We expected to find a wide choice of suitable products.

WOULD THE 'REAL' VITAMINS PLEASE STAND UP

What a blow! Our search led to a scandal. When we discovered many vitamin pills are worthless, the result was a nationally published exposé: the vitamin rip-off.

To sum up what we wrote: many vitamin products either contain far less nutrition than labeled, are old and have lost potency, or have been so badly mishandled throughout the production/distribution process, a jar of jelly beans would provide more nutritional value.

Our prime information source was Dr. Jeffrey Bland, formerly Associate Professor of Chemistry at the University of Puget Sound in Tacoma, Washington, currently on leave from his post as Professor of Nutritional Biochemistry at the University of Puget Sound, whose documented survey of off-the-shelf vitamins revealed:

- Consumers are often short-changed. More than one-third (36%) of the vitamins assayed, proved to have 25% less potency than was on the label;
- Supposedly identical products had widely diverse ranges of activity. Vitamin E products were particularly unreliable - many did not come close to providing what they were advertising;
- Vitamin C products labeled as including bioflavanoids, often did not include enough of this substance to be useful. The amount of bioflavanoids was insignificant in 62% of the products evaluated;
- The majority of Vitamin E supplements (52%) contained less than half of their specified potency; some showed up as having absolutely no value at all.
- Super "B's," commanding a premium price because of a claimed extra potency, turned out to have huge discrepancies between what was in the bottle and the promise on the label.

The evidence Dr. Bland furnished was good reason for people to throw up their hands in disgust and forget about vitamins. Much as you'd like to give the finger to dishonest purveyors, you can't dismiss your need for supplements.

DON'T GIVE UP YET

While self-manufactured and food-derived anti-oxidant systems may be sufficient to fend off free radical attack until we reach middlescence, from then on we need supplemental help. More so, depending upon how badly we've abused our bodies (by smoking, drinking, eating junk foods, taking drugs). Even under the best of circumstances, our natural store house of anti-oxidants is sure to decline by the time we've reached middle age.

Sooner or later - the sooner the better - we must locate a reliable source of nutritional supplementation. Once we are unable to replenish all that we require from food sources, we have no other choice.

What a drag! Read the vitamin ads, and you'll be further confused. Each manufacturer claims to be the most honest purveyors of nutritional supplements. Advertisements promise "guaranteed potency", "purity", "high quality", "free of fillers and additives."

Notice none mention impurities. As Dr. Harry Demopoulos, an acknowledged expert on free-radical pathology points out, there is no way of telling what contaminants have been used while turning many of the cheaper vitamins - (mass market, off-brand products) into tablets or capsules.

"Tree saps and gums may be added to hold the tablets together; shellac to coat the pills; talc and sand for stretchers or fillers. Worst of all, soaps and detergents such as magnesium stearate are often added as lubricants to help move the powders through the encapsulating and tableting machines in the factory," he writes.

Doesn't the FDA protect us? No. Manufacturers are not required to be specific and list all additives by name. They need not declare what type of raw materials they use - food grade or the more desirable USP pharmaceutical grade - and can add a sinister host of contaminants to the final product.

Where to turn? How then to choose a reliable product?

If you're under the care of a nutritionally-oriented physician, he'll probably have supplements to suggest. Most who resist the more noxious drug remedies, fashion each patient's supplement program based on the nutrient needs suggested by diagnostic testing.

When your doctor prescribes a vitamin/mineral formula is he interested in supplementing your health or his income? Chances are he's doing his best to guide you. A physician familiar with many manufacturers and their trade policies could be a close-at-hand authority on reliable brands.

If you are seeking nutritional insurance on your own, with the goal of balancing dietary deficiencies and to gain protection against free-radical aging, read labels carefully. Try to choose supplements designed to improve the heart's overall efficiency and to curb free-radical dirty work. Be on guard against extravagant claims. It is illegal for manufacturers of food supplements to allege their products cure or prevent disease, unless they have supportive research data.

A VITAMIN PRIMER

At the risk of presenting already familiar material, let us review the known health benefits of the most popular nutrients:

Vitamin A: an anti-oxidant, protective against some cancers, needed to grow and maintain skin and internal tissue linings, for vision, especially night vision and to fight infections;

Vitamin C: a potent free radical scavenger, needed to form and maintain collagen, help maintain teeth and gums, promote wound healing, extremely important for the production of T-cells and other components of the immune mechanism;

Vitamin D: under study as a possible treatment for osteoporosis and breast cancer, it regulates the metabolism of calcium and phosphorous and is used for healthy bones and teeth;

Vitamin E: a powerful free radical scavenger with strong anti-blood clotting action. It helps provide more oxygen and nutrients to the cells and strengthens and protects blood vessel walls and red blood cells, speeds the healing process, increases resistance to disease, and helps strengthen immune defenses;

Vitamin K: often used to speed up blood clotting;

Vitamin B1 (thiamine): the so-called 'happy vitamin', it aids in the conversion of the carbohydrates in starches, sugars and alcohols into glucose, maintaining a healthy nervous system and a good mental attitude;

Vitamin B2 (riboflavin): helps maximize the cells' use of oxygen, and maintains the mucous membranes, nervous system, skin and eyes, as well as releasing energy from proteins, carbohydrates and fats;

Vitamin B3 (niacin, niacinamide, nicotinic acid): may reverse narrowing and hardening of the arteries, helps release energy from proteins, carbohydrates and fats, improves blood circulation and reduces cholesterol levels, essential for the function of the central nervous system, the growth and health of the skin, tongue, sex hormones and digestive tissues;

Vitamin B6 (pyridoxine): plays an important role in the metabolism of protein, carbohydrates and fats, speeds conversion of stored glycogen into glucose to be burned as energy, promotes healthy functioning of the nervous system, and must be present during production of red blood cells and antibodies;

Vitamin B12 (cobalamin): needed for the nervous system and cells, the formation of red blood cells, the metabolism of protein, carbohydrates and fats;

CAUTION: Unless a specific deficiency in a single B vitamin has been identified, it is adviseable to take a supplement that is a complete B complex. Taking high doses of single B vitamins may produce deficiencies in the other B vitamins. Since the body tends to excrete all the B's at a similar rate, an overabundance of one will cause it to be dumped, dragging the others with it.

Biotin: plays a central role in making fatty acids in burning fatty acids and carbohydrates and enabling the body to utilize the B vitamins, folic acid and pantothenic acid;

Choline: helps burn fat and cholesterol, plays an important role in transmitting nerve impulses, and important for learning;

Folic acid; plays a key role in the formation and maturity of red blood cells, aids digestion and the liver, works with B12 in the production of genetic material and Vitamin C in protein metabolism;

Inositol: helps burn fat and reduce cholesterol, and also protects arteries, liver, kidneys and heart;

When it comes to the minerals, information is ambiguous and even harder to come by. The main problem to making wise selections is this is an area where a perfect working balance is critical. For instance: take calcium, magnesium and phosphorous. No question each is important for optimal heart health, but the ratio between these three is critical. If calcium and phosphorous are out of balance (frequently the case) magnesium intake may be too high or too low.

Copper and zinc are another pair of minerals where balance is important. What usually happens is copper is too high, and children react by becoming hyperactive and in women, pre-menstrual syndrome is the most common result.

Zinc is another essential mineral that is vital to ingest in the right balance with other minerals. The same holds true for selenium, so powerful a free radical scavenger, there have been reports of lower male cancer death rates in areas of the U.S. with high selenium levels in the soil.

Chromium has been shown to be useful to hypoglycemics and diabetics because it helps increase their ability to handle glucose, but only a minimal amount is needed. That is also true of many other equally essential minerals: **chlorine, cobalt, fluorine, iodine, iron, manganese, molybdenum, potassium, sulfur and vanadium,** not to mention those needed in such micro-mini levels, there's almost no way to determine need or assure availability or presence.

HEART HELPERS

The latest research suggests some supplements are potentially more useful than others when waging your private war against heart disease. The one you are most apt to be familiar with is the old standby: Vitamin E. Not that many years ago, critics belittled its worth, calling it a "vitamin in search of a disease." Today, mainstream researchers hail it as a first-line defense against the free radical chain reaction.

Focussing on E for the moment, researchers at recent Vitamin E conferences have suggested that the antioxidant properties of E may reduce plaque formation by one-half or more. French investigators at the Pasteur Institute recently presented research suggesting Vitamin E fights heart disease by preventing LDL's (the low-density lipoproteins generally assumed to be the 'bad' cholesterol) from becoming 'rancid'.

The January, 1991 issue of the *American Journal of Clinical Nutrition* noted that Vitamin E protects people against heart disease **regardless** of cholesterol levels. They based this conclusion on the findings of a large scale study of more than 100,000 people in 33 different population groups. The researchers hypothesized: "The antioxidant hypothesis is that Vitamin E prevents cholesterol from oxidizing in the artery walls, thereby preventing atherosclerosis.

Then there's the *Optimal Vitamin Study,* which provides persuasive evidence that "essential antioxidants, mainly

Vitamin E, may substantially counteract known risk factors for heart disease, especially elevated cholesterol and high blood pressure."

When William Mauer, M.D., a noted clinician, reviewed his 25 years of experience with Vitamin E in the treatment of blood clots and vascular disease, he added valuable insight. Reporting before the American Academy of Medical Preventics (now ACAM), Dr. Mauer told how he has routinely placed cardiac patients on a special brand of natural mixed tocopherols in dosage ranges of 1,600 to 2,400 units a day. At this dosage, he said, "I have observed dissolution of coronary scars, reversal of electrocardiographic abnormalities and dissolving of blood clots."

Dr. Demopoulos is among those who have pointed out Vitamin E also protects against abnormal blood coagulation, a particular danger for patients undergoing surgery. Vitamin E in doses of 800 I.U. helps prevent deep vein clots from forming, even in postoperative patients who have to remain immobile for long periods of time.

Since the body's nervous system is particularly vulnerable to attack by free radicals, researchers have been particularly interested in uncovering a link between Vitamin E levels and neurological disorders. Studies conducted at Albany (N.Y.) Medical College and Columbia University's College of Physicians and Surgeons, found that large doses of Vitamin E reduced the severity and delayed the progression of Parkinson's Disease.

People taking Vitamin E proved to carry out daily activities more easily, and had fewer complications of therapy. Another Columbia University researcher, testing a small number of people suffering from tardive dyskinesia (a nervous disorder often resulting from chronic use of antipsychotic drugs) found they could cut the severity of their symptoms in half when given large doses of Vitamin E.

Other studies conducted over the last decade show that Vitamin E is a lung protector. It helps us all breathe a little easier in ozone-laden polluted air. Vitamin E offers some protection to smoker's lungs and to those exposed to sidestream smoke.

Vitamin E is a fail-safe protector for "weekend warriors" - those periodically vigorous exercisers such as skiers, mountain climbers and others who work out at high altitude or to exhaustion, and out-of-condition sporadic exercisers. All of them are at great risk of lung damage, especially if they huff and puff in polluted air. During vigorous exercise, the body takes in and uses oxygen at a high rate - up to 10 to 20 times as much as in normal, day-to-day activity. The greater the use of oxygen, the more free radicals created and the higher the potential for cell damage, especially if Vitamin E levels are inadequate.

Can you overdose on E? Slim risk. An exhaustive review of the scientific literature revealed few side effects have ever been reported, even at doses as high as 3,200 International Units a day. The greater gamble, it appears, is too little rather than too much Vitamin E, should you rely on a product with so little antioxidant activity as to be virtually ineffective. When Dr. Mauer first heard we were writing this book, he made one request: "Spell out for your readers the difference in Vitamin E products. Steer them in the right direction."

Not only Dr. Mauer, but other knowledgeable physicians we respect, have pointed out that many commercial brands of Vitamin E contain only one of the seven or eight tocopherols found in natural Vitamin E, and thus have only 20 percent of the anti-thrombin activity and none of the anxtioxidant properties found in the natural, mixed tocopherols. Some inferior products are diluted with vegetable oil which can turn rancid (creating free radicals). The available anti-oxidant property of the Vitamin E is then consumed within the capsule before it is even ingested. Worse still, there might not be enough Vitamin E activity to neutralize more than a fraction of the rancidity produced by inexpensive additives. In that case, the net effect of taking one of these inferior capsules is you are subjected to more free radicals than if you had not taken the Vitamin E capsule in the first place.

The exceptional product, recommended by many holistic doctors (none of whom have any financial interest that we know of) is produced by the A.C. Grace Company (1100 Quitman Rd., Big Sandy, Texas 75755 1-800-638-8807.

What makes the Grace Company's Vitamin E unique? It is entirely natural, far more potent than chemically altered products, and Certified by Assay to have a reliably uniform dosage potency in each tablet. That's good enough for us.

THE VITAMIN C CONNECTION

No discussion of nutrient-bolstered free radical protection could possibly overlook the Vitamin C connection to healthy hearts. It's hardly 'new' news that this popular vitamin is a front-line defense against free-radical oxidation. The latest research to support belief comes from the University of California at Berkley, where researcher Balz Frei noticed that if he added oxidants - agents that create free radicals - to blood in a test tube, ascorbate (the chemical name for C) was the first substance to become oxidized. Damage to blood cells began only **after** ascorbate was used up. His most significant finding was that attacks on proteins and fats stopped as soon as additional ascorbate was added. This demonstrated one important way by which C may help to prevent many age-related diseases. No wonder Dr. Demopoulos calls Vitamin C the "anti-oxidant that prevents us from rusting." That's a vivid description of this nutrient's class act as a free-radical quencher.

Daily doses of 2,000 milligrams of Vitamin C (in combination with 200 units of Vitamin E) is what Dr. Anthony J. Verlangier recommends to help keep arteries unclogged. As Director of the Atherosclerosis Research Laboratories at the University of Mississippi, Dr. Verlangieri's research with lab animals led him to conclude that adequate amounts of these two nutrients inhibit the activity of a prime artery-damaging enzyme.

What else does C do? Whole books have been written on the subject, so let us just spotlight light the more relevant findings:

Ascorbic acid is now known to:

- Help control cholesterol;
- Stimulate collagen production for healthy tissues;
- Strengthen the immune system;
- Act like an antihistamine in fighting allergies;
- Increase iron absorption;
- Deactivate ingested carcinogens, by blocking the cancer-causing potential of nitrites found in salted, pickled and smoked foods;
- Help prevent glaucoma, by reducing intraocular pressure;
- Help you smarten up by playing a major role in brain function;
- Work well in conjunction with E when it comes to preventing blood clots, relieve circulatory disorders, and aid recovery from heart attacks.
- Be an antidote for hangovers by speeding clearance of alcohol from the bloodstream;
- Work well with Vitamin E when it comes to preventing blood clots, relieve circulatory disorders, and aid recovery from heart attacks.
- Prevent cancer.

The latest exciting possibility is Vitamin C may be a beauty cream. Research at Duke University into the topical application of the vitamin suggests a concentration of C in cream form will reverse the effects of skin aging better than Retin-A. If the research proves out, it will make C good for everything from colds to crinkles.

Despite all that's written and known about Vitamin C, chances are you're unaware all Vitamin C is not the same. "Bargain brands" are simple ascorbic acid and cannot be taken in doseages required - some 4 to 10 grams per day - to protect against aging, heart attack, stroke and cataract, without experiencing a diuretic reaction that results in heart-burn, nausea, bloating and flatulence.

There's good reason why Alacer Corporation's Supergram III is labeled "The Real Vitamin C", since each tablet provides 1000 mg. of mineral ascorbates, the only form of Vitamin C that can be taken in megadoses without negative side effects and without inducing the loss of such valuable minerals as potassium, calcium, magnesium, manganese, molybdenum, zinc and chromium. Furthermore, it is only as mineral ascorbates can Vitamin C be stored in vital organs: the adrenals, brain and heart.

If Supergram III mineral ascorbates are not available at your favorite health food store, complain to the manager or to Alacer Corporation through their 800 number: 854-0249.

BEYOND VITAMINS

No discussion of anti-oxidants should neglect two of the more exotic, lesser known supplements. The first of these is Coenzyme Q10 (CoQ10 for short), a natural substance originally synthesized from beef heart michocondria. It's been shown to be a remarkable aid in the recovery from heart disease as well as other serious ailments. Originally isolated in 1957 by a U.S. scientist, it languished unnoticed. For the next three decades, it was zealously developed, researched and marketed in Japan - where some ten percent of the population take it on a daily basis.

More recently, scientists worldwide have taken notice, and there are now hundreds of papers - most of them attesting to CoQ10's benefits - pouring forth not only from Japan, but also from Russia, Germany and Western Europe, and lately, from the United States.

Typical of the enthusiastic reports, are those released from the Free University in Brussels. These demonstrated CoQ boosts heart performance, even after cardiac disease has reached a serious, all but terminal, stage. In a case cited by the University of Bonn, a woman with a rapidly degenerating heart function, given just a few weeks to live, was totally recovered two years later thanks to treatment with CoQ supplements. Other studies show significant improvement in many patients with severe congestive heart failure after administration of CoQ.

Research published in the prestigious *American Journal of Cardiology* supported Japanese research claims that the substance is a "safe and promising" treatment for angina. Reports pour in that it has been found to boost the immune system, increase the strength of the heart without exercise, protect against heart attacks, lower blood pressure, and reduce weight naturally.

There's no lack of support for more extravagant claims: the most electrifying is the possibility that CoQ may be a life-extender. Dr. Richard Passwater, an internationally honored leader in vitamin research, considers CoQ to have exciting potential in this regard. When female mice were injected with CoQ, the oldest survivor lived 150 weeks - in human equivalent 140 years - and remained surprisingly 'youthful' to the very end, showing none of the usual signs of aging. Making the leap from mice to man is not easy, however it appears likely this nutrient's superb ability to counteract the bio-destructive effects of free radicals, does somehow impact on the most basic processes of aging.

Maintaining adequate levels of CoQ becomes more of a problem the older we get, Dr. Passwater points out. Although you can find this nutrient in a great variety of fresh foods - spinach, whole grains, beef, sardines, peanuts - it is fragile and easily destroyed during food preparation. To make things worse, the body's ability to 'extract' sufficient CoQ from food sources decline with age, and may 'turn off' completely at some point. All the more reason not to snatch the first handy-dandy brand off the closest store shelf. If CoQ10 is the 'miracle' nutrient many authorities believe it to be - noted researcher/physician/author Stephen Sinatra reveals that if he was to limit himself to just ONE nutrient, he would toss away all but CoQ10 - then it's essential to select the brand which can deliver maximum health benefits.

Which measures up? A hydrosoluble version manufactured by Physiologics using a patented technology boasting up to 300% higher bioavailability. It provides a six-fold increase in plasma CoQ10 levels over others (research documented results). This superior product is a real boon since traditionally, CoQ10 is poorly absorbed. If your physician cannot supply you with hydrosoluble CoQ10, call 1-800-638-8807.

GRAPE SEED EXTRACT - THE NEW KID ON THE ANTI-OXIDANT BLOCK.

Ten-to-one you've not heard of proanthocyanidins. Write it down - it's the one word to remember when shopping for the most powerful antioxidant discovered to date. How powerful? Believed to provide antioxidant activity at least 50 times stronger than Vitamin E and 20 times greater than Vitamin C (with which it works synergistically), proanthocyanidins have been used therapeutically for decades in Europe to alleviate circulatory disorders. All proanthocyanidins are not created equal.

Some confusion arises from the fact that virtually identical varieties come from pine bark, lemon tree bark, cranberries, hazel nut tree leaves and grape seeds. The best are extracted from grape seeds which is why grape seed extract is known world-wide as a premier anti-aging product. One of the other important differences between sources is in their varying concentrations.

The Grape Seed Extract that meets requirements yields a 95% concentration of Proanthocyanidin, 10% higher than the yield obtained from pine-bark derived Pycnogenol. It's worth being choosy - double-blind tests have documented this substance's ability to prevent and reverse such ailments as varicose veins, diabetic retinopathy, capillary fragility (easy bruising), high blood pressure and heart disease. Dr. P.P. Rothschild, a 1986 Nobel Prize nominee, explains: "It's the only antioxidant that can cross the blood brain barrier, providing extra protection from free radical damage throughout the nervous system."

If your doctor isn't up on the value of Proanthocyanidins, more information is available through the toll-free number: 1-800-638-8807.

DON'T NEGLECT MINERALS

While there's considerable awareness of the importance of vitamins, there's been relatively little attention paid to the role of minerals, active partners with vitamins in the maintenance of harmony and health.

That oversight is easily explained. The foundation for cellular biochemistry was laid down more than a century ago, yet few of today's most informed nutrition experts can explain the many ways in which organic and inorganic substances interact and cooperate with each other. The vast majority of pathways and biochemical interactions between vitamins and their mineral mates are yet to be discovered. Here's what we do know: the body has many hidden needs. Every human is to some extent a chemical factory with over 5,000 different chemical reactions known to the chemist taking place daily. Any deficiency of one or more minerals leads to cellular disturbance.

No argument. No wonder no one has a complete working knowledge of cellular medicine.

A recent literature review places two minerals in the spotlight. Magnesium, on its own, and in combination with potassium, has the potential, it's claimed, to save more than 900,000 heart disease victims a year.

Magnesium is vital for nerve conduction, muscular contractions and the transmission of impulses all along the nervous system. In combination with an appropriate amount of calcium, magnesium helps the heart maintain a steady beat. Marginal deficiencies have led to tics, tremors, slurred speech and other signs of neurological dysfunction, including cardiac arrhythmias and sudden death.

People with life-threatening arrhythmias have recovered their natural rhythm with no treatment other than magnesium supplementation. Dr. Hans Nieper of Hanover, West Germany claims to have demonstrated a 95% decrease in heart attacks among patients he's treated with a potassium/magnesium supplement.

When Dr. Gerhard Schurrmann of Burgsteinfurt, West Germany, tested this therapy with 150 of his own patients, he duplicated results, and declared: "They were all suffering from serious heart disease, and the majority were on the verge of heart attacks at the outset. Not a single one of them has had a heart attack since treatment started."

An American doctor, Dr. Garry F. Gordon of Sacramento, California also used the combination to treat over 700 of his cardiac patients over two years, "and 85 percent got dramatic relief of symptoms," he's said. Recently he confirmed long-term benefits of megnesium supplementation. "The more research that's completed, the more exciting the results. Magnesium does everything the high-priced drugs fail to do - and it does it cheaply and with no adverse side effects."

The latest news out of China is that many long-ignored trace minerals may be the key to longevity. Researchers at Nanjing Tie Dao Medical College gave a control group of 15 mice plain drinking water, and other groups drinking water supplemented with a different trace mineral in a concentration about five times that of normal tap water. They have reported striking results: manganese, copper, sodium and potassium supplements increased life spans by 84, 77, 54 and 24 percent, respectively, while chloride, zinc and calcium decreased life spans by 58, 41 and 20 percent. Obviously, what applies to mice may or may not apply to men. Even if it does hold true that some trace elements dramatically increase life while others shorten it.

Take care when self-medicating. Mineral supplementation is quite tricky, since the inter-relationships between the many trace elements is critical. For example, zinc - a popular supplement among oldsters eager to retard the progression of age-related macular degeneration - should never be taken without copper. As little as 50 mg. of zinc can impair copper absorption, and may result in anemia.

Unless you are a biochemist with a sophisticated understanding of your precise nutrient status, it is all too easy to throw vitamin co-factor systems and mineral utilization homeostasis out of synch. Avoid haphazard tinkering.

POTASSIUM, THE POWERFUL

Numerous studies have attempted to establish a link between strokes (the third leading cause of death in the United States), food and nutrients. The most recent review of the relevant literature infers that while it is difficult to come to firm conclusions, it is safe to say there is an inverse relationship between the ingestion of fruits and vegetables and stroke mortality rates (the more of the first, the less of the second) - and higher levels of dietary and urinary potassium have been linked to a significant (40%) - reduction in stroke-associated death.

The finding was consistent with a similar analysis from the 1988 Honolulu Heart Study in which rats fed a high-potassium (2.11%) diet demonstrated a 98% reduction in mortality rates at 8 months compared with rats fed a normal potassium (0.75%) diet. The beneficial effect of potassium on mortality rates appeared to be independent of blood pressure and was accompanied by a 95% reduction in brain infarcts in rats who survived for 1 year.

Nearly everyone 'knows' that high sodium intake (salt) is a major risk factor for high blood pressure. But very few persons are knowledgeable enough to pay serious attention to sodium's working partner, potassium. Because sodium (Na) and potassium (K) must be in balance to maintain osmotic pressure between the intra-cellular fluids (inside the cells) and the extra-cellular fluids (outside the cells), a potassium deficiency from any cause can lead to water-logged tissues, muscle and tissue damage and subsequent scarring.

Nonetheless, many academic nutritional texts dismiss potassium deficiency as rare, pointing out it is easily available in so many foods. They forget that a junk-food diet of high fat, refined sugars and oversalted foods is all that's needed to play havoc with the body's tenuous reservoir of potassium. In addition, potassium can be depleted by excessive sweating, protracted diarrhea, the use of diuretics, overzealous dieting or fasting, extreme stress or any number of abnormal conditions. Aspirin and other drugs, coffee and alcohol, are all known to leech potassium from the cells.

To quote Dr. Birger Jansson, a University of Texas oncology specialist, "Since Paleolithic times, the potassium/sodium ratio in the diet has been reduced by a factor of almost twenty." Dr. Jansson proceeds to note that even in today's primitive cultures, the K/Na ratios are 100 to 200 times as great as ours. The author believes there would be a significant reduction in cardiovascvular disease and cancer incidence if potassium/sodium ratios could be brought back into balance.

Given the possibility of substantial and widespread potassium deficiency, what are the dangers? Insufficient potassium is de-energizing. In one clinical study, healthy volunteers fed a potassium deficient diet for just one week suffered muscular weakness, lethargy and extreme fatigue.

Deprived of potassium, muscles get flabby, intestinal motility is reduced leading to constipation. Poor eyesight, throbbing migraine headaches, insomnia and bruises, cuts and injuries that resist healing are but a few of the more disheartening symptoms. Potassium deficiency has been related to kidney failure, and to tinnitus (ringing in the ears.)

It can be much more serious than that. Nerve conduction is largely dependent on there being a high concentration of potassium ions and a low concentration of sodium and chloride ions within the aqueous solution surrounding the myelinated fibers that form the bulk of human nerves. Inadequate potassium causes cardiac abnormalities and a slow, weak, irregular pulse and may be the primary cause of sudden death from heart attacks.

EVIDENCE FROM OUTER SPACE

How important is potassium to a regular heartbeat? Ask NASA's top medico, Dr. Charles Berry, who supervised the health of Apollo 15's astronauts David Scott and James Irwin. When both space travelers developed irregular heartbeats during their trip to the moon, Dr. Berry determined they'd been endangered by a potassium loss, caused by the low potassium over-refined "foods" necessitated by space travel. The solution? From Apollo 16 on, astronauts' hearts have been buttressed by a potassium-loaded pre-flight diet and they're supplied with potassium-enriched food and snacks while floating through space.

When it comes to heart disease, high blood pressure is the "biggie". Labeled the "silent killer," this ailment suffered by an estimated one in four adults, is a leading cause of strokes, heart attacks and deaths.

Drugs and diet are the usual prescription, with more emphasis on one or the other, according to the doctor's medical orientation. Doctors familiar with the most recent research are more apt to chuck drugs and rely on dietary potassium and potassium supplementation.

Several published studies show the addition of dietary potassium leads to lower stroke mortality in the black populations (African-Americans are three times as likely as whites to have severe high blood pressure) and has proven effective against hypertension in elderly Americans. The British Medical Journal has reported positive results (lowered blood pressure and a significant reduction in serum cholesterol) using potassium supplementation in 37 hypertensive adults in a double-blind placebo-controlled crossover trial lasting 32 weeks. A placebo-controlled trial conducted by cardiologists at the University of Nairobi also upheld the benefit of potassium supplementation, this time with patients suffering only mild hypertension.

Dr. William Castelli, director of the famed Framingham (Mass.) Heart Study and a lecturer in preventive medicine at Harvard Medical School, is pro-potassium, since he's found it lowers blood pressure, and reduces cholesterol. An equally prestigious cardiologist, Dr. Norman Kaplan, believes adults should consume at least 2,000 milligrams of potassium a day.

Should you be 'upping' your potassium stores? Probably so, but don't count on bananas (the most popular recommendation) to do it for you. Always thought to be the safest of fruits, bananas are now on the 'suspicious' list, possibly the most seriously pesticide poisoned. How come? Chemicals banned in the United States since the late 70's are routinely shipped to other countries, used on their crops, then come back in the foodstuff we import from other nations.

That's the case with bananas, according to a small band of consumer watchdogs who recently trumpeted news that a particularly potent pesticide, aldicarb, used by foreign fruit growers, seeps through tree roots, up into the fruit, contaminating all parts of the flesh. How do they know? Excessive levels of Temik (aldicarb's trade name) were recently discovered in bananas from test fields in Central and South America.

If bananas are a "no-no", what's left?

ORAL CHELATES?

Over the years, we've been repeatedly asked: "What about an oral chelate?" An understandable question. How much easier it would be - and more convenient - if we could pop an EDTA pill each morning, and avoid the hassle of the three hour infusion.

No such luck. EDTA doesn't work via the digestive tract. There are 'magnificent pretenders' on the market so don't be taken in by products advertised as an EDTA substitute.

Which is not to say an effective oral chelating formulation is impossible to concoct. Dr. Kurt Donsbach, the dean of nutritional medicine, is convinced that any compound combining all those ingredients known to reduce free radical activity as well as combining the specific nutrients necessary to keep heart and circulatory systems healthy, would fill the bill.

There's reason to believe he's on the right track. Long-time users of high levels of anti-oxidants are similar in many phsyiologic parameters to chelated patients. According to Dr. Donsbach, you can protect yourself against the possibility of heart disease (or restore your body to normalcy if you already have such a disease) by consuming all of the nutrients the body uses to abort or neutralize explosive free radical action on a daily basis.

More easily said than done. Tissue-specific antioxidants while important and effective, still leave much to be desired.

Studies have shown that supplements bound in a food matrix, the way nature intended, are superior to those composed of bare vitamins and minerals such as found in pharmaceutical products. Nature operates holistically, and this holds true for nature's foods. Taking supplements is in some sense 'unnatural', but the closer they resemble a natural product, the better the prospect they'll work synergistically with the body's systems to boost health.

BACK TO THE FUTURE

If you've been hearing a lot about herbs of late, it's because they're enjoying a renaissance in response to the 'back to nature' movement that's sweeping the health conscious. Are we reinventing the wheel? Yes and no.

It should come as no surprise that roots, seeds and leaves have the power to heal. Back at the dawn of time, the Chinese drank ginger tea for indigestion, which centuries later evolved into a British ginger-based stomach soother, which turned into today's ginger ale which modern American doctors still prescribe for mild stomach upsets.

Among the many remedies taken over by Western medicine from the ancient Chinese are rhubarb, castor oil, kaolin, camphor, and ginseng. Long before Hippocrates, primitive physicians knew about making vegetables into drugs. Derived from medicinal plants, many of these substances eventually found their way into western pharmacies, thanks to modern scientific methods.

America's medicine chests are crammed with drugs with herbal roots: aspirin, Sudafed, Metamucil. Despite the fact that a large percentage of U.S. prescription medications are still derived from plants, the average citizen seems more receptive to herbal remedies than the average doctor. No doubt a large segment of the population has lost faith with chemical drugs. They are properly fearful of side effects, and avidly seeking more natural alternatives.

Given the public's appetite for harmless ingredients, and their aversion to unsafe substances, we can appreciate the rapidly growing popularity of a 'new' - really 'old' - herbal formula that appears to be just what the public has been seeking. While writing this book several nutritionally-oriented doctors we'd been in touch with over the years, called our attention to a potassium-rich liquid, Km by name - (a 60 year old formula produced by Matol, Inc. of Canada). He recommended it as a reliable natural means of satisfying mineral requirements and 'upping' energy levels. A closer study of the ingredients that make up this unique botanical formula, suggests it provides much, much more.

According to the product literature, Km is concocted from 14 herbs: chamomile flower, saw palmetto berry, cascara sagrada, angelica root, thyme, passion flower, gentian root, licorice root, horehound root, senega root, celery seed, sarsaparilla root, alfalfa and dandelion root.

Check any recently published herbal guide, as we did, and you'll discover that the herbs mentioned are rich in the antioxidant Vitamins A, C and E; in the nerve-regulating B-complex nutrients; they're abundant sources of the essential minerals, calcium, magnesium, manganese and potassium, in iron, other trace minerals and indispensable oils as well as unidentified plant byproducts. All of which seems to add up to Km being the closest simulation yet to the "oral chelate" so many have been seeking for so long a time.

Make no mistake. The term 'oral chelate' is probably a misnomer, inasmuch as nothing but a genuine infusion of EDTA will systematically remove the heavy metals circulating through the blood stream. The intravenous procedure is surely preferable when heart health has deteriorated to the point where surgical intervention has been suggested, or there is some indication free-radical pathology has progressed to a point requiring strenuous remedies.

But if your health is not that far gone, or you are seeking

all-round supplementation to rejuvenate and revitalize your-self, Km is probably the most "user-friendly" nutritional product to be found. Its ingredients, being natural, work in harmony with each other and within the body. When herbal preparations are free of binders and fillers, more of their beneficial properties get into the bloodstream.

It's possible a superior concoction will emerge someday. Until it does, we take Km for the simplest reason - we haven't found anything better. We haven't found anything nearly as good. For more information, or the name of a distributor near you, the toll-free number: 1-800-638-8807.

No discussion of the importance of nutritional supple-mentation can possibly ignore the FDA's big vitamin crackdown, which threatens to severely restrict consumer access to health-food products. Things are getting tense, now that the FDA has adopted a super-aggressive stance, claiming that any supplement said to have a health benefit makes it a "drug", subject to federal regulation and illegal to sell until it's gone through years of multi-million dollar testing for safety and effectiveness.

Sending shock waves throughout the nutritionally-aware is H.R. 3642, the proposed Congressional legislation that's in-tended to beef up the FDA's enforcement powers, giving that agency gestapo-like authority over people's health.

Is this a wonderful country or what? Are we about to face off in the battle of the century? The vitamin-takers in one corner and the drug pushers in the other? Where does this controversy leave carrots? Apples? Grapefruit? All the foods known to lower cholesterol? What distinction can be made between recom-mending legumes such as chick peas and brown beans as a hearty appetitite-pleasing dish and the same vittles as a cholesterol-lowering food? If advocating vitamin pills can get one in big trouble, will recommending vegetables do the same?

If you have thoughts on the subject - we'll bet you do - wire your Congressman at once.

> *Our natures are the physicians of our diseases. This tendency to natural cure should be fostered, with all emphasis on diet and few drugs.*
>
> Hippocrates - 460BC

18

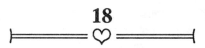

EATING TO YOUR HEART'S CONTENT

"Tell me what you eat, and I'll tell you what you are."

So said a famous 18th century physician. Translated into today's terms, that could mean:

If you're a calorie-counter, you are appearance, fashion and beauty-conscious, more interested in your looks than your health;

If you're a junk and/or fast food junkie, you're either so young you think you're immortal, or so old you think that what you eat no longer matters;

If you eat what you please with no consideration of health implications, you are either a space alien, or a Rip Van Winkle look-alike.

If you've recently switched from butter to margarine, from half-and-half to non-dairy creamers, from real eggs to 'egg beaters', and have made 'no-cholesterol' your primary food-buying standard, you're a well-intentioned individual who wants to do what's right, but have been misled into making unhealthy choices.

You may *think* you're eating properly, but not be nutritionally savvy. To find out whether you know enough to eat as well as you'd like, take this short quiz:

1: Rank the saturated fat contents of these oils (from lowest to highest): **(a)** canola; **(b)** coconut; **(c)** corn; **(d)** cottonseed; **(e)** olive; **(f)** palm; **(g)** peanut; **(h)** safflower; **(i)** soybean; **(j)** sunflower.

ANSWER: Canola is lowest, followed by safflower, sunflower, corn, soybean, olive, peanut, cottonseed, palm, coconut oils.

2: True or False? Most people can eat a dozen or more eggs a week without seriously increasing cholesterol levels?

ANSWER: True. In studies at Rockefeller University, two out of three subjects who ate three eggs a day had only a slight rise in blood cholesterol.

3: Rank these foods' fiber contents, highest to lowest: **(a)** 3 dried prunes; **(b)** 1/3 cup (before cooking) oatmeal; **(c)** 1/2 cup (cooked) kidney beans; **(d)** 1 potato with skin; **(e)** 1 apple.

ANSWER: Kidney beans are the highest with 7.5 grams of fiber, then apple 3.5; oatmeal 3; potato 2.5; prunes 2.

4: How do you rank these fresh foods' overall nutritional value, highest to lowest? **(a)** asparagus; **(b)** broccoli; **(c)** collard greens; **(d)** cucumber; **(e)** eggplant; **(f)** mushrooms; **(g)** sweet corn; **(h)** zucchini.

ANSWER: Collard greens are the highest, with 90 of a possible 100 points; then broccoli, 68; asparagus, 67; sweet corn, 41; zucchini, 22; eggplant, 18; mushroom, 9; cucumber, 6.

5: Rank these foods' calorie contents, lowest to highest: **(a)** 2 large eggs; **(b)** 1 cup chicken a' la king; **(c)** 1 cup popcorn, lightly buttered and salted; **(d)** 1 avocado;

(e) 8 ounces fruit-flavored yogurt; **(f)** 1 cup pecans; **(g)** 3 tablespoons sour cream.

ANSWER: Popcorn is lowest with 55 calories; then sour cream with 75; eggs with 150; yogurt 230; avocado 340; chicken a la king, 470; pecans, 720.

6: True or False? Carob candy bars are much more nutritious than regular milk chocolate bars.

ANSWER: False. Both candies are loaded with fat and sugar, and contrary to what you may have thought, the so-called 'healthy' carob bars are usually made with palm or coconut oil, highly saturated fats more conducive to heart disease than beef fat.

7: True or False? Most of the cholesterol in your body comes from the food you eat.

ANSWER: False. Eighty percent of the cholesterol in your body is manufactured by your liver. If you could eliminate *all* cholesterol from your diet, your liver would produce enough to satisfy cellular needs.

8: This question for label readers: Which of the following common additives are safe? which are not? **(a)** BHA and BHT; **(b)** MSG; **(c)** sulfites; **(d)** calcium propionate; **(e)** mono-and diglycerides; **(f)** EDTA

ANSWER: The first three (a), (b) and (c) are the ones to avoid. BHA and BHT are potentially carcinogenic shelf life extenders; MSG causes the allergic reaction better known as the "Chinese Restaurant Syndrome"; sulfites have been known to provoke fatal breathing difficulties in sensitive asthmatics; (d), (e) and (f) are the 'good guys'. Yes, EDTA as a food preservative has been given a high safety rating by the Center for Science in the Public Interest.

How did you do? If you flunked (didn't answer **every** question correctly), chances are your nutrition education has come from 'advertorials': the gratuitous dietary advice presented by the daily papers, TV news and other ad-supported media, and prepared by nutrition-illiterates: a high-paid horde of ad agency hired hotshot copywriters.

TRIMMING MISCONCEPTIONS OUT OF YOUR DIET

According to a recent Gallup Poll, most Americans really DO want to get their diets on target. We are no longer strictly meat-and-potato eaters. Chicken and broccoli are just as popular as main dish ingredients these days. More than three-quarters of those questioned said they'd pay more for produce that was tested and certified as being pesticide-free; 25 percent said they'd pay *double* the normal price for such assurance.

Despite such stated good intentions, the *American Journal of Public Health* reports that on an average day, 40 percent of Americans go without fruit, 20 percent eat no vegetables, and more than 80 percent pass up whole-grain breads and high-fiber grains and cereals.

But Americans do pay close attention to food news. Most have heard that bran can help lower cholesterol levels, that organic produce is more healthful, and that salt-laden diets can lead to high blood pressure. Also, we take scary food news seriously. Almost 75% of the respondents say they start cutting down immediately on any food linked to a health risk.

Where do we fall down? Much as we'd like to eat smart, we don't know how. More than half of those surveyed mistakenly said that high cholesterol - not fat, additives or nutrient-stripped foods - is the biggest problem with the American diet. Moreover, those who flunked this question believed they heard it from the Surgeon General.

We're also clogged with confusion when it comes to cholesterol. Two out of three erroneously said the way to go about lowering levels is to eat less cholesterol. Only one out of three understood they needed to reduce fat intake. Fewer still understood that high cholesterol levels are a symptom - not a cause - of disease.

Finally, we'd far rather cut back on simple staples - milk, meat, cheese - than give up rich desserts. Even those who suspect they ought to ditch the fat out of our diet, think they can do it without giving up cake, ice cream and similar treats.

CHOLESTEROLPHOBIA EXPOSED

No doubt about it. Americans are hooked on horror, obsessed with scare-you-silly diversions. We shell out big bucks for heart-stopping Stephen King novels and horror films. In every amusement park, the roller coaster ride that pushes nerves to the screaming limits boasts the longest ticket line.

If nightmare grade flicks are your idea of entertainment, no harm done. But if you've allowed "cholesterolphobia" to turn mealtime into a chilling experience, that's carrying fun too far.

You might suspect something's amiss when "cholesterol-free" is *the* buzz word in almost every food ad. Cashing in on public panic is so profitable, we expect to see claims for cholesterol-free coffee and cat food any day now.

Monitoring one's cholesterol has replaced baseball as the national pastime. "What's the score?" has been supplanted by "What's your number?" A new Gallup Poll finds that 32% of adults know their cholesterol level - up from 17% a year ago. School kids learn their HDL's and LDL's with their ABC's.

Leave it to America's fad-conscious merchandisers to spot a hot trend. Discount stores have installed cholesterol testing kiosks in place of other traffic-builders. They've proven popular despite published warnings that many sell inaccurate screenings, are unsanitary and improperly administered.

CHOLESTEROL. What do we really know about it? Consistently described as 'waxy' and 'fatty' and in other 'ugh' terms, there's not one kind word written about this natural substance, although it's essential to life, found in nearly every cell, and vitally needed to form cell membranes and to deliver essential fluids such as the sex hormones and bile acids to cells.

Hardly a mention that the body makes its own cholesterol, nor that body-made cholesterol is identical in every way to the kind you eat. Not so much as a whisper that it's been repeatedly shown that the less cholesterol a person eats, the more the body produces - that the body sets a cholesterol level for itself, in response to a multitude of biochemical and metabolic events, most of which we do not yet understand.

What we are fed instead is a strident, ever-escalating barrage of grim warnings naming cholesterol as the leading risk factor of heart disease and early death. Fueling the frenzy are hundreds of newspaper and magazine articles and of course best-sellers, prescribing a 'cholesterol cure'. The very promise is inaccurate, since cholesterol *isn't* a disease. Few understand that elevated cholesterol levels - like a high fever when a flu or other infectious virus attacks - is the body's effort to combat a disease process already taking place. Can you cure pneumonia by reducing fever with aspirin? No more than you can cure free radical disease by eliminating cholesterol-containing foods from your diet.

The result of misinformation? 'Cholesterolphobia' - best described as the needless and unfounded fear of dietary cholesterol. If you've been traumatized by the media-sustained anti-cholesterol campaign, you may be further horrified to learn that much of what you've read and heard has little scientific support.

CHOLESTEROLPHOBIA -
IS THERE CAUSE FOR CONCERN?

Here's one astute observer's opinion on cholesterol:
> *I really find it very droll-*
> *This fuss about cholesterol.*
> *The question now that's paramount*
> *Is 'Cholesterol? Why, what's your count?'*
> *And arteries devoid of fat*

Can make you an aristocrat.
While others shrink in perfect dread
For fear their lab tests will be read.
So 'ho' for oat bran, 'ho' for hype!
Fleece the suckers! Time is ripe.
Kellogg's stock is rising fast.
Make your profits. Have a blast.
Peddle muffins. Sell those pills.
Forget about the other ills.
Tell those doctors to endorse
All the food that suits a horse!"

Contrary to the impression given by ad campaigns, the jury is still out on whether there's any basis for the anti-cholesterol crusade. A three decades old controversy is raging in medical and nutritional circles, with the embattled authorities more at odds than ever before.

There are three distinct points of contention: **(1)** whether high serum cholesterol levels cause coronary artery disease; **(2)** whether the lowering of serum cholesterol levels will reduce the risk of heart disease and/or increase longevity; and **(3)** whether a low-cholesterol diet can have a beneficial effect on serum cholesterol levels and/or overall health.

The only issue on which you can extract almost universal agreement is this: Cholesterol's role is complicated and open to many questions; so is the part it plays in a not well understood disease.

WHERE DID IT ALL START

Much of the current anti-cholesterol hype is founded on an outmoded 1950's era theory - a theory, you ought to know, that has been contradicted by the very studies most frequently cited in support. At one time, physicians and scientists viewed the deposits that accumulate in arteries as caused by too much cholesterol in the blood. Thus, many jumped to the impulsive conclusion that this could only happen as the result of too much cholesterol in the diet. More thoughtful reviewers voiced their dissent, but were not well heard, though the famous Framingham study proved the 'cholesterol equals heart disease' notion wrong in 1970. **So eminent an authority as Dr. Michael E. DeBakey, prominent cardiologist at Baylor College of Medicine in Houston, reported in early 1977 that most heart patients he has operated on had "perfectly normal cholesterol levels."**

An early critic of the over-emphasis on cholesterol, Dr. Edward R. Pinckney, editor of the *Journal of the American Medical Association*, a Life Fellow of the American College of Physicians, author of five books on medicine and more than 100 scientific articles and books for the medical profession, wrote one of the first editorials blasting cholesterol-blamers.

In his 1973 book, *The Cholesterol Controversy,* he stated categorically: "There is no scientific evidence to show that a high blood cholesterol is the cause of heart disease or that lowering cholesterol - if such a thing is possible - will prevent heart troubles of any kind."

Almost twenty years later, there have been no new discoveries to refute him. Interviewed in 1987, he said: "I said it before, I say it today. The cholesterol controversy is a juggernaut based on no facts."

Almost totally ignored by the anti-cholesterol alarmists have been the findings of each of the following studies, **all showing that low-cholesterol diets DON'T reduce heart disease:**

- The St. Mary's Hospital Trial (1965)
- The London Research Committee Trial (1965)
- The Norwegian Trial (1966)
- The Anti-Coronary Club Trial (1966)
- The London Medical Research Council Trial (1968)
- The National Diet Heart Study (1968)
- The Finnish Mental Hospital Trial (1968)

- The Los Angeles Veteran's Trial (1969)
- The Framingham Study (1970)
- The Ireland-Boston Heart Study (1970)
- The St. Vincent's Hospital Trial (1973)
- The Diet and Coronary Heart Disease Study in England (1974)
- The Edinburgh-Stockholm Study (1975)
- The Minnesota Study (1975)
- The UCLA Study (1975)
- The Honolulu-Japanese Study (1975)

Additionally, the Coronary Drug Project in 1974 showed that drugs that reduced blood cholesterol were of no value in preventing heart disease.

Almost all new studies find no increased lingevity as reward for low cholesterol, and many raise uncomfortable concerns that there can be formerly unsuspected hazards. An ongoing study of 7,850 Hawaiian men reveals that those with cholesterol below 190 were twice as likely to have a cerebral hemorrhage; a large Japanese study came to much the same conclusion; so did the government's Multiple Risk Factor Intervention Trial (MRFIT); and an analysis of the health records of 12,000 American men and women showed a decided link between low cholesterol and higher rates of cancer of the lung, pancreas, bladder, cervix and blood.

If you've never heard of these studies, that's pleasing news to those hawking low-cholesterol foods. They would rather you didn't know that it's a myth that it's the cholesterol in your food that makes you sick. More to the point, since dietary cholesterol cannot and should not be totally avoided, it is unscientific, unfair and unhealthy to foster cholesterolphobia on the American public.

The ultimate irony is that as Americans become more health conscious and worry more about cholesterol, they inevitably switch to unhealthy foods. Eager to make sweeping dietary changes, the cholesterol-conscious rush to replace nutritious edibles with noxious substitutes. Many of the replacements chosen contain tropical oils and processed fats which break down into free-radical compounds proven to damage and destroy body cells. Wanting to do what's right, but not knowing the whole story, few consumers realize which items deserve to be carved out of the diet - by all rights, the foods containing excessive dietary fat and oxycholesterol (cholesterol damaged by oxidation).

THE NO CHOLESTEROL CRAZE - WHY NOW?

The current grandiose anti-cholesterol campaign began in 1987 with the formation of the National Cholesterol Education Program, which, in concert with the AMA, drug manufacturers, and cereal advertisers launched a major marketing scheme using books, videocassettes, study guides, pamphlets, round-the-clock publicity, national and local TV and all the media coverage they could round up to convince the public of the dangers of cholesterol.

Completely overlooked amid all the hoopla was the reality that the well orchestrated explosion of cholesterol condemnation was not triggered by any major scientific breakthrough. The cut-out-cholesterol crusade expanded despite the lack of new evidentiary findings or conclusive studies or any scientific proof whatsoever that the cholesterol-lowering mandate was based on solid factual data.

The hard sell was on, although experts with equally impressive credentials, looking at the same data, often came to far different opinions on the best method and/or desirability of lowering cholesterol levels. Critical inquiry in legitimate scientific journals received short shrift. Rockefeller University Professor Edward H. Ahrens, Jr. is one who has complained that the anti-cholesterol forces have made an unconscionable exaggeration of the data; no less a notable than former American Heart Association president Thomas N. James is among those who attempted to point out the public was being kept in the dark about the lack of unanimity or consensus among experts.

Indeed, the deeper scientists probe the diet question, the more diverse their opinions. There is no scientific evidence that any of the recommended strategies work - and considering the unpredictable vagaries of biochemical individuality, even less proof that what works for one will work for you.

Why then all this furor to promote a scientifically unsustainable position? Make no mistake - you have been the target of a concentrated commercial effort of groups more interested in your money than your life line.

Dr. Pinckney nailed it way back when, pointing out drug companies, food manufacturers and the medical world all had much to gain from scaring people out of their good sense. Prophetic words!

Today, the well-respected authority Fredrick J. Stare, Founder of the Department of Nutrition at the Harvard School of Public Health, has voiced the same charge in his book, *Balanced Nutrition*. In concert with co-authors Robert E. Olson, Professor of Medicine at SUNY and Elizabeth M. Whelan, President of the American Council on Science and Health, Dr. Stare minces no words when he states: **"The national obsession with cholesterol levels and the way to reduce them is a dangerous fad, aided by a hype-intensive media assault for the benefit of a number of fast-buck-minded food processors."**

As Dr. Stare and his colleagues point out, "Contrary to what many have come to believe, most Americans (86% or more) DO NOT have significantly elevated serum cholesterol levels, and the few who do, should be consulting a physician for advice, not advertisements, talk shows or magazine articles."

Dr. Stare's outrage at the way the public has been misled is shared by anyone well versed in nutrition. Unfortunately, not many enlightened spokespersons have had their say.

"The American Heart Association, the National Heart, Blood and Lung Institute, The National Cholesterol Education Program, and most recently, The American Medical Association are recommending sweeping changes in the American diet - changes that will have no positive effect on the risk of heart disease for most citizens. It's an ill-advised attempt to diagnose and treat 250 million Americans at once, with a diet that has never been shown to have any lasting effect on serum cholesterol levels."

That might sound like the ravings of a radical outsider, were not those strident words coming from a Harvard-based expert whose opinions cannot be easily dismissed.

DIET OR DIE?

Unlike scientific brawls that normally take place behind ivy-covered walls, this fracas is being fought in public, for the struggle is not for your mind, but your dollars. Ever since the anti-cholesterol troops manned their battle stations, the fight has been to increase profits.

The drug companies, understandably excited by the potential of a massive newly created market for cholesterol-lowering medications, have packed medical journals with ads, and sent record numbers of drug reps pounding on physician's doors to induce sales. Cashing in on the oft-repeated pronouncement that millions of Americans - an estimated 60 percent of the adult population - suffer from either "dangerously high" or "borderline high" cholesterol, and that all the rest have some cause for concern, the medical profession automatically assured themselves of an endless stream of new patients, all racing to their doctors for tests, drugs, and life-long treatments. What a deal!

The newest cholesterol-lowering drug on the scene is lovastatin (sold as Mevacor). It burst on the scene in November, 1991, with reports claiming it can shrink fatty plaque deposits in coronary arteries, based on a two-year study involving 270 people conducted at the University of Southern California for Merck & Company, the drug's manufacturers.

Following claims that the study 'proved' the drug would reduce risk of heart disease death, the first reaction came from the stock market - it went wild!

How should you react? Our suggestion is you call your broker instead of your physician. Chances are the stock will be more profitable to your bank balance than the drug to your health.

After checking with a number of authoritative sources, this is what we found out about this newest 'miracle' drug:

1: Since press releases failed to report the amount of plaque reduction or the magnitude of blood flow increase, the alleged pharmaceutical triumph is highly suspect.

2: The release reported that plaque reduction was determined by angiography, a totally inaccurate measuring technique.

3: Lovastatin chemically resembles the drug Clofribate which has been found to double the risk of gallbladder disease and cause liver cancer in rats.

4: The "good news" about lovastatin was trumped throughout the land before safety tests have even begun.

5: Reducing cholesterol levels does not deal with the underlying disease. Lowering cholesterol levels over an extended period of time with a toxic drug is apt to prove foolhardy, if not fatal.

PUT THE DIAPER SET ON DRUGS?

What other industry can create new business so easily? Late in 1988, the American Academy of Pediatrics, perhaps feeling left out, posed questions no one else had thought to ask: "Should children be tested for cholesterol levels? And when?"

Not surprising, they answered the questions themselves in a way that assured them a share of the cholesterol pie: "Any child two years or older should be tested if any close relative has high blood cholesterol or an 'early' heart attack."

And then what? They recommend a stringent low-fat diet, or a lifetime of cholesterol-lowering drugs.

"Wait just a minute!" says Dr. Stare.

"The idea of suggesting that a child of two years of age be placed on a low-fat, low-cholesterol diet . . . is incomprehensible. How on earth can small children benefit from such a diet?"

Benefit? How about the potential for harm? A recent study in the *American Journal of Diseases of Children* reported growth failure and severe weight loss in children placed on low-fat diets. No one knows how much damage might ultimately result from putting toddlers on so restrictive and artificial an eating regimen. Some alarmed scientists have warned of the possibility of brain damage.

Clearly the stakes are high when prudent voices are silenced. Even more alarming is that for the first time in history, Madison Avenue has taken charge of America's health. Slick ad agencies are the newly licensed authorities who have put the entire nation on a diet - the very diet, by the way, which was tried and FAILED as a heart disease prevention strategy back in 1971.

Who's paying the bill for all this advice? Not a hard question to answer: it's the companies with something to sell, of course. Open your paper and read a food-industry sponsored Sunday supplement entitled *The Truth About Cholesterol*. How inspiring. That's the 'truth' from the same wonderfulcorporations which once insisted smoking was sexy, sophisticated and safe. The major food conglomerates have spent millions of dollars to tailor and promote products for health-conscious shoppers. First they softened the market with anti-cholesterol propaganda; then they cashed in with products designed for consumers motivated to avoid the 'Big C'. A great marketing plan and one sure to benefit stockholders, but not much profit in it for innocent targets.

A margarine ad warns wives: "His heart is in your hands," suggesting women play Russian roulette with their mate's life if they don't switch to the advertised 'no cholesterol' product. Not true. What the ads don't tell you is this: margarines are as much as 35% 'trans' (the bad twisted molecules) fatty acids - free radical generators. Europe won't even allow the sales of our margarines because they are so high in trans-fatty acids. The ad-inspired margarine craze is profit-motivated, its benefits unsupported by science, and more harmful than the saturated fats they are designed to replace.

Similarly misleading life-saving claims are routine plugs for non-dairy creamers, whipped toppings, oat bran cereals and muffins, cookies, and crackers, mayonnaise and salad dressings, cooking oils and egg substitutes - the entire array of heavily advertised packaged and processed foods.

Major players race to develop new ways to capitalize on "cholesterolphobia." There's almost no end to the ingenious ways producers find to tinker with foods in the attempt to fatten profits. In the works now is a new technology said to remove as much as 90% of the cholesterol from egg yolks and to give eggs a longer shelf life.

The inventor is very secretive about the process, but is seeking venture capital with the promise that low cholesterol, long-lasting eggs will prove very valuable for food chains, nursing homes and hospitals, and potentially extremely profitable for the investors. Nowhere in the prospectus is there any indication that the new product will be good for consumers.

Every day brings a new contender in the race to jump on the profit bandwagon. Not too long ago, full page advertisements in major newspapers across the country trumpeted the benefits of Cho Low Tea, claimed to be "as effective as medically prescribed drugs" in reducing cholesterol. Dr. Harvey L. Alpern, the cardiologist quoted in the ad as having verified the tea's medical benefits, later admitted the product's claims were somewhat exaggerated, but "I don't think it would harm anyone."

True enough, if shelling out $29.85 for a 30-day supply of who-knows-how-it-tastes-or-what-it-does tea doesn't wreck your budget. Not true, if you're naive enough to follow the ad's advice to "Go ahead, eat your favorite foods" and you believe it's safe to pig out under the comfortable assurance the 'tea' will sweep your arteries clean.

IS THERE LIFE AFTER CHOLESTEROL?

The question remains: what are you to do while the experts are busily taking jabs at each other?

Don't misread the message. Food IS a health factor. Your diet DOES count. The point being, of course, you must change your eating habits in a way most apt to benefit you - not the pocketbooks of those advertisers whose claims are patently self-serving.

Use your common sense. This might be a good time to heed an old Wall Street aphorism: "When all the sheep are being herded in one direction, you can bet they're about to be fleeced."

Put your memory to work. If you're old enough to read this, you're old enough to remember that many of today's auspicious voices telling you how to diet to beat a heart attack were just a few short years back pooh-poohing Nathan Pritikin for claiming a diet and exercise program could reverse atherosclerosis. If they were wrong once, they can be wrong twice.

Be careful not to be flim-flammed into trading one poison for another. If you've given up breakfast doughnuts in favor of store-bought oat bran muffins, you could be consuming as much as 25 grams of the worst kind of fat (most commercial baked goods contain highly suspect partially hydro-genated soybean, cottonseed and/or palm, coconut or other tropical oils.)

We've bad news for margarine lovers. If you've switched from butter to margarine, you've swapped a natural, easily digestible fat with all the vital compensating nutrients for a far more deadly vegetable oil spread. A Dutch study shows that "transmonounsaturated fatty acids" are formed when polyun-saturated vegetable oil is converted into margarine that is solid or semi-solid at room temperature. If you cook with this processed fat - heat it, fry with it, or bake with it - there will be a chemical action between the polyunsaturates and the oxygen in the air that forms a polymer. Plastics are polymers. So is varnish and shellac. Think about this next time you're tempted to reach for any unnatural 'health' spread.

If you've given up eggs in favor of "egg-beaters", the yolks on you! How absurd to fall for the fiction that what Fleischmann's put in a box is healthier than what Mother Nature put in a shell.

The only time eggs get a good press is at Easter. The other 364 days in the year, they're maligned beyond all reason. We thought we were the only ones to remember eggs used to be called the "perfect food", until we heard the noted nutritionist Dr. Robert C. Atkins say so, too.

Dr. Atkins, whose unorthodox approach to diet and disease, often ruffles the feathers of the medical establishment takes the holistic view. If all doctors treated patients as he does, the drug industry would go bust, since he prescribes only 5% of the amount of drugs as his orthodox colleagues, treating patients with the same ailments, and gets better results!

As one of the more learned of the 'pro egg' physicians, Dr. Atkins explains: "Eggs contain a considerable amount of lecithin a cholesterol-lowering agent. They are an almost perfect protein."

Are eggs a health threat? Not according to the Tokyo Metropolitan Government's Institute of Gerontology, whose dietary survey of people aged 100 years or older revealed they now eat a variety of western foods, including daily servings of milk and eggs.

Dr. Hirotomo Ochi, director of research at the Institute for the Control of Aging in Shizuoka, says: "Eggs never seemed to harm Shigechiyo Izumi, who lived to be 120 years old. He ate eggs from the chickens he kept several times a week. Like other Japanese, he used eggs in a variety of ways - in soups custards and omelets, also by themselves."

If you're a terrified egg lover, and money is no object, you'll be a ready customer for the new "heart-healthier" eggs, produced in a way to insure higher levels of Vitamin E. Research conducted at the Medical College of Pennsylvania backs up the producer's claims that the new eggs, laid by hens fed E-rich canola oil, are a healthy strategy for cholesterolphobics. Be prepared, however, to pay two to three times as much as for 'normal' eggs.

WHAT IF THE DOCTOR SAYS: "TAKE THIS DRUG"?

If you've been prescribed a cholesterol-lowering drug, demand a complete list of the side effects and dangers before consenting to use it. Not long ago Mer/29 was advertised as a "breakthrough in anticholesterol" drugs and then had to be yanked off the market when it was found to cause dermatitis, changed hair color, loss of sex drive and a condition known as "alligator skin." There are twenty or more natural foods that can help normalize cholesterol levels safely and efficiently: carrots, apples, and other high fiber fruits and vegetables are good ones for starters.

Among the proven natural methods to lower cholesterol are these: fiber, which has the ability to increase the amount of cholesterol excreted in daily bowel movements; Vitamin B_3 (niacin) which is not only effective, but inexpensive; Vitamin C; calcium carbonate - two grams daily can reduce both cholesterol and triglyceride levels according to studies performed at St. Vincent's Hospital in Montclair, New Jersey; Vitamin E, selenium, avocados, lecithin, chromium, onions - cooked or raw; garlic, spirulina, pangamic acid (Vitamin B_{15}), black currents, yucca powder, olive oil, alfalfa tablets, and zinc supplementation. There are more - lots more.

To liberate yourself from "cholesterolphobia," learn how and when cholesterol can be a friend, not a foe. Sensible amounts of foods such as milk, cheese, butter, eggs, fish, beef, pork and lamb will not cause problems unless they're improperly cooked or carelessly stored - OR, if you consume too much.

Most important: do not allow yourself to be diverted or distracted from making the life style changes that have proven value. More on this in the chapters that follow.

THE FATS OF LIFE

Let's tackle the real rogue in your diet: fat overload. When your system becomes glutted with fat, the resulting free radical proliferation disrupts cellular homeostasis. In an effort to correct the imbalance, your body produces excessive amounts of cholesterol. **When you reduce fat consumption, you reduce free radical generation. As a consequence, your cells, given a chance to recuperate, will reduce their cholesterol requirements and cholesterol levels will drop.** In all but a few exceptions, this strategy works.

So fat is bad. Too much fat is very bad. But some fats are more evil than others. The most villainous of the lot are the adulterated fats, primarily because they are the most prolific free radical generators. This is an important distinction, especially since it means the saturated fats are far less offensive than the supposedly 'good-for-you' polyunsaturates, which are so zealously - and wrongly - promoted by the anti-cholesterol food mongers.

Sorting out the 'black hats' from the 'white hats' among the fats is not easy. Adding to the difficulty is the fact that often it's not the fats themselves but the way they're processed, stored, and used in the diet that makes for the difference.

Fats fall into four general classifications:

1: **Saturated fats** - (usually solid at room temperature) - are obtained primarily from animal sources and occur naturally in most meats, and butterfat products such as milk, cream, cheese and butter.

2: **Polyunsaturated fats** - (tend to be liquid at room temperature) - are derived from grains such as soy, corn, sunflower and safflower oils, and fish. Unsaturated fats in this category, however, are frequently converted into saturated fats by a commercial process called hydrogenation that food manufacturers use to give their products a longer shelf life. As a result many so-called 'polyunsaturates' - those prominent in bakery products, candies, margarine, salad dressings, vegetable shortening and mayonnaise - are highly saturated, and a prime example of a 'good' fat gone 'bad'.

3: **Monounsaturated fats** - found in olives and olive oil, almonds, peanuts, peanut butter and avocado - are generally applauded as the best of the lot. In recent years, research suggests that the mono-unsaturates have health-promoting properties;

4: **Hydrogenated fats and oils** - liquid fats made solid by adding hydrogen to the oil during processing - found in solid shortenings, margarine, baked goods, crackers, pie crust. Read labels carefully to avoid hydrogenated fats whenever possible.

If you're unclear as to which fats do what to your artery walls, no wonder. To a certain extent, it depends on whom you're talking to and when!

Going back a few years, almost no health authorities were alarmed that steak and butter-stuffed baked potatoes were a mainstay of the American diet. We ate what tasted good and no one thought much about it. Heart disease was something that just 'happened' and there wasn't a hint that what you ate made a difference. This complacent attitude was challenged in the 1950's when autopsies done on young American soldiers killed in the Korean War revealed a significant degree of arterial disease already in progress in men still in their early twenties. Scientists began to suspect something other than the aging process had to be responsible when autopsies on Korean soldiers did not show evidence of this disease.

Then, in 1961, came the startling news that being overweight wasn't the only consequence of fat in the diet. Dietary guidelines published by the American Heart Association urged everyone - not just would-be slimmers - to cut back. Since then, high-fat diets have been scientifically linked with a host of ailments - including cancer and heart disease - and low-fat eating has become a firmly established principle practically synonymous with good health.

For more than two decades now, the American public has been pestered, plagued, coaxed and wheedled to give up their porterhouse steaks and whipped cream desserts and urged to learn to love lean beans, veggies and fruits instead.

Good advice - as far as it goes. Most people know the foods that are rich in fat: meat, dairy products made from whole or 2% milk, oily spreads such as mayonnaise and salad dressings, chicken soup, gravy, fried foods, peanut butter and all nuts except the chestnut.

But to get on target, you need to know what makes one fat different from another, because reducing the amount of fat you consume may not be as crucial as eliminating the wrong kinds of fat from your diet.

Contrary to what television ads would have you believe, there's no evidence switching from butter to margarine prevents heart attacks. Quite the reverse. While both butter and margarine contain 80% fat, 1% protein and around 18% water (a teaspoon of each contains about 36 calories and 4.1 grams of fat, and when spread generously on a slice of bread contain about 40 calories) there's an important difference in the kind of fats found in each.

Margarine - which contains chemically altered fats - may be far more toxic to your heart's health than the natural fats contained in butter and other animal products.

Dr. Elmer Cranton explained why this is so in the book we co-authored, *Bypassing Bypass,* when he said: "Contrary to current popular mythology, it is not the saturated (animal) fats that are the 'bad guys' and the polyunsaturated fats (liquid oils of vegetables or seed origin) that are the 'good guys'. It is exactly the reverse if the oils have been exposed to light, heat and air in the extraction, bottling and food preparation process."

The point made is that the natural saturated fats (as found in butter, eggs, beef, etc.) can be eaten more safely than the (unnatural) commercially manufactured polyunsaturated fats, which become peroxidized (rancid) during processing. When food manufacturers hydrogenate fats to give their products longer shelf life - as they do with margarine, vegetable shortenings, non-dairy creamers and non-dairy toppings - they have turned these items into destructive substances the body cannot metabolize normally.

That's because the real problem with fats is not just the number of calories they add to your diet, but the health dangers they pose from free radical activity. Unless you've a Ph.D. in biochemistry, you're going to find it tough to understand the deadly effects of oxidized fats.

JACK SPRAT ATE NO FAT. HOW DID HE DO IT?

You can't begin to cut down on fats unless you're aware of all the 'hidden' fats in foods. The typical American diet actually puts the average individual at risk of consuming, over a lifetime, more than a TON (5,000 to 7,000 pounds) of pure fat.

For instance, while you don't see any fat on pound cake and brownies, the fact remains, more than thirty percent of the cakes and pastries commonly sold in American supermarkets either prepared or as mixes consist of fat. Ironically, the worst culprits are often products labeled 'light' - 63% of the calories in the instance of one nationally advertised product. The same holds true for candy bars - their main ingredients: sweet chocolate, dried coconut and nuts are all high-fat foods.

Worse still, the more fats you eat, hidden or not, the hungrier you get. Tests have shown animals and humans eat the most when offered their free choice of a cafeteria-style diet that contains large amounts of fats and sugars. Fats make foods taste good. Restricting intake of fats makes foods less tasty, so people eat less.

Cutting the fat out of your diet is easier said than done. If you eat at fast food restaurants, good nutrition becomes that much more difficult. On the average, 40 to 60 percent of the calories in fast foods come from fat. A double-beef Whopper with cheese at your local Burger King contains about 13 and a half teaspoons of fat; a Big Country breakfast with sausage at Hardee's is equally lethal with 15.9 teaspoons of fat. And while many people think that chicken and fish items are the best choices, they can be really bad when they're coated with batter and deep-fried. Even 'salad' options are not necessarily recommended for good health. Hard to believe, but it's a fact, that the fattiest food you can buy at a Taco Bell is a salad! Within the shell, their taco salad with ranch dressing, packs 1,204 calories and 20.6 teaspoons of fat (that's over 110 percent of the fat and 115 percent of the saturated fat the average adult should eat in an entire day).

Think you know your fast foods? Let's see. Guess which of these McDonald's desserts has the least fat?

(A) Cinnamon Raisin Danish; **(B)** Apple Pie; **(C)** Soft Serve Cone; **(D)** Chocolate Chip Cookies?

If you chose (C), you're right on target. All the others have three times as much.

An occasional meal at a fast-food spot won't do you in, but if you dine at such places regularly, here are some guidelines:

- **"Hold the sauces"** - skip the tartar, mayonnaise and cheese;
- **Forego 'fried'** - or discard the breading;
- **Cut out croissants** - they're high in calories and fat;
- **Pick 'plain'** - an ungarnished baked potato is nourishing, filling and virtually fat free. With a topping, such as sour cream, butter, bacon or cheese adds 640 calories and 6 teaspoons of fat; a plain roast beef or French dip sandwich is lower in fat than a hamburger, but not so once you top it with bacon, cheese and sauces; salad bars offer low-fat meal choices, provided you avoid high-fat toppings such as regular dressings, bacon, and cheeses, and side-step items mixed with dressings such as potato, carrot or macaroni salads;
- **Try eating a little 'dessert' first** - choose fresh fruit. It is a creative way to curb your appetite and avoid overeating.

It's just as important to be informed and creative when dining at home. Here are some practical suggestions offered by the American Holistic Medical Association:

1: In general, decrease the amount of beef and pork you eat. Serve beef in smaller portions (small portions in casseroles, smaller steaks, etc.). Avoid roasts and other large cuts of meat. Always use the leanest meat available. When a recipe calls for hamburger, always pre-cook it and drain off the fat before adding it to the dish.

2: As you eat less meat, eat more fish and lean fowl, since these are lower in total fat. Remove as much of the skin and subcutaneous fat as possible before eating fowl.

3: Use the dairy products with the lowest fat content, such as 1% fat cheese and cottage cheese. Use 1% low-fat or skim milk instead of whole milk.

4: Add as little oil, butter, milk or cream as possible to dishes and sauces. Use oil-free salad dressings or cut the fat content by mixing a low-fat dressing with equal parts of low-fat yogurt. Lemons or herbs may be used as an oil-alternative.

5: Limit your intake of ice cream, cakes, pies and pudding since these contain excess fats.

We assume that by now you're convinced that cutting down on fat makes sense. But how much you are willing - or able - to cut down depends on your motivation. Scaring people about the health consequences of their action rarely works. All too often, folks justify self-destructive behavior by telling themselves: "I know I should stop smoking, eat a healthier diet, exercise regularly, wear my seat belt – and someday I will. In the meantime, nothing bad is going to happen to me."

How else to explain why sales of super-fatty gourmet brands of ice cream are enjoying ever increasing popularity? Potato chip, candy, chocolate and croissant sales are also bringing fat profits. Despite all the publicity given to the health risks of eating such foods, their popularity has soared at the very time Americans are supposedly becoming more health conscious.

If you've been listening, but done more worrying than changing, one solution to switching to a more healthful diet is to develop a backlog of recipes that you'll really enjoy. The first thing most people think when they hear 'low-fat' is "Awk!" Calvin Trillin might have been speaking for the multitudes when he said, "Health foods make me sick."

Heart-saving foods need not be bland and unsatisfying. They can be tantalizing and delicious. Visit your bookshop or library. There are dozens of really good cookbooks on the market to help you prepare nutritionally sound-delicious-meals.

Meals that heal make dinnertime a real joy. To help you find fat-free fun-to-eat food, you'll find a sampling of our family's favorite recipes in a later chapter.

There are some foods which are extremely detrimental
and it is proper for men never to eat them,
such as large salted old fish,
old salted cheese, truffles, mushrooms,
old salted meat, wine must,
and a cooked dish which has been kept
until it acquired a foul odor.

Moses ben Maimon (1135-1204)

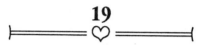

THE WORLD'S OLDEST AND HEALTHIEST DIET

"How come my doctor knows so little about nutrition?"

Good question. It's one that mystifies many who find it hard to believe so many doctors were raised by food-illiterate mothers. A possible explanation is that despite what good eating habits the young would-be M.D. learned at home, he is educated in med school to embrace an anti-nutrition stance.

A study published in the *American Journal of Clinical Nutrition* found that although most (74%) matriculating freshmen rate nutrition important at the outset, few (13%) retain that view after two years of medical schooling. Of the 125 medical schools in the U.S., only 30 have even one required course in nutrition; the average U.S. med student receives a total of 2.5 hours training in nutrition during 4 years of medical school. Why are doctors systematically discouraged from considering nutrition significant?

The pharmaceutical industry, which influences med school curriculum (by providing the research funds to support university labs), would rather young docs learn to depend on drugs than natural cures. Once graduated, most doctors receive ongoing medical education via the drug detailmen who visit their offices periodically to provide literature and inform them of medical advances - (translated into English that means an update on their firm's newest FDA-approved drugs) - or if they are avid followers of the medical journals, they'll read 'advertorials' - research reports favoring the very drugs promoted in the periodical's ads.

Nor do physicians smarten up after they've been in practice long enough to think for themselves. As Dr. Jean Mayer, the distinguished medical professor from Harvard University, discovered: **"We have just completed a study to find out what the average doctor at Harvard knows about nutrition. What we found is this: the average doctor knows a wee bit more about nutrition than his secretary, unless his secretary has a weight problem, in which case the average secretary knows a wee bit more about nutrition than the average doctor."**

If you want to solve your health problems with food, you're on your own. However, no matter how strongly you resolve to 'eat better', you'll have to sift through contradictory advice from a variety of sources. If watching the experts squabble leaves you confused, take heart. There is a treasure trove of reliable dietary philosophy you may have overlooked.

THE BIBLE

You needn't be religious to recognize the Good Book as an excellent source of nutritional counsel. While some biblical diet dictums are not easy to follow, since modern food processing does things to foods the good Lord never intended, the general principles are worth heeding. Without benefit of scientific research, writers of the scriptures recorded healthful and life-promoting nutritional wisdom.

To refresh your memory - many Biblical notables enjoyed long and productive lives. Physically vigorous, with amazing mental clarity, they were fertile into their eighties and beyond. If diet had anything to do with their extraordinary good health, we'd do well to follow their example.

What does the Bible recommend?

- **An abundance of whole grains.** In Biblical days, flat leaves of fragrant, coarse brown bread were a diet mainstay. Nowadays, you have to explore farmer's markets and health food stores to find whole grain bread without additives and preservatives. However, you can bake bread at home, or buy whole grain pita bread, or try matzo.

   Baked by the Israelites' when they were fleeing Egypt, matzo is for sale in most supermarkets and is an excellent cracker or bread substitute. Whole wheat matzo is made from whole-wheat flour, wheat bran and water. One large piece has 110 calories, and is fat and salt-free. If you find matzo unappetizing - (Marilyn Monroe once asked: "Isn't there any other part of the matzo you can eat?") - pita bread is a tasty possibility, providing you read the package label carefully.

- **Beans and peas ('legumes') along with other high fiber foods.** Today we know that beans are longevity-boosters. Scientists at the University of Alabama recently confirmed that soybeans are a woman's best defense against breast cancer. Some agent in soybeans appears to mimic the action of a drug called tamoxifen, blocking tumor development. Only one in 50 to 80 Chinese and Japanese soybean-eating women develop breast cancer, as against one in ten among American females.

- **Artery-cleansing foods.** While in Egypt, the Israelites survived primarily on such fruits and vegetables as melons, cucumbers, leeks, onions and garlic - the very items since found to elevate blood levels of HDL (the helpful form of cholesterol), bring down LDL (the dangerous form), to keep fatty deposits in the blood stream under control, and prevent excessive clotting.

- **Seafood.** In the Old Testament, the ancients recommended fish: they specifically named fish with fins and scales, such as mackerel, salmon, bluefish, mullet, rainbow trout, butterfish and pompano. These are the same ones currently recommended for their high content of the fish oils that lower blood triglyceride (fat) levels.

- **Honey.** Solomon, writing in Proverbs said: "My son, eat honey, because it is good." Moses ate honey in the fields; the Promised Land was called a "land of milk and honey," symbolizing a place of eternal youth. Current scientific research confirms that honey contains many nutrients not present in other sweeteners. More recently, researchers have discovered that Propolis, a substance derived from honey combs, enhances immunological function.

- **Meatless, low-fat meals.** In Leviticus 3:17, the scriptures state: "It shall be a perpetual statute for your generations throughout all your dwellings that ye eat neither fat nor blood."

This was an easy statute for the Israelites to obey since there were no fast-food drive-ins in the wilderness serving up fatty burgers and deep-fried chicken, fish and potatoes.

TAKE TWO ONIONS AND CALL ME IN THE MORNING

The ancient idea of food as medicine is suddenly coming back into vogue. In November of 1991, CBS devoted an entire week to a *Meals That Heal* series spotlighting the National Cancer Institute's Designer Foods Research Project. The telecast indicates the race is on in the nation's labs to concoct "superfoods" that will fight, even prevent, heart disease and cancer - this time with the blessing of the FDA and the U.S. Government.

High-tech diets loaded with the phytochemicals locked inside common fruits, vegetables and other edible plants such as herbs, grains and spices, are proclaimed as the wave of the future. How strange that what the "health nuts" have been saying for years - and biblical wise men testified to centuries ago - is now hailed as the new medical frontier.

While the Bible does not mention vitamins, calories or minerals, it clearly recognizes that poor eating habits result in disease that good foods cure. Health professionals now looking at foods the same way agree with the ancient prophets. More than 5,000 scientific studies have confirmed the food-disease connection, and the amazing curative powers of common everyday foods.

For example, take garlic, now considered a first aid food. For many people the mention of this herb conjures thoughts of exotically - and possibly excessively - seasoned dishes. But for some medical mavens, garlic means healing. Modern studies have credited raw garlic with myriad benefits. Among them: lowering blood cholesterol, killing the viruses that cause cold sores and one form of influenza, breaking down blood clots that can cause heart attacks and strokes, and neutralizing agents that can cause stomach cancer. Three different studies have linked high garlic consumption with lowered stomach and colon cancer risk.

The compound responsible for both garlic's smell and its medicinal abilities is allicin, which forms when two substances within garlic react when a clove is crushed, sliced or minced. Allicin is said to fight bacterial infection and acts as a heavy duty antibiotic. Cooking destroys allicin, but enhances another healthful compound, ajoene, which is also a potent anti-clotting agent with the ability to prevent heart attacks. A 1986

Japanese study found that ajoene is also a powerful anti-fungal agent, impeding the growth of two common fungi, including the candida albicans that is responsible for yeast infections.

Other components of garlic help the body eliminate toxins such as food preservatives, dyes and additives. Still others hunt for free radicals. These findings and others make garlic a leader in the world of medicine. The *Journal of the National Medical Association* has called garlic "the best example of the philosophy that your medicine should be your food and your food should be your medicine."

POWER TO THE PEPPER

We think it astonishingly prophetic that many Bible-favored foods are the very ones with a super-supply of the newly discovered free-radical fighting anti-oxidants (namely vitamins A, C and E). For example, citrus fruits, high-carbohydrate vegetables, whole grains, beans, high-fiber fruits, peppers, onions, the garlic group, berries, nuts and seeds.

Let's look at flaxseed, currently receiving much attention. It contains two major classes of compounds linked with anti-cancer activity, one of which is a fiber that curbs dangerous estrogen activity on vulnerable tissues. This could explain why women who are strict vegetarians have the lowest breast cancer rates, according to Dr. Herbert Pierson, an NCI toxicologist.

Dr. Pierson is also a citrus fruit cheerleader, and points out that chemically speaking, citrus fruits are powerful free radical fighters, and thus important in cancer-preventive activity. The same holds true, for cruciferous vegetables which contain indoles, such as cabbage, broccoli and kale, and for the umbelliferous vegetables: celery, parsley, parsnips and beta-carotene rich-carrots.

Finally, there's the lowly soy bean, which NCI investigators believe contains compounds called isoflavones which have a natural affinity for inhibiting an enzyme that gets overproduced in precancerous stages, says Dr. Pierson.

While we applaud NCI's new devotion to the food pharmacy concept, we are disappointed with their single-minded focus on cancer. It stands to reason that foods that shield you from one dread disease will also protect you from others. It's highly unlikely that if eating broccoli will keep you out of the clutches of an oncologist, it will not also safeguard you from the cardiovascular surgeon, the rheumatologist, allergist, internist . . . No need to name all the specialties.

COLOR ME HEALTHY

The Christmas colors - dark red and green - have a special significance for the nutritionist. According to Brian Morgan, Ph.D., acting director of the Institute of Human Nutrition at the College of Physicians and Surgeons of Columbia University, the deeper the color of fruits and vegetables, the more nutritious they are and the greater their anti-oxidant potential.

For example: pink grapefruit contains 30 times more Vitamin A than white grapefruit; cantaloupe has 510 milligrams of Vitamin A versus honeydew's meager 7; Romaine lettuce has far more calcium, iron and Vitamins A and C than paler iceberg lettuce; brown bread (or rice) is more nutritious than white. The highest levels of beta carotene are found in the dark-green, yellow-orange and red vegetables and fruits - broccoli, spinach, Brussels sprouts, lima beans, peas, asparagus, sweet potatoes, apricots, carrots, beet greens, red bell peppers, tomatoes, and squash - all deep-color foods.

According to a University of Wisconsin-Madison researcher, Beta III, a new and improved deep-orange super-carrot, with two to four times more beta-carotene than the ordinary grocery store variety, may help you live longer. Developed at the USDA's Human Nutrition Center in Beltsville, Md., the carotenoids contained within this colorful vegetable act to prevent cancer, slow aging and pep up the immune system by suppressing free radical activity.

The same chemicals that give fruits and vegetables their deep color also stifle the uncontrolled and dangerous growth of cancerous cells according to recent studies in Kyoto, Japan conducted by biochemist Michiaki Murakoshi and his coworkers at the department of biochemistry at Kyoto Prefectural University of Medicine. When they added either alpha-carotene or beta-carotene to cancer cells in the laboratory, they found alpha carotene shut down cell growth even at minute concentrations. Beta-carotene produced the same results though at higher levels.

New confirmation of the legitimacy of ancient food codes is pouring forth. The floodgates have opened, but since it's difficult to make use of each specific research finding as it becomes known, we've developed the K.I.S.S. plan to help you put the proven Biblical imperatives into practice.

K.I.S.S. HEALTH PROBLEMS GOOD-BYE

"K.I.S.S." - an acronym for "Keep It Short and Simple" - is not a diet per se but a set of health-promoting guidelines. Fad diets come and go. They work for a while, later replaced by new ones. Many structured eating regimens make promises they cannot deliver. The more rigid a diet, the more difficult it is to follow.

"K.I.S.S." gets back to basics. It's based on easy-eating ideas you can live with over the long term. You can 'kiss off' diet-related health problems with these ten rational eating commandments.

1: THOU SHALT NOT EAT ANYTHING THOU CAN NOT PRONOUNCE OR SPELL.

To borrow a phrase from Nancy Reagan, "Just say 'No'" to foods that are chemical concoctions. Trust your instincts. If it doesn't sound like food, it probably isn't. Check for "mysterious ingredients." When was the last time you sent your child to the store for xanthum gum? Know what you are eating. Common preservatives such as BHT, BHA and TBHQ are made from petroleum and are better suited for filling your car's gas tank than your stomach. Follow these guidelines and you will turn down approximately 90% of the chemically-laden nutritionally bankrupt convenience foods so prominent on supermarket shelves. Here's one example of a product you'll have to reject - according to the label, it includes: sugar, modified corn starch, dextrose, citric acid, partially hydrogenated soybean oil, carrageenan, pectin, potassium sorbate, mono&diglycerides, calcium lactate, agar, calcium propionate, whey solids, ammonium bicarbonate, sorghum grain flavor and BHT (shorthand for `butylhydroxytoluene'.

Can you name the product you'll be passing up? If you didn't guess 'lemon meringue pie' (the right answer), no surprise, since there are neither lemons nor cream among the ingredients, but an alarming array of chemicals, most of which are cheap sweeteners, starch modifiers, artificial soap-like fats, and preservatives designed to extend shelf life - not yours. Among the tongue-twisters are two additives judged as "unsafe" or "very poorly tested" by the Center for Science in the Public Interest. Several others are "suspect" - carrageenan, for example, has harmed test animals' colons; artificial colors can cause allergic reactions in aspirin-sensitive people.

2: THOU SHALT LEAN TOWARD THE LEAN

No question but fat - (especially processed fat) - not cholesterol, is your heart's real enemy. If you're over forty, your body's ability to metabolize and digest fats efficiently has already begun to diminish. A sixty-year old, for example, requires several hours to clear the same fat content of a meal from the blood that a thirty-year old metabolizes in a fraction of the time. Excess fats cause many health problems, not the least of which is obesity. Of equal concern are studies linking fat intake with colon, breast and other kinds of cancer. Even more alarming is evidence that improperly processed fats trigger free radical damage.

Your best bet is to limit daily fat intake to twenty-five percent or less of total caloric consumption. If you can get down to twenty percent, all the better. Ask the household cook to put your favorite recipes on a low-fat diet by making the following substitutions:

- Use ground turkey as a substitute for ground beef in meat loaf and spaghetti sauce recipes;
- Use an equal amount of low fat yogurt or buttermilk to replace sour cream, milk or butter;
- Use skinless chicken breasts when a recipe calls for chicken parts;
- Saute vegetables in water or broth instead of oil;
- Eliminate cooking oils by using a nonstick pan or non-stick spray;
- Pick the leanest meats. Turkey, chicken and Cornish hens are much leaner than ducks and geese; at the beef counter, the leanest cuts are the parts of the animal that get the most exercise - the neck, shoulder, and legs;
- Prepare sauces and dips with a base of non-fat plain yogurt;
  Use water-packed tuna.
- Say farewell to surface cooking grease with a new fat-absorbing pad now available in supermarkets nationwide that skims fat from the top sauces, gravies and soups. Developed by food scientist Dr. Carol Costello. a package of six costs about $1.50.

A word to the wise: Be wary of food manufacturers who try to fool the public into thinking their products are low in fat by using deceptive food labels. Robert Abrams, the Attorney General of the state of New York has stopped Kentucky Fried Chicken, Dunkin' Donuts and Nestle from tricking the public with misleading product names and misleading cholesterol-free claims. Nestle's Carnation Coffee-Mate Liquid, for example, contains twice the fat as found in whole milk. Rich Products non-dairy creamer claims that it is 100% cholesterol-free when it gets 100% of its calories from fat. Hebrew National 'Lite Beef Franks' claim they contain less fat when they get 81% of their calories from fat. Perdue Farms' Chicken Franks claim they are lower in fat when they get 71% of their calories from fat.

3: THOU SHALT NOT EAT LIKE A PIG.

"Pigging out" is `out'; "grazing" is `in'. Three square meals a day, with no between-meal nibbling is NOT where it's at. Eating four, five - even six - mini-meals a day is an excellent way to lose weight, get the most nutritional benefit from your food, and may even help ward off heart disease.

A Pennsylvania State University weight loss specialist finds people burn more calories 'nibbling' than consuming the same amount of food in three meals. Men placed on a 'nibbling diet' of 17 snacks a day by Dr. David J. A. Jenkins, professor of medicine and nutritional sciences at the University of Toronto showed "lowered concentrations of the bad types of cholesterol (LDL) and lipoproteins (apolipoprotein B), both associated with increased risk for heart disease, without lowering levels of HDLs (high density lipoproteins) that are recognized as beneficial."

The new research confirms findings from similar studies conducted 25 years ago, when investigators first learned 'nibbling' places less of a strain on the digestive system - and the heart - than a large meal. The less food the body must cope with at once, the more efficiently it can metabolize it.

To be a healthy nibbler:

- Space small frequent meals throughout the day *WITH-OUT* eating more than you normally would.
- Be careful what you nibble on - fresh fruit, vegetables, low-fat cheese, low-fat yogurt - are all O.K. Potato chips, crackers, ice cream, candy and cake are not.

4: KEEP THY FOOD SAFE FROM ADULTERATION.

For food to be nutritious, it must not be contaminated - that's a given. However, food poisoning strikes millions of people every year. Too bad, since you can keep your edibles safe by following six simple rules:

- Keep food very hot or very cold. Bacteria multiply most rapidly when food is at room temperature (between 40 and 140 degrees Fahrenheit). Refrigerate foods to be stored at once instead of setting it out on the kitchen counter to cool. Slow cooling is the perfect environment for bacterial growth.
- Since raw meat can be contaminated with salmonella and campylobacter, cook all meats, seafood and poultry thoroughly. Don't taste while cooking. One undercooked contaminated bite can make you sick.
- Wash hands before handling food. Wash all food thoroughly (including packaged meats) before cooking or serving.
- Scrub utensils, cutting boards and cooking equipment thoroughly before storage and rinse before re-using.
- Discard dated foods. Check 'use before' dates on all packaged and canned foods.
- If power fails, or your refrigerator or freezer begins acting up, do not open doors unnecessarily. Do not keep thawed frozen food for more than two days. Do not refreeze thawed frozen foods.

5. THOU SHALT CHOOSE FRESH FOOD OVER DEAD FOOD.

Confine food shopping as much as possible to the produce department. Whenever you can, go with Mother Nature. Peas in the pod beat peas packaged or canned. When it comes to frozen against fresh, no contest.

In keeping with the times, many supermarkets now boast 'health food sections'. Think on that. What does it say about the foods stocked in other aisles? Avoid 'prepared' foods that have had their natural goodness destroyed - the overprocessed, over-concentrated, over-salted, over-sweetened, overcooked, scraped and devitalized. A good rule of thumb to follow is this. the prettier the package, the less edible its contents.

Even so-called 'fresh' foods can be suspect. By the time a vegetable lands on your plate, it's been picked, packed, shipped and stored. The longer the time span between garden and gullet, the more food value lost. Then the cook contributes to the damage with the ordinary kitchen knife and a pot of boiling water.

To master the art of fresh cooking:

- When boiling, use just enough water to keep the pot from scorching. Better yet, use a steamer. Less contact with cooking water means less leaching of water-soluble vitamins;

- Bring the water to a boil before dropping in vegetables. Do not overcook. The longer you cook, and the more mushy the vegetables get, the more nutrients lost. Quick hot, and dry - as when stir-fried in a Chinese wok - works best.

- Cook vegetables whole or in big chunks. Cut them up after cooking, wherever possible. Slicing and dicing exposes vegetables to oxidation - allowing nutrients to vanish more rapidly.

- Cook vegetables unpeeled. The natural covering protects potatoes, squash and cucumbers against leaching and oxidation and preserves nutrient content.

- When buying frozen food, check the temperature in your supermarket's freezer. If it reads higher than 5°F., it's not cold enough to prevent vitamin loss. If there's no thermometer, pick up a frozen food package and squeeze - if there's *any* give, give up and shop elsewhere.

- Push your shopping cart quickly past all the food displays that greet your entry into the supermarket. Head directly - as fast as you can - to the produce aisle. Limit your shopping, as much as possible, to the unboxed items found there.

- Collect quick and easy 'cook-from-scratch' recipes. Build a personal library of fast and fabulous concoctions that you can put together in minutes from items already in your cupboard. One of our favorite 'quickie' meal-in-a-minute dishes is salmon croquets. A one pound can of salmon, 1 egg, chopped dried onions, horseradish and seasoned bread crumbs, mixed together is all you need to form and brown patties in a non-stick pan (no oil, no fat.) Serve with a salad and vegetable side dish and take your bows. For many more easy-fix dishes, consult the wonderful *Four Ingredient Cookbook* created by Shirley Atwater and Marilyn Meich two busy ladies who are creative cooks.

6: THOU SHALT NOT COVET SUGAR AND SALT

Many nutritionists consider sugar to be Public Enemy Number One - with salt a close second. Sugar is murder on teeth, and on blood sugar levels, and has been voted the "most likely to cause disease" by noted nutritionist Dr. E. Cheraskin, who has linked the following health problems to excess sugar consumption: cavities and gum disease; high blood pressure; atherosclerosis - (sugar in the diet stimulates the liver to produce more cholesterol); infections; slowed bowel transit time; decreased immune system functioning; bone thinning. Sugar is also associated with such unfavorable personality changes as increased irritability, anger and impatience.

How quickly can reduced sugar intake bring about beneficial change? In a double-blind study of healthy young persons, the heart rates of the group that consumed less sugar decreased in just three days.

What can we say about salt? Not much good.

"If salt were a new food additive, it is doubtful it would earn a 'safe' classification." So says Dr. Mark Hegsted, former chief of the USDA Human Nutrition Center. His objections to salt? We need very little and consume too much. Almost all epidemiological research has shown that populations with the lowest salt consumption have the lowest incidence of hypertension, heart attack, stroke, and kidney failure.

The solution: Make friends with your spice cabinet. Mustard, Cajun-style spices, paprika, red pepper and parsley are great spicy salt substitutes.

7: THOU SHALT NOT EAT FOODS ROBBED OF NUTRIENTS.

When the label on a box, can or wrapper boasts "enriched" or "vitamin fortified," what does that really mean? The best that can be said is that of everything stripped away, some four to ten elements have been put back. That's a very poor bargain by any standard.

8: THOU SHALT RESPECT BREAKFAST AS THE DAY'S MOST IMPORTANT MEAL.

It's unlikely we're the first to remind you that the earliest meal of the day - breakfast - is your best defense against stress. Eating a nutritious breakfast is absolutely vital, according to Brian Morgan, an assistant professor at the Institute of Human Nutrition at the College of Physicians and Surgeons of Columbia University, who recommends: orange juice, whole grain cereal and a slice of buttered high-fiber bread as an excellent example of a breakfast that gives you an odds-on chance of starting and ending your day calm and relaxed.

When under time pressure, grab a banana, an orange, a slice of whole wheat bread, a glass of low-fat milk. The combination will provide you with a balanced amount of protein and carbohydrates, also essential vitamins and minerals.

9: THOU SHALT DRINK ALCOHOLIC BEVERAGES SPARINGLY.

Does alcohol shorten or lengthen life? That's the debate of

the day, with equally learned opinions to be found on both sides of the aisle. Most authorities agree, moderate drinking - no more than two ounces a day - is usually safe.

Be cautious. Besides the oft-repeated dangers of drinking and driving, there is the hazard of alcohol conversion into acetaldehyde (a close relative of embalming fluid) that enhances free radical production and cell damage.

10: THOU SHALT HONOR THY KITCHEN.

. . . and keep it busy.

Equally important to WHAT you eat is HOW you prepare food. A potent defense against free radical activity and degenerative disease can be cooked up in your kitchen. Easy to say - hard to do if you don't know how to go about it. Since most of us have little time to shop and cook, we've turned into the 'heat and eat' generation - a serious dilemma because, as previously stated, quick-fix foods are either loaded with fats and chemicals or nutrient depleted, or both.

Despite strict time limitations, you can do better thanks to new wonder appliances. 'Cooking from scratch' is no longer the arduous, time-consuming chore it once was. For starters, we've a prime example: you can wake up to the mouth-watering aroma of fresh baked bread. It's no longer a luxury.

If you can make ice cubes, you can make bread with the newest machines that turn out a perfect loaf in four hours or less, doing everything automatically from kneading to baking. You only need five minutes to toss in the ingredients, close the lid and turn the switch on.

Bread bakers used to be expensive, but now can be bought many places for less than $150.00.. (We bought ours from Dak, the catalog supplier, for under $200 two years back.) Regardless of the cost, a breadmaker pays for itself by producing bread unsullied by such unappetizing ingredients as corn syrups, hydrogenated oils, colorings, additives and the preservatives common in commercially prepared baked goods.

For pennies a loaf, you can produce a healthy, tasty alternative to store-bought versions.

The same goes for pasta: pasta makers are not a luxury if you value your health. Here again, it's cheaper to make whole grain noodles at home from buckwheat or semolina flour than pay health food store prices. With the newest models, you can prepare homemade pasta from scratch in just twenty minutes.

Is pasta healthy? Sophia Loren said it best when she remarked: "Everything you see, I owe to spaghetti."

To cut down on the dangers of free radical production, prepare meals in a wok, a crock pot, a slow cooker at low heat, or a microwave oven and foods will not exceed the 212 degree range where lipid peroxidation takes place. A steam cooker provides a quick and easy way to prepare nutritious, flavor-packed meats, vegetables, fish and poultry. The newest models let you 'set it and forget it'.

Equally valuable: the pressure cooker. It makes food more digestible, enhances flavors and preserves nutrients. Today's pressure cookers do not "blow up." They are self-regulating and safe, provided you follow manufacturer's instructions.

When it comes to speed, health and convenience, nothing beats the microwave oven. Microwaving enhances flavors of foods such as fish, poultry, vegetables and fruit by keeping them moist without added oil or salt. The shorter cooking time required by a microwave means fewer nutrients are lost to heat than by conventional methods.

As an added bonus, according to a USDA study, microwaved meat contains less fat and fewer calories than meat cooked by electric broiling, roasting, convection baking, or frying - no matter how much fat in the pre-cooked meat.

Nearly three out of four U.S. households have microwave ovens, but many of their owners are still a bit uneasy. No need to worry: your microwave will not 'nuke' your food; you don't need to wear a lead apron; you're not apt to set off a Geiger counter when you microwave.

There are causes for concern you may not have thought of: some of the containers and packages designed for microwave cooking, including some cling-wraps, special 'browning packages' and a few 'microwave safe' cookware products, may be releasing potentially harmful substances into your food. Many of these products are exempt from government regulation so your only protection is to check carefully before use.

What are backyard barbecue devotees to do now that it's suspected that grilled foods may promote cancer? If the bad news caused you to lose your taste for grilling, you can grill away with a clear health conscience by changing your cooking style in a way to avoid the noted dangers. With conventional grilling, the fat that drips from the meat onto the heat source - gas, electric or charcoal - is converted into PAH (Polycyclic Aromatic Hydrocarbons). These substances are known to cause cancer.

Carcinogenic-free grilling IS possible. To keep your grilled food free of PAH, prevent the fat from dripping on the fire. You can do this with by using a vertical grill, which holds the meat in a metal basket or wire holder sandwiched between heat sources placed on each side of the meat. With this method, the pan beneath the meat remains cold, and fat drippings are not converted into cancer-causing chemicals.

Simpler still, invest in a smokeless stove-top grill (available in most hardware and discount stores for $5 to $20) that sits on top of a conventional range (gas or electric) and sports a water-filled outer ring that catches fat and juices during cooking, eliminating smoke and spattering.

Here are a few more inexpensive additions to turn your kitchen into a 'health center':

- A clay cooker: Cooking in clay is a centuries-old method of preparing food without the addition of water, oils or fat. Meat, fish and poultry all stew in their own juices, insuring wholesomeness and digestibility. A modern twist is to cook with clay in your microwave - you retain all the benefits of clay cookery and add the speed of the microwave;

- Food processor: A great appliance if it encourages you to prepare fresh salads and vegetables. If you're short of cash, a good set of kitchen knives, an old-fashioned grater and a hand chopper will do;

Then there are some excellent health-enhancing products costing $20.00 or less:

- A hot-air corn popper: No oil needed to turn out a wholesome high-fiber, low-calorie, low-cost snack in minutes;
- Egg poacher: Eggs are healthiest soft boiled or poached, with no added fat and without exposure to high heat;
- Yogurt maker: Have a consistent supply of low-fat yogurt by making it from scratch with natural ingredients. The most popular yogurt maker makes one full quart (5 individual portions) of yogurt overnight or while you're at work.

And the following are inexpensive 'good-for-you' gadgets:

- Non-stick pans: Their non-stick surface permits you to prepare foods without the addition of fat; when desperate for a 'spritz' of grease to saute onions, mushrooms and the like, use a no-stick spray made from lecithin.;
- A plastic colander: Buy one large enough to stand on its own feet and use it in your microwave to brown chopped beef for meat loaf, chili and spaghetti sauces. It's a neat way to render fat out before combining the meat with other ingredients.
- Oven bags. No muss, no fuss, no added fat when you cook your favorite foods - alone or in combination - in oven bags. Use them in your conventional oven , or in your microwave. Either way, they keep food moist and savory and minimize clean-up time.

- Green plantain leaves: No health-conscious cook should be without this Caribbean touch of cooking wizardry. Fresh plantain leaves (available in most oriental food stores) make possible pseudo-'fried' foods with no fat whatsoever. Wrap small pieces of cubed or sliced potato in the banana leaves, bake until tender and crisp and they'll rival French fries. The same method works well with chicken and fish.

Keeping a healthy kitchen is simplified once you have the proper tools on hand. If you're on a budget, start small and build gradually.

20

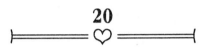

RECIPES FOR HEALTHY PLEASURES

Give up French fries! Swear off fried chicken! No more banana splits, beer parties, back-yard barbecues, pig-outs at the pizza parlor! Yuk! We can hear you complaining now.

"What good is it to be healthy if you can't have any fun? I might live longer - or it might just *seem* longer!"

Right you are. There must be more to life than 'eat this', 'work up a sweat', 'swallow these vitamins'. It's certainly true that enjoying life should be an important part of any prescription for good health. Here's why: healthy people are happy. The reverse is even truer: happy people are healthy. The latest research shows that having a good time is not only pleasurable, but health-enhancing, as well. Our immune system works better when we're in an upbeat mood. Playfulness and laughter trigger beneficial biochemical reactions. Vitamin 'W' does exist. It is the `will to be well' and can help you ward off everything from colds to cancer. You can develop this powerful nutrient by making a clear commitment to experiencing pleasure as often as you can.

So how about a healthy diet? Can foods that are 'good' for you taste 'good' too? Good question. Individuals newly introduced to the importance of sound nutrition often fear they have to give up eating for pleasure in the pursuit of eating for health.

Not so. Our family advocates the Pleasure Diet - getting as much joy as you can from every calorie. Fortunately, following that principle is also extremely good for you. According to one researcher, boosting the flavor - but not the calories - of what you eat, helps you lose weight. Another study showed that spicing up your meals not only gives a lift to your palate, but also beefs up your metabolism, enabling your body to burn up calories faster.

Never overlook the power of eye appeal. In Vietnam, they have a proverb; "You don't eat just with your mouth, but with your nose and eyes, too." When you bring out the soup bowl, it should be hot and steamy; every dish served should look beautiful - fresh and inviting; a sprig of greens can give the simplest platter the gourmet touch.

Remember this: the dining table is the very center of our social existence. It's where we bond our most intimate relationships, meet and create new friends, start a romance, end an argument, and carry on family rituals and traditions. Given mealtime's significance to our emotional lives, it's appropriate to do all we can to enhance eating pleasure.

You've lots of help now: thousands of cookbooks to suit every nutritional requirement, ethnic preference and taste; hundreds of articles in newspapers and magazines offering innovative ways to satisfy your taste, health requirements and pocketbook. Discover what suits you best by trial and error, testing and tasting. Use high quality ingredients that reflect the seasons and market conditions and discover new ways to have fun with food.

COOKING WITH 'C'

In consideration of the evidence that Vitamin C is one of our prime defenders against free radical attack and an important antioxidant, it makes good sense to place emphasis on Vitamin C-rich foods that also help keep arteries from clogging. Cooking with 'C' can be a health-saving strategy and pleasurable as well.

To become a C-conscious cook, start your shopping in the produce department, and include at least one or two of the following in each day's meals: broccoli, Brussels sprouts, cabbage, cantaloupe, cauliflower, citrus fruits, currants, green and/or red peppers, guavas, honeydew, kohlrabi, papaya, persimmon, pimentos, strawberries, tomatoes, and dark, green leafy vegetables. Try to include five - (yes, FIVE) - servings of fresh vegetables and/or fruits every day.

Now for some innovative ways to use them. The first is a favorite with our daughter.

SHARON'S SPINACH SOUP

2 quarts boiling stock	1/2 cup diced carrots
or vegetable water	2 cups cooked chopped spinach
1/2 cup chopped onion	2 tablespoon olive oil
1 tablespoon chopped parsley	2 cups cooked brown rice
1/2 cup thinly sliced celery	Salt and pepper to taste
4 coarsely cut tomatoes	1/4 cup Parmesan cheese
(or 1 can whole tomatoes)	

Add onion, parsley, celery, tomatoes and carrots to boiling stock. Simmer until celery is just tender (12 to 18 minutes). Saute spinach in olive oil 2 minutes. Stir into simmering stock. Add rice and seasonings. Cook 5 minutes. Serve with a light garnish of grated cheese.

(6 to 8 servings)

♥   ♥   ♥

We have Sharon to thank for another favorite dish. She concocted this one - Yum Ba Mee, a Korean noodle salad - to entice fellow real estate agents to view houses she'd listed for sale - but we revised it for an easy-fix card-players' lunch.

THE BRIDGE BUNCH LUNCH

1/2 to 3/4 cup fresh shelled and deveined shrimp (cut in half) or an equal amount of cooked chicken (cut in small pieces)

1/2 lb. fresh egg noodles - or 2 and 1/2 3 oz. packages of oriental noodles

2 quarts hot water or chicken stock

2 tbsp. garlic oil or sesame oil

2 cups (1/2 lb) cut up iceberg lettuce or 2 cups thinly sliced celery

1/2 lb. bean sprouts, parboiled 1 minute and rinsed in cold water, then drained - OR - 2 cups sliced carrot sticks, boiled for 3 minutes, then cooled and drained

1/2 to 1 tsp. chili powder

2 tbs preserved cabbage

3 tbs fish sauce (or thin soy sauce)

3 tbs lime juice (more or less to taste)

1 tbs sugar

4 spring onions, cut up in fine pieces

Using high heat, cook noodles about 3 minutes in boiling water. Drain and rinse with cold water. Cook shrimp in boiling water for 2 minutes and rinse with cold water (if using chicken, cook about five minutes, then chill.) Using large salad bowl, add noodles and garlic/sesame oil, stir. Add meat, lettuce, and carrots. Add chili powder, fish/soy sauce, lime juice, sugar and spring onions. Mix together well and serve immediately. Stand back and graciously accept the applause.

♥   ♥   ♥

Vegetables need not be confined to side-dish status. Here are three good examples of ways to elevate them to main dish rank. The first is one our son favors.

JERRY'S LASAGNA

Make the filling first, by mixing together the following ingredients.

1 cup low-fat large curd cottage cheese	1/4 tsp. oregano
1 small clove minced fresh garlic	1-1/2 cups chicken stock (skim off the fat) or vegetable water

Set the above aside. Next, assemble the rest of the ingredients:

2 cups thinly sliced zucchini	1/2 fresh lemon
1 cup sliced mushrooms	1 tsp. paprika
1 cup chopped onion	freshly ground pepper
1 cup diagonally sliced green beans	10 curled edge lasagna noodles
1/4 red or green bell pepper, cut in 1/4" strips	

Preheat the oven to 350 degrees. Saute the onions, zucchini, mushrooms, green beans and pepper until just tender in a large skillet that has been lightly coated with nonstick spray. Season with lemon juice, paprika and pepper to taste.

Lightly coat the bottom of a square 8x8 inch glass casserole dish with nonstick spray. Arrange one layer of lasagna noodles (dry) in the bottom of the dish, breaking as necessary to fit. Cover with half the vegetable mixture. Add another layer of noodles. Spread all the filling on top. Add another layer of noodles, covering them with the balance of the vegetable mixture. Pour chicken stock over the top. Cover and bake for 45 minutes; then uncover and bake for 15 minutes more.

❤   ❤   ❤

PAPA JOE'S HOT-TO-TROT CHILI

1/2 tbsp. olive oil
4 garlic cloves, minced
1 medium onion, chopped
1-1/2 tbsp. chili powder
1/2 tsp. ground cumin
1 tsp. leaf oregano
3/4 tsp. leaf thyme
1/4 tsp. freshly ground pepper

1 green pepper, chopped
2 cups fresh tomatoes, chopped
(or 1 16-ounce can whole tomatoes)
1 (4-ounce) can chopped chilies,
drained ('mild' for tender palates)
1 15-1/2-ounce can red kidney beans,
undrained
1/2 cup water
1/2 cup coarse bulgur

Combine oil, garlic, onion and seasonings in a 2 quart microproof casserole. Cover and microwave on HIGH 1 minute; stir and add remaining ingredients, mixing well to combine. Cover and microwave on HIGH 6 to 8 minutes or until boiling. Continue to microwave on MEDIUM (50 percent power) for 15 minutes. Let stand five minutes before serving. If desired, serve with shredded cheddar cheese or non-fat yogurt, or sprinkle with dried Parmesan cheese and serve over macaroni for the vegetarian version of Chili-Mac.

❤ ❤ ❤

POP'S MEATLESS STUFFED CABBAGE

12 large cabbage leaves
1 beaten egg
1/4 cup water
2 cups cooked brown rice
1 onion, grated
1 carrot, grated

Salt and pepper to taste
1/4 tsp. dried, crushed
thyme leaves
1 cup tomato sauce, canned
1/4 cup lemon juice
2 tbsp. honey

Blanch cabbage leaves by covering them with boiling water for 2 or 3 minutes. Drain and set aside to cool.

Combine rice, egg, onion, carrot, salt, pepper and thyme in a large bowl. Divide into 12 equal portions and place one portion in the center of each cabbage leaf. Roll it up, envelope style, tucking the ends in securely. Place close together in a heavy skillet.

Combine the tomato sauce, lemon juice and honey, and pour over the cabbage rolls, adding enough water to cover. Cover tightly and cook over moderate heat 30 minutes. Bake in the oven another 30 minutes at 350 degrees to brown on top, turning once to brown under sides. Hot water may be added in small quantities if necessary during the baking period.

♥ ♥ ♥

MAGNOLIA EGG PLANT

This recipe comes to us by courtesy of Mrs. Helen Hensley, who runs the Magnolia Cafeteria in Little Rock, Arkansas.

2 lb. eggplant	1/4 lb. American cheese, diced
1 egg	or, low-fat mozzarella, shredded
2 tbsp. olive oil	1 medium onion, chopped
1 #2 can tomatoes	Salt, pepper to taste

Peel and slice eggplant. Boil until tender. Drain well. Saute in small amount of olive oil. Place in mixing bowl, and fold into eggplant mixture the pulp of canned tomatoes, egg, diced cheese and seasonings. Mix well with wire whip. Add enough cracker meal to tighten mixture.

Pour in a baking dish and sprinkle the top with a layer of cracker meal. Dribble with a bit more oil, additional grated cheese, and bake in 400 degree open 20 minutes. Serve hot out of the oven to 6 lucky people.

♥ ♥ ♥

Vegetables are also a great way to spice up a meal. Back in the 'old country', Harold's grandmother, Rifka Lattner, was a professional pickler. Here are two favorites this wonderful Polish lady passed down.

RIFKA'S PICKLED BABY EGGPLANTS

2 lbs. baby eggplants	1/2 tsp. cayenne pepper
Salt to taste	4 cloves garlic, crushed
3/4 lbs. ground walnuts	brine to cover made with
	white wine vinegar

Wash eggplants and make an incision in each one. Poach covered in salted water for five to ten minutes until soft. Mix walnuts, cayenne and garlic into a paste and stuff each eggplant through incision. Pack in jars and cover with brine. Refrigerate. Eggplants should be ready to eat in about one week.

♥ ♥ ♥

RIFKA'S MIXED PICKLES

1/2 lb. green beans, poached in	1/2 lb. turnips, sliced
salted water for five minutes	1/2 lb. hot peppers, whole
1/2 lb. Jerusalem artichokes or	3 cloves garlic per jar
sun chokes, peeled and sliced	3 sprigs fresh dill per jar
1/2 lb. carrots, sliced	3 whole peppercorns per jar
1/2 lb. cauliflower, separated	4 coriander seeds per jar
into flowerets	2 stalks celery per jar
	brine made with red wine vinegar

Wash vegetables. Place garlic, dill, peppercorns, coriander, and celery in jars. Layer vegetables. Pack tightly and fill to brim with brine. Refrigerate. Pickles should be ready in two weeks.

♥ ♥ ♥

President George Bush might not have bad-mouthed broccoli if he'd ever tasted our version. It's good enough to serve White House guests, so we've now renamed it:

BUSH'S BROCCOLI BASH

1 lb. thin spaghetti	1/4 cup Virgin olive oil
1 lb. fresh broccoli spears,	2 small cloves garlic
or 2 packages (9 oz. each) of	dash hot red crushed pepper
frozen broccoli	salt, to taste
2 small tins flat anchovies	pepper, to taste

Boil pasta and broccoli according to directions, omitting salt in boiling water. Meanwhile, empty the anchovies into a small frying pan, add olive oil, press the garlic cloves into the mixture, add hot pepper flakes. Saute together gently until anchovies disintegrate (about 2 or 3 minutes). Set aside until pasta and vegetables are done and then mix all three together in serving bowl. Add salt and pepper and serve immediately to 6 hungry or 8 finicky people.

♥ ♥ ♥

If you've gone in for gardening, you're a winner on two health fronts. Gardening is excellent exercise *and* a wonderful source of food you can trust.

Gardening is good therapy, say researchers in the Netherlands who have found that people who lovingly tend their plants have significantly fewer heart attacks than those who never work the soil. Gardening lowers blood pressure, increases the body's resistance to stress and even might harden your bones.

Beginning gardeners would do well to plant proven producers: tomatoes, cucumbers, green and red peppers and radishes - no green thumb magic needed to enjoy a bounty harvest.

Now for ways to make good use of what you've grown:

PHYLLIS' HEALTH SPA SALAD

1 cup mung sprouts
1/2 cup adzuki sprouts
1/2 cup cabbage sprouts
1/2 sweet red pepper, thinly sliced
6 thinly sliced radishes
2 thinly sliced ripe tomatoes
15 snow pea pods, quartered
1 scored and thinly sliced unpeeled cucumber
4 medium stalks Chinese cabbage, chopped
1/2 celery stalk, cut into matchsticks
2 garlic cloves, pressed
1/4 cup scallions, chopped
1/4 cup tamari
3 tbsp. lemon juice, fresh
1/4 cup spring or filtered water

Marinate sprouts and vegetables for two to four hours in a mixture of tamari, lemon juice and water. Stir occasionally so that all the vegetables are equally soaked. Serve on a bed of fresh crisp chopped lettuce and top with fresh avocado cubes.

♥ ♥ ♥

LISA'S LONGEVITY SOUP

1 large onion, diced
1 tbsp olive oil
3 cups chicken stock
2 carrots, diced
1 large sweet potato, diced
1 stalk celery, diced
1 zucchini, chopped
1 cup sliced green beans
1 tomato, diced
1 bay leaf
1/2 teaspoon dried thyme
1/2 tsp dried basil
1 cup shredded spinach
1 cup cooked millet
1 cup skim milk

In a 3-quart saucepan, saute the onions in the oil until translucent. Add the stock, carrots, potatoes, celery, zucchini, beans, tomato, bay leaf, thyme. and basil. Simmer for 30 minutes. Stir in the spinach, millet and milk. Simmer for 5 minutes. Discard the bay leaf.

The key to this health-promoting dish is to load the soup pot with immunity-upping, disease-fighting ingredients. Vary it as you like, but be sure to include at least one vegetable from each of the following nutrient groups. *Carptempoids*: carrots, butternut squash and sweet potato; *cruciferous vegetables*: broccoli, cauliflower, cabbage; *Vitamin C*: green peppers, Chinese cabbage, Brussels sprouts; *Vitamin E*: leafy greens, spinach, kale, Swiss chard; *fiber*: lentils, kidney, or any other dried beans; *sulfur compounds*: onions, leeks, shallots, garlic.

If you've always relied on store-bought tomato sauce and catchup, these home-made varieties will spoil you for all time.

GLEN'S FRESH-FROM-THE-GARDEN TOMATO SAUCE

2 pounds home grown tomatoes -
(plum tomatoes are preferable
but any kind will do)
1 mild chili pepper, seeded
and coarsely chopped
4 green onions, coarsely chopped
1 tbsp. chopped celery leaf

2 tsp. olive oil
1 tsp. red-wine vinegar
1 bay leaf
1 tsp. mixed Italian seasonings
(basil, thyme, rosemary, oregano,
sweet sage)

Combine all ingredients in food processor and process very briefly. DO NOT OVERMIX. When ingredients look well combined, transfer to a 10 inch pie plate, and microwave, uncovered on high for about 6 or 7 minutes, rotating 3 times during cooking time. Discard bay leaf, and store in clean, covered glass jars in refrigerator.

♥ ♥ ♥

ARLINE'S HOME-ON-THE-RANGE CATCHUP

10 pounds tomatoes	1/4 cup salt
3 medium onions, cut up	1/2 tbsp. celery seed
2 medium red or green peppers, cut up	1/2 tbsp. paprika
	1 tsp. hot pepper sauce
1 large garlic clove	3/4 tsp. fresh ground pepper
1-1/3 cups sugar	3/4 tsp. allspice
1-1/4 cups vinegar	3 1-pint canning jars with caps

Remove stem ends from tomatoes, and cut tomatoes into chunks. Fill food processor or blender about 3/4 full at a time, and process tomatoes at a high speed until they're very juicy, but not pureed. Press tomatoes through a coarse sieve, discarding skin and seeds, and put in large pot, preserving and setting aside 1/2 cup of tomato liquid.

Next use a blender to process one half of the onions, peppers and garlic with 1/4 cup of tomato juice until very smooth; add to tomatoes in pot. Repeat with remaining half of vegetables and tomato liquid. Add sugar to entire mixture and cook on high heat to boiling. Reduce heat to medium and cook uncovered 4-1/2 hours or until desired consistency is reached, stirring occasionally. Volume should be reduced in half.

Follow standard canning procedures to store, sterilizing and sealing jars as manufacturer suggests. Fresh leftover catchup can be stored in refrigerator and used safely for about 1 month.

❤   ❤   ❤

The secret to making the most of fresh vegetables is to gather basketfuls before summer's end - if not from your backyard, then from local markets and roadside stands. Then turn your creative urges loose. Don't fall back on the tried-and-tired - mix and match new combinations, seasoned with fresh herbs, spices, garlic, chilies, vinegars. Serve them raw, or lightly cooked, and process, freeze, can and store the excess for future joy.

❤   ❤   ❤

How about those favorite dishes for which there seems no acceptable replacement? The recipes that have been handed down from one generation to another when the cook only cared if it tasted good, not if it were good for you?

Use your ingenuity and you'll find a way to retain traditional fare - and your health, as well. For example: for years, Brecher family feasts always included a chopped chicken liver appetizer - the first tasty delicacy of a holiday meal. But that was in our younger days, before Pop had his heart attack, and before we all learned that the schmaltz (chicken fat) that made this dish so delicious could be a deadly pleasure.

So when we nixed this time-honored appetite-pleaser from the menu, it was with great reluctance to lose such a well-loved standby. Leave it to my mother-in-law to come up with a savory solution. If we didn't know it for a fact, we'd never suspect this tasty substitute is a healthful, vegetable-based 'fake'.

❤   ❤   ❤

MAMA'S MOCK CHOPPED LIVER

1-1/2 cups finely chopped or ground cooked green beans (packed tight)	1 chopped onion
	1 tbsp. canola oil
1 hard cooked egg	salt and pepper to taste

Mash hard cooked egg with the beans. Lightly brown chopped onion in the oil and add seasoning to taste. This should wind up as a compact mass, that looks - and tastes - just like chopped beef or calf's liver.

♥ ♥ ♥

And what do we serve non-Jewish guests before dinner? Easy. We toast cut up fat-free pita bread, and offer a big bowl of our favorite Mid-East dip. We cherish this recipe, as it's been a closely held secret of our friends at the International Gourmet and Delicatessen in Herndon, Virginia.

TARLAN'S HUMUS (HOMMOS) DIP

Boil 6 oz. raw chic peas 30 minutes or use 6 oz. of canned pre-cooked chic peas. Drain and mash with blender or hand masher. Mix in the following:

2 tbsp. Tahini sauce (sesame paste)	1 tbsp. olive oil
2-3 minced fresh garlic cloves	salt and pepper to taste
1 tbsp. lemon juice	

♥ ♥ ♥

"What good is bread without butter?" is a common complaint. Among the complainers: husband Harold. Our answer to him, and others like him, is this ingenious substitute, courtesy Drew Alan Kaplan, President of Dak Industries.

HAROLD'S BETTER-THAN-BUTTER SPREAD

1 16 ounce package low fat	2 packages *Butter Buds*
(1/2% milkfat) cottage cheese	(natural butter flavored mix)
1/4 cup water	1-3 packages Sweet 'n Low
4 Tbsp. nonfat dry milk	

Pour all ingredients into your blender. Mix on low, increasing speed until the mixture is smooth. Then pour/scrape the mixture back into the empty cheese container and refrigerate. With just 7 calories per tablespoon (as compared with 100 for butter and margarine) you can spread freely and enjoy, guilt-free.

❤ ❤ ❤

If you're fearful of fats, and suspicious of sweets, you've got a problem. The answer is to be found in these two delicious, fruit-based spreads, both of which provide lots of fiber, and are delicious on muffins, scones, pancakes and waffles also on plain or toasted bread.

MAMA ROSE'S APPLE BUTTER

2 cups unsweetened applesauce	1/4 tsp. ground cloves
1 tsp. ground cinnamon	1/4 tsp. ground nutmeg

Combine ingredients and heat quickly, stirring frequently, until mixture begins to boil. To tell if it's done, take a big cooking spoonful of the apple butter and put it on a saucer. Turn the saucer upside down over the pot, and if the apple butter stays on there in a lump, it's finished. If there's liquid seeping from the mound of apple, it indicates more cooking and stirring are required. When done, by this test, pour into sterilized glass jars. Cover and cool. Refrigerate.

MAMA ROSE'S PRUNE BUTTER

2 cups soft or soaked pitted prunes	1 tsp. vanilla
1-3/4 cups apple juice	1/2 tsp. fresh lemon juice
1/4 cups raisins	1 tsp. unsulfured molasses

Simmer in a large saucepan over low heat for 30 minutes, stirring frequently. Let the mixture cool, then transfer to a food processor or blender and process on low speed until smooth. Store, covered, in refrigerator.

❤ ❤ ❤

What about desserts? Is it possible to top off your meal with something delicious without destroying your health?

Absolutely. Adopting the appropriate attitude is most important. Resist throwing discretion and good nutrition to the wind, succumbing to the notion that since you've been virtuous up to this point, you can afford to eat a 'little poison'.

Admittedly, dessert-time is what separates those 'serious' about good nutrition from those who talk a good game. There's often much family pressure to overcome as well. In many households, the idea of fresh fruit for dessert is as welcome as receiving new underwear for Christmas.

Stand your ground - no need to resort to broiled grapefruit and stewed prunes, risking divorce and desertion. Here are the family's favorite light and luscious end-of-the-meal delights:

COUSIN DONNA'S APPLE AND RAISIN PUDDING

6 or 8 apples	1 tbsp. cornstarch
1/2 box raisins	1 tbsp. butter
2 cups water	1 tbsp. honey

Wash apples, core and cut into eighths. Arrange in baking dish, filling in open spaces with raisins. Cover with liquid made by boiling the water, cornstarch, butter and honey together for a few minutes. Place in oven and bake until apples are tender.

❤ ❤ ❤

COUSIN JOYCE'S TROPICAL MERINGUES

First, prepare the meringues:

4 egg whites	3/4 cup sugar
1/8 tsp. salt	1/2 tsp. vanilla
1/4 tsp. cream of tartar	1 tbsp. grated orange peel

In large bowl, beat egg whites, salt and cream of tartar until foamy. Gradually beat in sugar, 1 tbsp. at a time, until stiff peaks form when beater is withdrawn. Fold in vanilla and orange peel.

Spoon 6 mounds onto greased baking sheet and make a depression in center of each mound. Bake at 225 degrees for 45 minutes, or until lightly browned. Remove and cool.

For the filling:

3 tbsp. cornstarch	1/2 cup pineapple juice
1/3 cup sugar	juice of 1/2 lemon
1/4 tsp. salt	1 tsp. grated orange rind
3/4 cup water	3 bananas
1/2 cup orange juice	

In medium saucepan, mix cornstarch, sugar and salt. Gradually stir in water, orange juice, pineapple juice and lemon juice. Simmer over low heat, stirring constantly until mixture thickens and comes to a boil. Cook for 1 minute, continuing to stir. Remove from heat; stir in orange peel. Cool. Peel bananas; slice Fold in. Chill about 3 hours. Just before serving, fill meringues.

❤ ❤ ❤

And finally, a master stroke, a dessert not to be trifled with:

AUNT ELIZABETH'S LIGHT BUT LUSCIOUS TRIFLE

2 packages vanilla pudding and pie-filling mix	1 package (3 oz.) ladyfingers
1 quart low-fat milk	1/3 cup pure fruit (no sugar) strawberry preserves
2 tsp. sugar	1/2 cup macaroon or vanilla wafer crumbs
1 tsp. pure vanilla	

Combine pudding mix, milk and sugar in a saucepan and cook over a medium heat, stirring constantly, until mixture

thickens and comes to a boil. Stir in vanilla. Split ladyfingers
Fill with preserves and put them together again.

Layer a 2 quart serving dish with one-fourth the ladyfingers,
cookie crumbs and pudding. Repeat three more times, ending
with pudding. Refrigerate at least three hours. Garnish with
additional dots of strawberry fruit preserves before serving.
You should have to make ten dessert-lovers contented.

♥ ♥ ♥

Whatever happened to the joy of dining out? It went the
way of the dinosaur - doomed to obsolescence by the "fear of
food."

"Restaurant anxiety" is a common syndrome among many
who fear restaurant eating means relinquishing control over
their diet to some crazed chef who lacks knowledge of, or
interest in, good nutrition.

Does restaurant food have to be life-threatening? Of course
not. Here are some guidelines to help you avoid the soggy,
greasy, unwholesome and worse.

- CALL AHEAD.

  No reason to wait until you're handed the menu to
  discover whether the restaurant's meal choices meet
  your requirements, when a phone call allows you to
  check things out ahead of time.

- ENLIST THE AID OF YOUR FOOD SERVER.

  Tell your waiter or waitress about your nutritional
  concerns. If you want to be certain the dishes you order
  are low fat, without salt, have no added MSG, are not
  fried, say so. Ask for your server's recommendation for
  a healthful offering. Usually, your server will be eager to
  help you stay on your diet - your tip pays her salary.

- BE MENU-WISE.

  Learn to interpret menu items correctly. Foods 'sauteed'
  have added butter; 'tempura' means fried in batter; 'au

gratin' could mean anything - but for sure suggests a cheese sauce added that might contain unwanted ingredients. Beware such 'buzz words' as 'buttery', 'crispy', 'creamed', 'in its own gravy', 'hollandaise', 'pan-fried', 'escalloped', 'marinated' and 'braised' descriptions of dishes that could contain lots of fat. Watch out for pickled or smoked foods.

- ORDER 'CLEAN' FOODS.
  Request salad dressings 'on the side', baked potatoes without toppings - (or with a scoop of cottage cheese or a small dish of yogurt) - bread or toast served 'dry', chicken, fish and meats without added gravies or sauces.

- WATCH OUT FOR THE SALAD BAR.
  Most salad bars load up with items best shunned: mayonnaise-laden macaroni and potato salads, bacon bits, croutons, sugar-laced gelatin-fruit combos, oil-heavy dressings. Choose wisely and the salad bar can be the healthy main event; be careless and you'll have been taken in by a clever merchandising scheme.

- CONSIDER SHARING.
  Not only in Chinese restaurants is it a good strategy to split meals. Ordering two appetizers plus one entree that two people can share is a good way to pare down portions. When dining alone, ask for 'children's size' or 'half-size' servings.

- SEEK OUT NO-FAULT FAST FOOD.
  Yes, there is such a thing. Healthy fast food is not an oxymoron. There are worse meals than lean roast beef sandwiches (hold the French fries), and lightly dressed (or better still, undressed) salads, a baked potato sans rich toppings, and a citrus juice drink. If you're stuck - and starving' - at a drive-in that serves nothing but deep-fried chicken and fish, remove all the skin and outer crispy layer before eating.

- AVOID DINING ROOMS DECORATED IN RED, OR-
ANGE OR YELLOW.
The color of your surroundings can affect your appetite,
according to noted nutritionist Dr. Maria Simonson,
Professor Emeritus at Johns Hopkins Medical Institutions
and Director of the Health, Weight and Stress Clinic. Dr.
Simonson's studies have shown red, yellow and orange
are appetite-stimulating colors, and will encourage you
to eat more than you'd like when they're prominent in
your eating environment - walls, chairs, tablecloths,
plates, napkins. To keep your appetite in check, seek out
restaurants with a 'cool' decor - light green, light blue,
pale mauve.

❤   ❤   ❤

Once you've mastered feeding your body, what else can
you do? Learn to feed your soul. One last chapter coming up.

> *"Forty is the old age of youth;*
> *Fifty is the youth of old age."*
> **Victor Hugo**

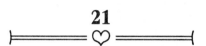

21

FORTY-SOMETHING FOREVER: A LONGEVITY PRIMER

"When I was *your* age, I was *MUCH* older," the elder generation likes to say. And it's true. The meat-and-potatoes generation faction worked very hard, ate fried steak, fried chicken, fried potatoes, fried bread and gravy, didn't know any better and expected to be 'old' long before they qualified for Social Security.

So what have we learned? What are the chances that you can put the brakes on aging with what we know now about youth-promoting nutrition, body-improving exercise, antioxidant supplementation? And what's the truth about chelation therapy? Will a course of EDTA infusions *really* keep you from looking or feeling your age well into your sixth, seventh, eighth, ninth decade even longer?

There's no doubt there are no more youth-obsessed individuals than can be found in the entertainment industry, where almost all the well-known routinely shave off years.

Donna Mills, for example, told interviewers she was 40 in 1986 . . . and in 1987 . . . and in 1988. Joan Rivers once boasted to her TV audience that she "didn't feel like 50" - certainly the truth, since she was 56 at the time! Jack Benny, of course, never made it to 40, since he jokingly insisted on being 39 until he died in his eighties.

What do active, long-lived celebs like Bob Hope, George Burns and Zsa Zsa Gabor do, so that like Duracell's Energizer bunny, they just go on - and on - and on? Would it surprise you to learn that the one place in America chelation therapy as a youth-sustaining modality caught on first and furious was Hollywood?

A CLOSER LOOK AT WRINKLE-FREE CELEBS

Our first indication that EDTA infusions might be the Fountain of Youth came in 1975 when, on assignment from a national mag, we went to Hollywood to complete in-depth interviews with Dr. Harold Harper, then billed as the "diet doctor to the stars." What neither we nor our editors knew at the time, was that the good doctor was a chelation specialist as well as a weight-control expert. Among his famous patients was Zsa Zsa Gabor.

If ever a woman has defied the passage of time, it is 70-something Zsa-Zsa. She's beautifully ageless. Viewed up close, her unlined face and time-stopped-still appearance is mind-boggling. Even if she was a bride at six, she doesn't look her age. Forget the biography and carefully doctored Hungarian birth certificates. Can you believe what you see?

"Has she had a face lift?" we asked Dr. Harper.

"I can guarantee she hasn't," he assured us, adding "a nose job, yes. A face lift, no." Dr. Harper then went on to explain that many of his celebrity clients were receiving chelation treatments. Careful as he was not to violate doctor-patient confidentiality, the message was clear: La-la land had a jump start on the rest of the country by relying on EDTA to curb the clock and the calendar.

Who else visited Dr. Harper regularly and surreptitiously for their EDTA 'booster' shots? Hard to say, since Dr. Harper's files have died with him, but it's tempting to speculate. Ronald Reagan? Nancy? Frank Sinatra? Perhaps. One thing for sure. Several California physicians have admitted they treat many celebrities. At this point in time, as Richard Nixon liked to say, there are more chelation doctors per capita in the Los Angeles area than any place in the world.

Why be chelated and keep it a secret?

That's a tough question to answer. Most people can't say enough about the difference chelation therapy has made in their lives. On the other hand, celebrities *are* different. Most seem to believe their careers hinge on keeping their chelation treatments top secret. We know of one individual - a well-known talk show host - who was 'bypassed' several years ago. He bragged, bragged, bragged on this wonderful life-saving operation. He's not bragging any more. Three years ago he discovered, as many bypassed patients do, that his 'miracle' had back-fired. Arteries clogged once more, worse than ever, he refused to be re-bypassed. His choice this time? Chelation therapy. How do we know? His doctor told us. Has the celeb broadcast these facts to his vast listening audience? No. Why not? You'll have to ask him.

AN OVERLOOKED LIFE-LENGTHENING STRATEGY: EAT LIKE A BIRD; POOP LIKE A PARROT

Anyone needing an incentive to live as long and healthily as possible should consider the purchase of the ultimate in life-prolonging pets: a parrot. Since psittacines normally live at least seventy years, even in captivity, adopting one presents a health-promoting challenge - how to outlive your feathered friend.

An in-residence parrot can teach you a lot about the habits that contribute to exceptional longevity. Watch your long-lived buddy carefully and you'll note he nibbles, instead of gorging. Human 'grazers' live longer also, we're told by many longevity scientists, including Roy Walford, professor of pathology at UCLA. Dr. Walford believes cutting back on calories and spreading consumption more evenly throughout the day can add 25 to 50 years to our life span.

What else do parrots do that enable them to outlive their human housemates? When given a choice of foods, they invariably prefer live, fiber-rich items. Our yellow-cheeked Amazon carefully selects grapefruit seeds, raw cranberries, carrot greens and crunchy pine nuts over less fiber-intensive edibles. One positive result, we suspect, is foods race through his system - he 'poops' regularly and frequently, and never suffers a digestive upset. Keep this in mind when you hear physicians say two or three bowel movements a week are normal and adequate. Don't you believe it. Evidence is accumulating that two to three bowel movements *a day* are more in order.

How come? The toxic wastes that accumulate in the colon include the leftover fragments from incompleted digestive processes, remnants from improper foods, refined products, and harsh chemical additives. These combined noxious materials become prime free radical generators, result in auto-intoxication and trigger many fatal diseases. Not only colon cancer, but *all* forms of cancer, including breast cancer have been linked to constipation. One study confirming this, and reported in *Lancet*, found that women having two or fewer bowel movements per week are at four times the risk of breast disease (benign or malignant) as women who have one or more bowel movements a day.

To assure or restore normal bowel movement, rely on diet and exercise - not laxatives. Eat cabbage, stewed prunes, raw fruits and vegetables, bran and other fiber-rich foods, also herbal remedies known to be internal cleansers.

Your bowel's best friend may turn out to be potassium, which in combination with Vitamin A (abundant in many herbs including celery seed, dandelion root and alfalfa) stimulates the enzymatic process, which then melts down the wastes, dissolves the blockages and propels them through elimination channels.

LIGHT: THE FORGOTTEN NUTRIENT

Dr. Jacob Liberman makes a good case for light being the medicine of the future. In his new book by the same name, he points out what many former researchers have discovered, natural full spectrum light is essential to optimal health. We are all in danger of mal-illumination, thanks to such modern technological advances as fluorescent lighting, sunglasses, tanning lotions and indoor lifestyles, all of which block natural light, an immune system booster.

Many years ago, we recognized the impact of natural light on health when we detailed Dr. John Ott's work in *Psychodietetics*. Dr. Ott, a pioneer researcher in the therapeutic benefits of natural light, early discovered that living in artificially lit environments, as most of us do, contributes to cellular break-down, immune deficiency and has a detrimental effect on all vital biochemical functions, also mood and behavior.

Dr. Liberman has now carried these initial findings several steps further by describing the many ways in which full spectrum (natural) light affects human functioning:

- The pineal gland, known as the body's prime regulator, is totally dependent on an adequate supply of natural light;
- Vitamin D is manufactured in the body in response to sunlight;
- Natural light improves learning, by increasing attention span, visual and auditory memory and visual field;

- Natural light is a potential disease-preventative: lab animals living under artificial light are the first to develop abnormal conditions such as loss of fur, toxic symptoms, abnormal weight, digestive problems, sterility, pathological bone development, cataracts and cancer;
- Light aids longevity: cellular damage caused by ultraviolet radiation has been reversed by full spectrum exposure;
- Light is a blood cleanser: lab tests have shown light can decontaminate blood for transfusions eliminating the risk of infections such as herpes and AIDS;
- Light has successfully healed sexual dysfunction, seasonal depression (SAD), jet lag, neutralized stress, alleviated PMS (premenstrual syndrome), AND increased the efficiency of the heart, improved EKG readings and blood profiles of people with atherosclerosis and reduced cholesterol.

If that's not good enough reason to get outdoors for two or more hours a day (or replace all indoor lights with full spectrum bulbs), Dr. Liberman can provide more.

MORE NATURAL RESOURCES: FEED YOUR SOUL

The latest research assures us our thoughts and emotions have a huge impact on our health. Although the field of psychneuroimmunology is still in its infancy, there is good evidence we can literally 'worry' ourselves sick, or become self-healers by practicing mind-power medicine.

Here's what science knows now about 'mood medicine':

- **Exercise your mind.**
  Mental workouts are as important as muscle-boosting exercises, say researchers who have found that actors, lawyers, public speakers and others who remain healthy and vital into their nineties do so by keeping their wits about them and their memories intact. Assume your brain will atrophy if you don't use it. Stay mentally fit by

reading, memorizing, studying and playing mind-stretching games: bridge, Scrabble and Trivial Pursuit are a few that come easily to mind.

- **Positive thinking pays off.**

  People who see themselves and the world through rose-colored glasses are healthier than those who are more realistic. Great expectations boost the immune system. Fear of the future raises the blood pressure, invites invasion by opportunistic infections, encourages the growth of unwanted cells, leads to muscular degeneration and cardiovascular failure.

- **A 'hurting' heart hurts you.**

  Harsh feelings are physically destructive as well as emotionally painful. Carrying a grudge, feelings of hostility, anger, disgust, and contempt for others appears to have lethal consequences. Angry people who have walled themselves off from loved ones - despite the reason - have more heart attacks and more blockage of the coronary arteries than those who can forgive and forget.

- **Listen more than you talk.**

  Poor listeners are at higher risk of getting sick, says a University of Maryland study that found those who like to talk a lot and listen very little are at increased risk of developing high blood pressure. "Hyper-talking" - a term coined by Dr. James Lynch, author of *The Broken Heart* - can be a serious health hazard. Shut your mouth and open your ears and you'll come out years ahead.

- **Destressing your life can be a heart saver.**

  What does stress do to you besides making you nervous, irritable and 'antsy'? It boosts your cholesterol and throws your blood fats out of balance. To cope better with what life hands you, recognize that *you* are usually the principal generator of stress in your life. Other people and circumstances cannot cause you stress if you do not allow it. When you can't change something, change your attitude toward it.

- **Good Samaritans reap health benefits.**

Do-gooders do themselves much good, suggests studies from Harvard University and elsewhere where they're finding altruism gives a boost to the immune response. Good Samaritans are not only happier - they live longer. In one ambitious survey of 2,770 people conducted by the University of Michigan Survey Research Center, it was found there was a 2.25 times greater incidence of death among men who did no volunteer work compared with men who did at least one hour per week of community service.

"People who help others seem to get helped at least as much as the people they help," is the way psychologist Steven J. Danish puts it. Other researchers who have noted the real health benefits of volunteerism explain that altruism gives a `lift' to the heart. Laboratory tests suggest that doing good deeds raises the germ-fighting substances (immunoglobulin) in the blood and lowers those substances that suppress immune activity, further supporting the notion that being good-hearted pays off in heart health.

- **'Networking' reduces health risks.**

According to a University of California study of 5,000 people, a rich social life significantly prolongs life. Developing a solid network of friends, relatives and links with community organizations offers real health protection. Those with good social supports were two times less likely to die during the study period as those without a social network.

The more sociable you are, the longer you may live, agrees Richard Hessler, professor of sociology and family and community medicine at the University of

Missouri-Columbia School of Medicine who has found, "despite health problems, people with formal social networks are more likely to remain independent and survive."

In his landmark twenty year study of 1,700 elderly that began in 1966, Dr. Hessler found that the most significant factor to whether a person lived or died during the research period was social involvement.

"When there are people counting on you, you have a reason to get up in the morning," he says. "Stimulation is the key to longevity."

- **Be more trusting.**

A fifteen-year study at Duke University makes it clear that trusting individuals are significantly less prone to premature death than the mistrustful.

- **Try the 'Laughing Cure'.**

Long before Norman Cousins' testified to the life-saving benefits of a 'laugh-a-day', old-timey health experts recognized the connection between laughing and health. In the 1800's American physicians advised: "Indulge in good, hearty, soulful laughter at stated periods and when the opportunity offers, and it will send new tides of life and good health to the person." In recent years, laugh researchers such as Dr. William Fry have confirmed the health-promoting aspects of enjoying a good laugh.

- **Pleasuring yourself pays off.**

Everywhere science looks, they find new evidence there's no better prescription for good health and longevity than enjoying life every day just as it comes.

For one thing, enjoying life fully strengthens the desire to live, which in turn increases your commitment to life-promoting activities and encourages you to give up life-damaging habits.

Put another way, those who find life unenjoyable, and thus feel they have less to live for, tend not to start long-term projects - career goals, friendships, develop new hobbies and skills - that in turn, makes life even less fulfilling and enjoyable.

♥ ♥ ♥

So where do you go from here?

Enjoy yourself. Read the books that intrigue you. See the movies that sound entertaining. Listen to your favorite music.

Avoid people who grate on your nerves. Goof off when you feel like it. When you talk to yourself - (we all do it all the time) - take care to tell yourself good things.

Pursue health and happiness as though your life depends on it. It does!

APPENDIX A

STANDARD CPR and DOUBLE-PUMP CPR

CPR (cardiopulmonary resuscitation) is administered when someone's breathing or pulse, or both, stop. When both stop, it spells sudden death - the usual cause is a heart attack.

The most common signal of a heart attack is uncomfortable pressure, squeezing, fullness, or pain in the center of the chest behind the breastbone. Other signals may be sweating, nausea, shortness of breath, or a feeling of weakness.

Should someone be felled by a heart attack, there are two CPR procedures - standard CPR and Double-Pump CPR (DP-CPR).

Standard CPR forces the heart to pump blood by applied rhythmic pressure to the lower half of the victim's breastbone.

DP-CPR, developed by David Bergman, M.D., chairman of St. Joseph's Hospital and Medical Center's department of surgery, is a counter-propulsion technique which pumps arterial blood back toward the heart when the heart is between beats. The action forces blood from the aorta into the coronary arteries to furnish the heart muscle blood in addition to the blood it receives with each chest compression. When used in conjunction with standard CPR, DP-CPR has proven almost twice as effective as standard CPR used alone.

DP-CPR, however, has one drawback - it ordinarily requires two people to administer. Standard CPR, requires but one person.

When using Standard CPR alone or in conjunction with DP-CPR, the first 4 steps are identical.

1. Call, or have someone call the local emergency number, usually 911.
2. Determine whether the collapsed victim is unconscious by gently shaking a shoulder and shouting "Are you all right?" If there is no response, and the victim is not lying flat on his or her back, roll the victim over, moving the entire body as a unit.

3. Check for breathing by looking for chest movement, listening for breathing sounds, or feeling breath on your cheek. If the victim is not breathing, provide rescue breathing by:
   - tilting the head back by lifting up the chin gently with one hand while pushing down on the forehead with the other. [see fig. 1]
   - While maintaining pressure under the chin to sustain head tilt, pinch the victim's nose shut.
   - Give two full breaths while maintaining an air-tight seal with your mouth on the victim's mouth.
4. Locate the victim's carotid artery to determine if the heart is beating. (The carotid pulse is located in the groove [C - fig. 1] beside the Adam's apple.) If you cannot feel a pulse, provide artificial circulation (CPR) in addition to rescue breathing.

STANDARD CPR [Fig. 2 & 3 - A]

Kneel at the victim's side near the chest. With the middle and index fingers of the hand nearest the victim's legs, locate the notch where the bottom rims of the rib cages meet in the middle of the chest. Place the heel of one hand on the sternum next to the fingers that located the notch. Place your other hand on top of the positioned hand, keeping fingers up off the chest wall.

Bring your shoulders directly over the victim's sternum as you press downward, keeping your arms straight. Depress the sternum about 1 1/2 to 2 inches for an adult victim. Then relax pressure completely, allowing chest to return to its normal position between compressions. Relaxation and compression should be of equal duration.

Compressions are applied at 80 to 100 times per minute. If you must provide both rescue breathing and CPR, provide 2 breaths after every 15 chest compressions.

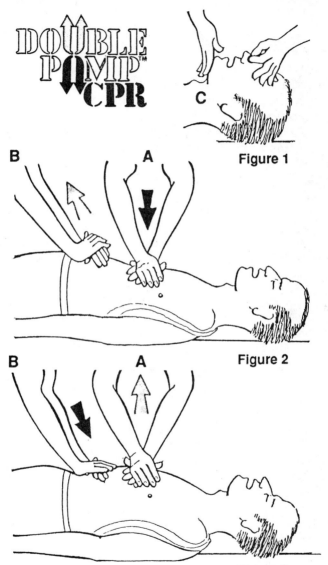

DOUBLE PUMP™ CPR

Figure 1

Figure 2

Figure 3

DOUBLE-PUMP CPR [Fig. 2 & 3 - B]

While one person is administering standard CPR to the chest, another straddles the victim's legs and applies pressure to the stomach, synchronizing pumping action to chest compressions.

Pressure is centered on an area 1 1/2 to 2 inches above the navel and is applied to alternate with chest compressions - that is, when the chest is compressed the stomach is relaxed; when the stomach is compressed, the chest is relaxed. The stomach is compressed 2 to 3 inches.

As with chest compressions, stomach compressions are applied 80 to 100 times per minute.

Stomach compressions are stopped momentarily when rescue breathing is administered.

APPENDIX B
CHELATION PHYSICIAN DIRECTORY

Since you can't turn to the Yellow Pages to find a chelating physician, we're providing the following directory. Entries include members of ACAM (American College for the Advancement of Medicine, 1-800-532-3688) and GLCCM (Great Lakes College of Clinical Medicine, 1-800-286-6013) as well as non-affiliated doctors who administer EDTA chelation therapy.

For a more complete list, check MedSearch™ on our website - http://arxc.com/search.htm. (See page 367 for details)

NOTE: Inclusion in this directory does not signify the publisher's endorsement of a physician's expertise or competence.

ALABAMA
Gus Prosch, MD
  759 Valley St., **Birmingham**, AL 35226 .... (205)823-6180
George P. Gray, MD, ND
  2227 Drake Ave., Bldg 5, **Huntsville**, AL 35805 .... (256)885-4495

ALASKA
Sandra C. Denton, MD
  3201 C St., #602, **Anchorage**, AK 99503 .... (907)563-6200
Robert J. Rowen, MD
  615 E. 82nd Ave, Ste #300, **Anchorage**, AK 99518 .... (907)344-7775

ARIZONA
Charles D. Schwengel, DO, MD
  1927 N. Trekell Rd. **Casa Grande**, AZ 85222 .... (602)668-1448
Lloyd D. Armold, DO
  4901 West Bell Rd., Ste. 2, **Glendale**, AZ 85308 .... (602)939-8916
William W. Halcomb, DO, MD
  4323 E. Broadway, Ste. 109, **Mesa**, AZ 85206 .... (602)832-3014
Charles D. Schwengel, DO; MD
  1050 E. University #4, **Mesa**, AZ 85203 .... (602)668-1448
Alan K. Ketover, MD
  10565 North Tatum Blvd., Ste. B115, **Paradise Valley**, AZ 85253 . (602)381-0800
Linda C. Wright, MD
  10565 North Tatum Blvd., **Phoenix (Paradise)**, AZ 85253 .... (602)483-8986
Jeff Baird, DO
  1413 16th St., **Parker**, AZ 85344 .... (520)669-8982
Stanley R. Olsztyn, MD, PC
  4350 E. Camelback Rd., Ste B220, **Phoenix**, AZ 85018 .... (602)840-8424
Gordon Josephs, MD
  7315 E. Evans Rd., **Scottsdale**, AZ 85260 .... (602)998-9232
  405 S. Beeline Hwy #D, **Payson**, AZ 85541 .... (520)474-0442
  315 W. Goodwin St., **Prescott**, AZ 86303 .... (520)778-0169
Marcia Coyle. Denton, MD
  2490 Country Lane, **Yuma**, AZ 85365 .... (602)726-6381

ARKANSAS
William Warren, MD
  4737 Central Ave., (Hwy 7 South), **Hot Springs**, AR 71913 .... (501)525-7765
Melissa Taliaferro, MD
  101 Cherry St., **Leslie**, AR 72645 .... (870)447-2599
Doty Murphy, MD
  326 N. Bloomington, **Lowell,** AR 72762 .... (501)659-0111
Merl R. Cox, DO
  1613 Hwy 62 East, **Mountain Home**, AR 72653 .... (870)424-5025

CALIFORNIA
David A. Howe, MD, DC
505 N. Mollison Ave, Ste. 103, **El Cajon**, CA 92021 .... (619)440-3838
Mack B. Drucker, MD
4403 Manchester Ave., Ste #107, **Encenitas**, CA 92024 .... (760)632-9042
Ratibor Pantovich, DO
560 East Valley Pkwy, **Escondido,** CA 92025 .... (760)480-2880
David Edwards, MD
360 South Clovis Ave., **Fresno,** CA 93727 .... (209)251-5066
Hitendrah H. Shah, MD
229 W. 7th St.,**Hemet,** CA 92583 .... (909)487-2550
James J. Julian, MD
1654 Cahuenga Blvd., **Hollywood,** CA 90028 .... (323)467-5555
Francis Foo, MD
10188 Adams Ave, **Huntington Beach**, CA 92646 .... (714)968-3266
Robert L. Harmon, MD
43-576 Washington St., **Indio,** CA 92201 .... (760)345-2696
Richard Shapiro, MD, George Weiss, MD
8950 Villa La Jolla Drive, Suite 1162, **La Jolla**, CA 92037 .... (800)450-1707
Hitendrah H. Shah, MD
22807 Barton Rd., **Loma Linda**, CA 92313 .... (909)783-2773
H. Richard Casdorph, MD
1703 Termino Ave., Ste. 201, **Long Beach**, CA 90804 .... (562)597-8716
Hans D. Gruenn, MD
2211 Corinth Ave., Ste. 204, **Los Angeles**, CA 90064 .... (310)966-9194
Murray Susser, MD
2211 Corinth Ave., Ste. 204, **Los Angeles**, CA 90064 .... (310)966-9194
Julian M. Whitaker, MD
4321 Birch St., **Newport Beach**, CA 92660 .... (949)851-1550
Robert Neal Rouzier, MD, David Freeman, MD, Daniel Johnson, MD
2825 Tahquitz Canyon Way, Ste. B200, **Palm Springs**, CA 92262 (760)320-4292
Bessie Jo Tillman, MD
2787 Eureka Way, Ste. 1-1, **Redding**, CA 96001 .... (530)246-3022
Michael Kwiker, DO
3301 Alta Arden, Ste. 3, **Sacramento**, CA 95825 .... (916)489-4400
Richard Shapiro, MD, George Weiss, MD
2667 Camino Del Rio S., Plaza Suite A, **San Diego,** CA 92108 .... (619)294-7911
Nolan Higa, MD
221 Town Center West #107, **Santa Maria**, CA 93458 .... (805)929-3063
Luigi C. Pacini, MD, Gilbert Greene, DO
1307 N. Commerce St., **Stockton,** CA 95202 .... (209)464-7757
Salvacion M. Lee, MD
15243 Van Owen St., Ste 406, **Van Nuys**, CA 91405 .... (818)785-7425

COLORADO
Ron Rosedale, MD
7490 Clubhouse Rd., Suite 103, **Boulder**, CO 80301 .... (303)530-5555
George Juetersonke, DO, James Fish, MD
3525 American Drive, **Colorado Springs**, CO 80917 .... (719)528-1960
Terry Grossman, MD
2801 Youngfield St., #117, **Denver**, CO 80401 .... (303)233-4247
3150 S. Peoria St., **Denver**, CO 80014 .... (303)338-1323
Gary B. Clark, MD, MPA
PO Box 591, 205 Lopp Dr., Unit 1, **Georgetown**, CO 80444 .... (303)569-0164

CONNECTICUT
Alan R. Cohen, MD
67 Cherry St., **Milford**, CT 06460 .... (203)877-1936
Jerrold N . Finnie, MD
333 Kennedy Drive, **Torrington,** CT 06790 .... (860)489-8977

DELAWARE

Jeffrey K. Kerner, DO, D/C
200 Bassett Ave., **New Castle**, DE 19720 .... (302)328-0669

DISTRICT OF COLUMBIA

Lance S. Wright, MD
5039 Connecticut Ave. N.W., **Washington**, DC 20008 .... (202)686-7130

FLORIDA

Ross N. Clark, MD
20335 Biscayne Blvd., Suite L-11, **Aventura**, FL 33180 .... (305)705-0106
Marc M. Kesselman, DO, FA.CC; Michael Braun, MD
2845 Aventura Blvd., Suite 250, **Aventura**, FL 33180 .... (305)932-8441
Leonard Haimes, MD
7300 N. Federal Hwy., Suite 100, **Boca Raton**, FL 33487 .... (561)995-8484
Eteri Melnikov, MD
116 Manatee Ave. East, **Bradenton**, FL 34208 .... (941)748-7943
Joseph T. Witek, MD; Bach McComb, DO
3957 Cortez Rd. West, **Bradenton**, FL 34210 .... (941)727-4842
George O. Brick, MD; Edward D. Scanlan, MD
425 S. Kings Ave., **Brandon**, FL 33511 .... (813)685-1220
Donald Carrow, MD
4908 Creekside Drive, **Clearwater**, FL 33760 ....(727)573-3775
David I. Minkoff, MD
129 Garden Ave. N., **Clearwater**, FL 33755 .... (727)466-6789
Susana T. Donaire, MD
730 S. E. 5th Terrace, **Crystal River**, FL 34429 .... (352)564-8620
Richard Hill, MD
2581 S. University Dr. **Davie**, FL 33324 .... (954)474-8030
Bruce R. Dooley, MD
2583 E. Sunrise Blvd., **Ft. Lauderdale**, FL 33304 .... (954)564-8888
George Graves, MD
P.O. Box 2220, 11512 E. Hwy. 316, **Ft. McCoy**, FL 32134 .... (352)236-2525
James F. Coy, MD
13141 McGregor Blvd., #7, **Fort Myers**, FL 33919 .... (941)415-9355
Robert A. DiDonato, MD
3443 Hancock Bridge Pkwy., Ste 301, **Fort Myers**, FL 33903 ...... (941)997-8800
John R. Pletnicks II, MD
6314 Whiskey Creek Dr., **Fort Myers**, FL 33919 .... (941)433-1221
Gary Pynckel, DO
3840 Colonial Blvd., Ste. 1, **Fort Myers**, FL 33912 .... (941)278-3377
Hanoch Talmor, MD
4400 N.W. 23rd Ave., Suite B, **Gainesville**, FL 32607 .... (352)377-0015
Carlos F. Gonzalez, MD
7989 S. Suncoast Blvd., **Homosassa**, FL 34446 .... (352)382-2900
Norman S. Cohen, MD
4063 Salisbury Road, Suite 206, **Jacksonville**, FL 32216 .... (904)296-0900
Stephen Grable, MD
7563 Philips Hwy, #206, **Jacksonville**, FL 32256 .... (904)296-9355
Neil A. Ahner, MD
1080 E. Indiantown Rd., **Jupiter**, FL 33477 .... (561)744-0077
Sam Baxas, MD
50 W. Mashta Dr., #3, **Key Biscayne**, FL 33149 .... (305)361-3956
Nelson Kraucak, MD
8985 NE 134th Ave., **Lady Lake**, FL 32159 .... (352)750-4333
Peter R. Holyk, MD
2500 W. Lake Mary Blvd., Ste 210, **Lake Mary**, FL 32746 .... (407)328-0014
Sherri Pinsley, MD
2290 10th Ave. North, Suite 605, **Lake Worth**, FL 33461 .... (561)547-2770
Azaci P. Borromeo, MD
2653 N. Lecanto Hwy., **Lecanto,** FL 34461 .... (352)527-9555

Joya Schoen, MD; Jack Young, MD
341 N. Maitland Ave., Ste 200, **Maitland,** FL 32751 .. .. (407)644-2729
Richard A. Saitta, MD
1010 N. Barfield Dr., **Marco Island**, FL 34145 .... (941)642-8488
Neil A. Ahner, MD
1270 N. Wickham Road, **Melbourne**, FL 32935 .... (407)253-2009
Rajiv Chandra, MD, PhD, FACC
20 E. Melbourne Ave., **Melbourne,** FL 32901 .... (407)951-7404
Joseph G.Godorov, MD
9055 S.W. 87th Ave., Suite 307, **Miami**, FL 33176 .... (305)595-0671
Bruce R. Dooley, MD
975 Imperial Golf Course Blvd., Suite 107, **Naples**, FL 34110 ...... (941)594-9355
David Permutter, MD
800 Goodlette Rd. N., Suite 270, **Naples**, FL 34102 .... (941)649-7400
Koussay Baaj, MD
8720 S.W. State Road 200, Suite 12, **Ocala**, FL 34481 .... (352)237-2244
Travis L. Herring, MD
106 Weat Fern Drive, **Orange City,** FL 32763 .... (904)775-0525
Hana T. Chaim, DO
595 W. Granada Blvd., **Ormond Beach**, FL 32174 .... (904)672-9000
Naima Abdel-Ghany, MD, PhD
340 W. 23rd St., Suite K, **Panama City**, FL 32405 .... (850)872-8122
Cris Enriquez, MD
767 South State Road 7, **Plantation**, FL 33317 .... (954)583-3335
Joseph T. Witek, MD; Bach McComb, DO
2828 S. Tamiami Trail, **Sarasota**, FL 34239 .... (941)957-0200
Peter R. Holyk, MD
600 Schumann Dr., **Sebastian,** FL 32958 .... (561)388-5554
Calin V. Pop, MD
5327 Commercial Way, Suite B 108, **Spring Hill**, FL 34606 .... (352)597-2240
Neil A. Ahner, MD
705 N. Federal Hwy., **Stuart**, FL 34994 .... (561)692-9200
Martin Dayton, DO
18600 Collins Ave., **Sunny Isles Beach**, FL 33160 .... (305)931-8484
Jean M. Allen, DO
1502 S. MacDill Ave., **Tampa**, FL 33629 .... (813)679-1525
Eugene H. Lee, MD
1804 W. Kennedy Blvd**., Tampa**, FL 33606 .... (813)251-3089
Nelson Kraucak, MD
204 N. Texas Ave., **Tavares**, FL 32778 .... (352)742-1116
Neil A. Ahner, MD
717 17th St., **Vero Beach**, FL 32960 .... (561)978-0057
John Song, MD
1360 U.S. Hwy #1, **Vero Beach**, FL 32960 .... (561)770-2070
Antonio L. Court, MD
2260 Palm Beach Lakes Blvd.,#213, **W. Palm Beach,** FL 33409 (561)478-3777

GEORGIA
Stephen B. Edelson, MD
3833 Roswell Rd., Ste. 110, **Atlanta**, GA 30342 .... (404)841-0088
Milton Fried, MD
4426 Tilly Mill Rd., **Atlanta**, GA 30360 .... (770)451-4857
Susan Kolb, MD; Daniel Greenberg, MD
4370 Georgetown Square, **Atlanta**, GA 30338 .... (770)390-0012
Bernard Mlaver, MD
4480 N. Shallowford Road, **Atlanta**, GA 30338 .... (770)395-1600
William Richardson, MD,
1718 Peachtree St. NW, Suite 360, **Atlanta**, GA 30309 .... (404)607-0570
Oliver L. Gunter, MD
24 N. Ellis St., **Camilla**, GA 31730... (912)336-7343

John L. Givogre, MD; Kathryn E. Herndon, MD
530 Spring St., **Gainesville,** GA 30501 .... (770)503-7222
James T. Alley, MD
2518 Riverside Dr., **Macon,** GA 31204 .... (912)745-3727
Donald Ruesink, MD; Earl Alderman, MD
5000 Peachtree Industrial Blvd., **Norcross,** GA 30071 .... (770)734-0101
E. Glynn Taunton, DO
100 Riverview Lane, **Oglethorpe,** GA 31068 .... (912)472-2550

HAWAII
Fred M. K. Lam, MD
1270 Queen Emma Bldg., #501, **Honolulu,** HI 96813 .... (808)537-3311
David I. Miyauchi, MD
1507 South King St., Suite 407, **Honolulu,** HI 96826 .... (808)949-8711
Ronald Sorenson, MD
2919 Kapiolani Blvd., Suite #7, **Honolulu,** HI 96826 .... (808)739-6060
Clif Arrington, MD
Honalo Business Center, P.O. Box 649, **Kealakekua,** HI 96750 ... (808)322-9400

IDAHO
Stephen Thornburgh, DO
824 17th Avenue, South, **Nampa,** ID 83651 .... (208)466-3517

ILLINOIS
William J. Mauer, DO
3401 N. Kennicott Ave., **Arlington Heights,** IL 60004 .... (847)255-8988
Thomas L. Hesselink, MD
888 South Edgelawn, #1743, **Aurora,** IL 60506 .... (630)844-0011
6413 Logan Ave, #104, **Belvidere,** IL 61008 .... (815)547-8187
Alan F. Bain, DO
30 N. Michigan Ave., Suite 1410, **Chicago,** IL 60602 .... (312)236-7010
Ross A. Hauser, MD
715 Lake St., Suite 600, **Oak Park,** IL 60301 .... (708)848-7789

INDIANA
Harold Sparks, DO; Larry W. Banyash, MD
3001 Washington Ave., **Evansville,** IN 47714 .... (812)479-8228
Thomas J. Ringenberg, DO
941 Etna Ave., **Huntington,** IN 46750 .... (219)356-9400
David A. Darbro, MD
7168 Graham Rd., **Indianapolis,** IN 46250 .... (317)913-3000
David R. Decatur, MD
8925 North Meridian St., Ste. 150, **Indianapolis,** IN 46260 .... (317)818-8925
David Chopra, MD
428 South Main, **Lynn,** IN 47355 .... (765)874-2411
Oscar J. Ordonez, MD
400 South Oak St., **Winchester,** IN 47394-2104 .... (765)584-6600

KANSAS
Roy N. Neil, MD
105 West 13th St., **Hays,** KS 67601 .... (785)628-3215
John R. Toth, MD
2115 S.W. 10th St., **Topeka,** KS 66604 .... (785)232-3330

LOUISIANA
Lawrence Giambelluca, MD
8200 Hwy. 23, Suite B, **Belle Chasse,** LA 70037 .... (504)392-8691
Carol Chaney, MD
5101 West Esplanade Ave., Ste. 8, **Metairie,** LA 70006 .... (504)885-5234

MAINE
Joseph G. Cyr, MD
  62 Main St. **Van Buren**, ME 04785-0448 .... (207)868-5273

MARYLAND
Binyamin Rothstein, DO
  2835 Smith Ave., #203, **Baltimore**, MD 21209 .... (410)653-8155
  101 Marlboro Road, #25, **Easton**, MD 21601 .... (410)770-5900
Bruce Rind, MD
  11140 Rockville Pike, Suite 550, **Rockville**, MD 20852 .... (301)816-3000
Norton L. Fishman, MD; Ali Safayan, MD
  11140 Rockville Pike, Suite 600, **Rockville**, MD 20852 .... (301)816-0500

MASSACHUSETTS
Ruben Oganesov, MD
  39 Brighton Ave., **Allston**, MA 02134 .... (617)254-2500
Carol Englender, MD
  1426 Beacon St., **Newton**, MA 01776 .... (617)965-7770
Barry D. Elson, MD
  52 Maplewood Shops, Old South St., **Northampton**, MA 01060 .. (413)584-7787

MICHIGAN
Paul A. Parente, DO; Albert J. Scarchilli, DO
  30275 W. 13 Mile Rd., **Farmington Hills**, MI 48334 .... (248)626-7544
William Bernard, DO; Kenneth Ganapini, DO; Janice Shimoda, DO
  1044 Gilbert St., **Flint**, MI 48532 .... (810)733-3140
Tammy Guerkink-Born, DO
  3700 52nd St. S.E. , **Grand Rapids**, MI 49512 .... (616)656-3700
James M. Nutt, DO
  420 S. Lafayette, **Greenville**, MI 48838 .... (616)754-3679
Eric E. Born, DO
  100 Maple St., **Parchment**, MI 49004 .... (616)344-6183
Vahagn Agbabian, DO, PC
  28 North Saginaw St., **Pontiac**, MI 48342-2144 .... (248)334-2424
James Ziobron, DO
  71441 Van Dyke, **Romeo**, MI 48065 .... (810)336-3700
S. J. Judge, MD
  2550 Niles Road, **Saint Joseph**, MI 49085 .... (616)429-1085
Ole C. Kistler, DO
  12100 Dix-Toledo Rd, **Southgate**, MI 48195 .... (734)284-7140

MINNESOTA
Jean R. Eckerly, MD
  13911 Ridgedale Drive, **Minetonka**, MN 55305 .... (612)593-9458
  216 E. Main St., **Albert Lea**, MN 56007 .... (612)593-9458

MISSISSIPPI
George H. Ellis, MD
  1540 E Beach Blvd., **Gulfport**, MS 39501 .... (228)871-5433
  2659 Lakeland Dr., **Jackson**, MS 39208 .... (601)664-0133

MISSOURI
Lawrence E. Dorman, DO
  9120 E. 35th St., **Independence**, MO 64052 .... (816)358-2712
Harvey Walker, MD; PhD
  138 North Meramec Ave., **St. Louis**, MO 61305 .... (314)721-7227

MONTANA
Daniel J. Gebhardt, MD
  P.O. Box 338, **White Sulphur Springs**, MT 59645 .... (406)547-3603

NEVADA

Frank Shallenberger, MD
896 West Nye Lane, Suite #103, **Carson City**, NV 89703 .... (775)884-3990
Robert D. Milne, MD
2110 Pinto Lane, **Las Vegas**, NV 89106 .... (702)385-1393
Phillip Minton, MD
1515 S. Virginia St., **Reno**, NV 89502 .... (775)324-5700

NEW JERSEY

Alan Magaziner, DO
1907 Greentree Rd. **Cherry Hill**, NJ 08003 .... (609)424-8222
Richard B. Menashe, DO
15 South Main St., **Edison**, NJ 08837 .... (732)906-8866
Robin Leder, MD
235 Prospect Ave., **Hackensack**, NJ 07601 .... (201)525-1155
Robert J. Peterson, DO
Hamilton Township Area, **Hamilton**, NJ .... (888)290-9355
Sharda Sharma, MD
131 Millburn Ave., **Millburn**, NJ 07041 .... (973)376-4500

NEW MEXICO

Ralph J. Luciani, DO
2301 San Pedro NE, Suite G, **Albuquerque**, NM 87110 .... (505)888-5995
Gerald M. Parker, DO; John T. Taylor, DO
9577 Osuna Rd., Suite M, **Albuquerque**, NM 87111 .... (505)271-4800
John Laird, MD
1 Camino Altito, **Santa Fe**, NM 87501 .... (505)989-4690

NEW YORK

Kenneth A. Bock, MD, CCN; Steven J. Bock, ND
10 McKown Rd., Suite 224, **Albany**, NY 12203 .... (518)435-0082
Jose B. Llorens, MD; Charles A. Krieger, DO
38-04 31st Ave., **Astoria**, NY 11103 .... (888)787-8432
Kalpana D. Patel, MD
65 Wehrle Drive, **Buffalo**, NY 14225 .... (716)833-2213
Robert F. Barnes, DO
3489 E Main Rd., **Fredonia**, NY 14063 .... (716)679-3510
5225 Southwestern Blvd., **Hamburg**, NY 14075 .... (716)649-0225
Ronald Santasiaro, MD
5451 Southwestern Blvd., **Hamburg**, NY 14075 .... (716)646-6075
Dariusz J. Nasiek, MD
71 Prospect Ave., **Hudson**, NY 12534 .... (518)828-8307
Serafina Corsello, MD
175 East Main St., **Huntington**, NY 11743 .... (516)271-0222
Monica Winefryde Furlong, MD, DC
921 W. Boston Post Rd., **Mamaroneck**, NY 10543 .... (914)381-7687
L. Titus Parker, MD; Patricia L. W. Nash, RPA-C
220 Steuben St., **Montour Falls**, NY 14865 .... (607)535-7154
Richard N. Ash, MD
800A & B Fifth Avenue, **New York**, NY 10021 .... (212)758-3200
Serafina Corsello, MD
200 W. 57th St., **New York**, NY 10019 .... (212)399-0222
Richard J. Ucci, MD
521 Main St., **Oneonta**, NY 13820 .... (607)432-8752
Kenneth A. Bock, MD, CCN; Steven J. Bock, ND
108 Montgomery St., **Rhinebeck**, NY 12572 .... (914)876-7082
Michael B. Schachter, MD
Two Executive Blvd., Suite 202, **Suffern**, NY 10901 .... (914)368-4700
Julio Epstein, MD; Levi Lehv, MD
78 Virginia Rd., **White Plains**, NY 10603 .... (914)428-8400

NORTH CAROLINA
John Wilson, Jr., MD; Stephen Blievernicht, MD; Eileen Wright, MD; John Laird, MD
1312 Patton Place, **Asheville**, NC 28806 .... (828)252-9833
Keith E. Johnson, MD
1009 N. Lake Park Blvd., Suite C-5, **Carolina Beach**, NC 28428 . (910)458-0606
Tyler I. Freeman, MD
1005 South Kings Drive, **Charlotte**, NC 28207 .... (704)373-2444
Rashid A Buttar, DO
20721 Torrence Chapel Road, Ste. 101, **Cornelius**, NC 28031 .... (704)895-9355
Dennis W. Fera
1000 Corporate Drive, Ste. 209, **Hillsboro**, NC 27278 .. .. (919)732-2287
Anthony J. Castiglia, MD
206 N. Cannon Blvd., **Kannapolis**, NC 28083 .... (704)933-2342
Tyler I. Freeman, MD
9623-D E. Independence Blvd., **Matthews**, NC 28105 .... (704)849-8266
Clarence E. Norris, MD
13024-F Idlewild Road, **Matthews**, NC 28105 .... (704)846-6071
Keith E. Johnson, MD
1852 US Hwy. 1 South, **Southern Pines**, NC 28387 .... (910)695-0335
John Wilson, Jr. MD; Stephen Blievernicht, MD;Eileen Wright, MD; John Laird, MD
Plaza 21 North, US Route 21, **Statesville**, NC 28687 .... (704)876-1617

NORTH DAKOTA
Brian E. Briggs, MD
718 SW 6th St., **Minot**, ND 58701 .... (701)838-6011

OHIO
Josephine C. Aronica, MD
1867 West Market St., **Akron**, OH 44313 .... (330)867-7361
L. Terry Chappell, MD
122 Thurman St., Box 248, **Bluffton**, OH 45817-0248 .... (419)358-4627
Leonid Macheret, MD
375 Glensprings Drive, Suite 400, **Cincinnati**, OH 45246 .... (513)851-8790
John M. Baron, DO
4807 Rockside Road, Suite #100, **Cleveland**, OH 44131 .... (216)642-0082
Ronald B. Casselberry, MD
2132 W. 25th St., **Cleveland**, OH 44113 .... (216)771-5855
840 Brainard Rd., **Highland Hts.**, OH 44143 .... (440)460-1880
John Coppinger, DO
3484 Cincinnatti Zanesville Rd., **Lancaster**, OH 43130 .... (740)653-0017
William D. Mitchell, DO
10401 Sawmill Pkwy., **Powell**, OH 43065 .... (614)761-0555
John P. Heilman, DO
3703 Columbus Ave., **Sandusky**, OH 44870 .... (419)625-8085
Jay W. Nielsen, MD
4607 Sylvania #200, **Toledo**, OH 43623 .... (419)882-9626
James Ventresco, Jr., DO
3848 Tippecanoe Rd, **Youngstown**, OH 44511 .... (330)792-2349

OKLAHOMA
Charles H. Farr, MD, Phd
5419 South Western, **Oklahoma City** OK 73170 .... (405)634-7855
Adam Merchant, MD
3535 N.W. 58th St., Suite 750, **Oklahoma City**, OK 73112 .... (405)942-8346
Charles D. Taylor, MD
4409 Classen Boulevard, **Oklahoma City**, OK 73118 .... (405)525-7751
Gordon P. Laird, DO
304 Boulder, **Pawnee**, OK 74058 .... (918)762-3601
Adam Merchant, MD
717 South Houston, Suite 402, **Tulsa**, OK 74127 .... (918)583-6364

R. E. Zimmer, DO
602 N. Dalton St., **Valliant**, OK 74764 .... (580)933-4235
Douglas B. Cook, MD; Lance B. Hightower, MD
1108 N. Washington, **Weatherford**, OK 73096 .... (580)774-2214

OREGON
John Gambee, MD
86 Club Road #140, **Eugene**, OR 97401 .... (541)686-2536
J. W. Fitzsimmons, MD
591 Hidden Valley Rd., **Grants Pass**, OR 97527 .... (541)474-2166
Paula R. Bickle, PhD
9310 S.E. Stark St., **Portland**, OR 97216 .... (503)256-9666
Richard C. Heitsch, MD
177 N.E. 102nd , Bldg. V, **Portland**, OR 97220 .... (503)261-0966
Jeffrey R. Tyler, MD
163 N.E. 102nd Ave., **Portland**, OR 97220 .... (503)255-4256

PENNSYLVANIA
Robert J. Peterson, DO
2169 Galloway Road, **Bensalem**, PA 19020 .... (216)579-0330
Dennis J. Courtney, MD
446 McMurray Rd., **Bethel Park**, PA 15102 .... (412)835-4679
Erik Von Kiel, DO
9331 Hamilton Blvd., **Breinigsville**, PA 18031 .... (610)398-8310
Robert J. Peterson, DO
Chadds Ford, PA 19317 .... (888)287-0636
Donald Mantell, MD
6505 Mars Rd., **Cranberry Township**, PA 16066 .... (724)776-5610
Lance S. Wright, MD
112 South 4th St., **Darby**, PA 19023-2809 .... (610)461-6225
Karl J. Falk, DO
4234 Buffalo Rd., **Erie**, PA 16510 .... (814)899-7777
Harold H. Byer, MD, PhD
5045 Swamp Rd., Suite 101, **Fountainville**, PA 18923 .... (215)348-0443
Nicholas J. D'Orazio, MD
736 Baltimore Pike, Suite 6, **Glen Mills**, PA 19342 .... (610)558-3600
Conrad E. Maulfair, Jr. DO
600 Haverford Rd., Suite 200, **Haverford**, PA 19041 .... (610)658-0220
Jule Jenkins, Jr., MD
New Garden Plza, 747 W.Cypress St, **Kennett Square**, PA 19348(610)444-1424
Mamduh El-Attrache, MD
20 East Main st., **Mt. Pleasant**, PA 15666 .... (724)547-3576
Andrew Lipton, DO
822 Montgomery Ave., Suite 315, **Narbeth**, PA 19072 .... (610)667-4601
Rober J. Peterson, MD
1614 Wrightstown Road, **Newtown**, PA 18940 .... (215)579-0370
George L. Danielewski, MD
142 Bellevue Ave., **Penndel**, PA 19047 .... (215)757-4455
7927 Fairfield St., **Philadelphia**, PA 19152 .... (215)338-8866
P. Jayalakshmi, MD; K.R. Sampathacar, MD
6366 Sherwood Rd., **Philadelphia**, PA 19151 .... (215)473-4226
John G. Wassil III, MD
92 W. Connelly Blvd. **Sharon**, PA 16146 .... (724)346-6500
Conrad G. Maulfair, Jr., DO
403 N. Main Street, **Topton**, PA 19562 .... (800)733-4065

SOUTH CAROLINA
Connie G. Ross, MD; Mack S. Bonner, Jr., MD
1000 East Rutherford Rd., **Landrum**, SC 29356 .... (864)457-4141
Arthur M. LaBruce, MD
9231A Medical Plaza Dr., **N. Charleston**, SC 29406 .... (843)572-1771

James C. Scheer, DO, MS
  7510 Northforest Drive, **North Charleston**, SC 29420 .... (843)572-1600
Connie G. Ross, MD; Mack S. Bonner, Jr., MD
  2915 Cherry Rd., **Rock Hill**, SC 29732 .... (800)676-7542
James M. Shortt, MD
  2500 Winchester Place, Suite 107, **Spartanburg**, SC 29301 .... (864)595-2552
  3901 Edmund Hwy., Suite 107, **W. Columbia**, SC 29170 .... (803)755-0114
Connie G. Ross, MD; Mack S. Bonner, Jr., MD
  2222 Airport Rd., **W. Columbia**, SC 29169 .... (800)676-7542

SOUTH DAKOTA
Hal Fletcher, MD
  4601 South Techlink Circle., **Sioux Falls**, SD 57106 .... (605)362-8256

TEXAS
Albert Kincheloe, DO
  5200 Buffalo Gap Rd., Bldg. F, **Abilene**, TX 79606 .... (915)698-0006
Gerald M. Parker, DO; John T. Taylor, DO
  4714 S. Western, **Amarillo**, TX 79109 .... (806)355-8263
Charles R. Hamel, MD
  4412 Matlock Rd., **Arlington**, TX 76018 .... (817)468-7755
R.E. Liverman, DO
  801 W. Road to Six Flags, Suite 147, **Arlington**, TX 76012 .... (817)461-7774
V. Rizov, MD
  911 W. Anderson Ln., #205, **Austin**, TX 78757 .... (512)451-8149
Theodore Tuinstra, DO
  5757 Lovers Ln., #300, **Dallas**, TX 75209 .... (214)352-1590
J. Robert Winslow, DO
  14900 Landmark Blvd., **Dallas**, TX 75240 .... (972)702-9977
Ricardo B. Tan, MD
  3220 N. Freeway, **Ft. Worth**, TX 76111 .... (817)626-1993
Robert M. Battle, MD
  9910 Long Point Rd., **Houston** TX 77055 .... (713)932-0552
John Karl Blum Do
  1618 West 18th St., **Houston**, TX 77008 .... (713)802-4357
John Parks Trowbridge, MD
  9816 Memorial Blvd., Suite 205, **Humble**, TX 77338 .... (281)540-2329
Donald R. Whitaker, DO
  210 E. Elizabeth St., **Jefferson**, TX 75657 .... (903)665-7781
John L. Sessions, DO
  1609 South Margaret, **Kirbyville**, TX 75956 .... (409)423-2166
Rudy Rivera, MD
  5068 W. Plano Pkwy., Suite 272, **Plano**, TX 75093 .... (972)930-0111

UTAH
Dennis W. Remington, MD; Judith Moore, DO
  1675 No. Freedom Blvd., #11-E, **Provo**, UT 84604 .... (801)373-8500
Dennis Harper, DO
  2046 E. Murray Holladay Rd., #100, **Salt Lake City**, UT 84117 .... (801)277-5000

VIRGINIA
Norman Levin, MD
  39070 John Mosby Hwy. (Rt 50), **Aldie**, VA 20105 .... (703)260-3484
E. Aubrey Murden, MD
  4020 Raintree Road, Suite C, **Chesapeake**, VA 23321 .... (757)488-9900
David G. Schwartz, MD
  101 Woolfolk Street, **Louisa**, VA 23093 .... (540)967-2050
Joan M. Resk, DO
  5249 Clearbrook Lane, **Roanoke**, VA 24014-6637 .... (540)776-8331
Elmer Cranton, MD; Eduardo Castro, MD
  P.O. Box 44 - 799 Ripshin Road, **Trout Dale**, VA 24378-0044 ...... (540)677-3631

Robert A. Nash, MD; FACM
    5589 Greenwich Rd., Ste 175, **Virginia Beach**, VA 23462 .... (757)490-9311
James B. Hutt, Jr.; MD; Robert M. Hutt, MD
    550 Broadview Ave., Suite 202, **Warrenton**, VA 20186 .... (540)347-9983

WASHINGTON
Jon R. Mundall, MD
    PO Box F, 111 North Columbia Ave., **Connell**, WA 99326 .... (509)234-7766
Jonathan Collin, MD
    12911 120th Ave NE, #A -50, PO Box 8099, **Kirkland**, WA 98034 (425)820-0547
    911 Tyler St., Port **Townsend**, WA 98368 .... (360)385-4555
Patrick Scott, MD
    216 S. 23rd St., **La Crosse**, WA 54601 .... (608)785-0038
Elmer M. Cranton, MD
    503 First St. South, Ste. 1, P.O.Box 5100, **Yelm**, WA 98597-7510 (360)458-1061

WEST VIRGINIA
Prudencio Corro, MD
    251 Stanaford Rd., **Beckley**, WV 25801 .... (304)252-0775

WISCONSIN
Carol Uebelacker, MD
    700 Milwaukee St., **Delafield**, WI 53018 .... (414)646-4600
Eleazar M. Kadile, MD
    1538 Bellevue St., **Green Bay**, WI 54311 .... (920)468-9442
Patrick J. Scott, MD..
    3456 Losey Blvd. South, **La Crosse**, WI 54601 .... (608)785-0038
J. Allan Robertson, Jr., DO
    1011 North Mayfair Rd., Suite 301, **Milwaukee**, WI 53226 .... (414)302-1011
Carol Uebelacker, MD
    5404A N. Lovers Lane Rd., **Milwaukee**, WI 53225 .... (414)466-2002
Robert S. Waters, MD
    320 Race St., **Wisconsin Dells**, WI 53965 .... (800)200-7178

WYOMING
Rebecca Painter, MD
    201 W. Lakeway Rd., Suite 300, **Gillette**, WY 82718 .... (307)682-0330

❤   ❤   ❤

Now that there's **MedSearch**™, finding a holistic physician in your area who utilizes natural medicine has never been easier. Fire up your Internet connection and access the world's most complete directory of doctors who practice many forms of alternative care including physicians, dentists, naturopaths, chiropractors, nutritionists and others. The keyword searchable data base allows you to locate a choice of health professionals by name, city, state, and specialty - and in many cases, a direct link to the clinician's website provides additional information. Nothing could be easier. Bookmark this site for easy reference: http://arxc.com and click on the **MedSearch**™ icon. Best of all, it's **FREE**.

Does chelation therapy work? What about other forms of alternative medicine? Now it's your turn. We want to hear from you. If you've had an experience with chelation therapy and/or other forms of alternative medicine you'd like to share, we can help you tell the world. **P.I.E.-in-the-SKY (Patient Information Exchange)** on the Internet has been set up to give patients' testimonials the attention they deserve. Just e-mail your story to abrecher@arxc.com (or mail to PIE, PO Box 683, Herndon, VA 20172) and we'll take it from there.

SELECTED REFERENCES

Abraham, A.S., *Potassium Magnesium Status in Ischemic Heart Disease*, Magneisum Res, 1988(1)53-57

Alsleben, H.R., Shute, W.E., *How to Survive the New Health Catastophies*, Survival Publications, 1973

Archer, E.A., *Cooking Methods, Carcinogens, and Diet-Cancer Studies*, Nutr Cancer, 11, 75-79, 1988

Baim, S., Ignatius, E.J., *Use of Percutaneous Transluminal Coronary Angioplasty: Results of a Current Survey*, Am J Cardiol, Vol 61, 3G-8G, 5/3/1988

Bliznakov, E.G. ET AL, *The Miracle Nutrient Q10*, Bantam, 1987

Blumer, W., et al, *Leaded Gasoline - A Cause of Cancer*, Envir Int J 3: pp 465-471

Braunwald, E., *Coronary Artery Spasm*, JAMA, 246:17, 10/17

Casdorph, H.R., "EDTA Chelation Therapy: Efficacy in Brain Disorders", J Adv Med, 2:1/2, Spring/Summer 1989

Castleman, M., *The Healing Herbs*, Rodale, 1991

Collin, J., *90 Percent Reduction in Cancer Mortality After Chelation Therapy with EDTA?*, Townsend Letter, May, 1990

Cross, Carroll E. et al, *Oxidative Stress and Abnormal Cholesterol Metabolism*, J of Lab and Cl Med, 1990; 115(4); 396-404

Dean, W., Morgenthaler, J., *Smart Drugs & Nutrients*, B&J Pub., 1990

Donsbach, K.W., *Oral Chelation Therapy*, Int Ins Nat Hlth Sci, 1983

Eaton, S.B., Konner, M., *Paleolithic Nutrition*, NE J Med, 312:5, Jan 31, 1985

Faxon, D.P., *Current Status of Coronary Angioplasty*, Hospital Practice, 3/30/1987, P. 59-71

Fuenmayor, A.J., *Vitamin E and VEntricular Fibrillation ...*, Jap Circulation Jrnal, October 1989; 53(10):1229-1232

Finci, L., Meier, B., *Advances in Coronary Angioplasty*, Cardio, 9/1987, P. 53-57

Goldstein, J., *Demanding Clean Food and Water*, Plenum, 1990

Hahn L.J., et al, *Dental 'Silver' Tooth Fillings: A Source of Mercury Exposure Revealed...*, FASEB J, 3, 12/1989

Halstead, B.W., *Free Radical Pathology and Its Immunological Halstead, B.W.*, The Scientific Basis for EDTA Chelation Therapy, *Golden Quill Publishers, 1979*

Harper Index, Survey Result, *1991*

Consequences, J Adv Med, 4:2, Summer 1991

Hedding-Eckerich, M., *Effect of Potassium and Magnesium Aspartate on CArdiac Arrhythmias..*, Magneisum Res., 1988;(1):105

Huggins, H.A., *It's All In Your Head*, Life Sciences Press, 1989

Inlander, C.B. ET AL,*Medicine On Trial*, Prentice Hall, 1988

Jansson, B., *Potasium to Sodium RAtios...*, Cancer Detection and Prevention, 1990; 14(5):563-565

Johnsgard, Keith W., *The Exercise Prescription for Depression* Plenum Press, 1989

Kim, A.H.Y., *Discover Natural Health*, Kim's, 1988

Kindness, G., *The Role of Blood Platelets In Vascular Disease*, J Adv Med, 2:4, Winter 1989

Kitchell, J.R., et al *Treatment of Coronary Artery Disease with Disodium EDTA*, J Amer Card, 4/1983

Kronhausen, E. et al, *Formula for Life*, Morrow, 1989

Kunin, R.A., *Mega-Nutrition*, McGraw Hill, 1980

Lawton, Wm., J., et al, *Effect of Dietary Potassium ...*, Circulation, Jan 1990; 81(1):173-184

Lucaire, Ed, *Ther Celebrity Almanac*, Prentice Hall, 1991

McDonagh E.W., Rudolph, C.J., Cheraskin, E., *Effect of (EDTA)...Blood Cholesterol...* J Int Acad Prev Med, 7:5-12, 1982

The Psychotherapeutic Potential..., J Orthom Psychiat 14:3, 214-217, Third Quarter 1985

'Clinical Change' in Patients Treated with EDTA... J Orth Psych 14:1, 61-65, 1985

An Oculocerebrovasculometric Analysis ... J Hol Med, 4:1, Spring/Summer 1982

Effect of EDTA Upon Renal Function... J Holist Med, 4:2, Fall/Winter 1982

Glycohemoglobin (HbAlc) Distribution in EDTA-Chelation- Eligible Patients, J Orth Psych, 12:1

Nutrition-Prevention Connection, Osteo Annals 11:3, 3/1983

Effect of EDTA..Upon Reported Fatigue, J Orth Psy 13, 1984

Psychotherapeutic Potential of EDTA.., J Orth Psych 14:3

Effect EDTA...Systolic Blood Pressure, J Orth Psych 13, 1984

Masuelier, J. et al, *Flavonoides et pycnogenols* Int J Vit Nut Rsch, 49:3, 1979

Men's Health, *Breaking the Age Barrier*, June 1991

Moore, T.J., *Heart Failure*, Touchstone, 1989

Ochi, Hiorotmo, *East Meets West: Super Nutrition From Japan*, Ishi Press International, 1989

Olszewer, E., Carter, J.P., *EDTA Chelation Therapy: A Retrospective Study of 2,870 Patients*, J Adv Med, 2:12, Spring/Summer 1989

Pinckney, E.R., *The Cholesterol Controversy"* Sherbourne, 1973

Podrid, p.J., *Potassium and Ventricular Arrhythmias*, Am J of Card, Mar 6, 1990; 65:33E-4E

Radner, Gilda, New England Journal of Medicine, November, 1988

Rothfeder, J., *Heart Rhythms*, Little, Brown, 1989

Rudolph, C.J. et al, *A Nonsurgical Approach ...* J Adv Med, 4:3, Fall 1991

Observation of Effect of EDTA... J Adv Medicine, 3:3 Fall 1990

Effect of Intravenous Upon Density Levels", J Adv Med, 1:2, Summer 1988

Chelation Carrier Solution: An Analysis of Osmolarity and Sodium Content", J Int Acad Prev Med, VIII: 1, Winter 1983

Russell-Manning, B., *Silver (mercury) Fillings and the Immune System*, Greenwald Press, 1985

Schwartz, J.,et al, *The Second National Health and Nutrition Examination Survey*, Am J of Epid, 1990;132-(1):67-76.

Singh, R.B., *Dietary Modulators of Blood Pressure and Hypertension* , Eur J of Cl Nut, 1990;44:319-327

Siskin, Bernard et al, *What Are the Chances?*, Crown Publishers, 1991

Stare, Fredrick J., et al *Balanced Nutrition*, Bob Adams, Inc., 1989

Trivoni, D. et al, *Suppression of Ventricular Arrhythmias...*, Am J of Card, June 1, 1990; 65:1397-1399

Tufts University Diet & Nutrition Letter, Vol. 7, No. 10, December 1989

Uchinda S., et al *Condensed Tannins Scavenge Active Oxygen Free Radicals*, Med Sci Res, 15, 1987

Kern, B., *Three Ways to Cardiac Infarction*, Int Assoc Inf Cntrl, 1971

University of California, *Berkeley Wellness Letter*, August 1989, Volume 5, Issue 11

Vimy, M.J., Takahashi, Y., Lorscheider, F.L., "Maternal-Fetal Distribution of Mercury Released From Dental Amalgam Fillings", Amer Phys Soc J, 0363:6119, 1990

Vitamin E Fact Book, Veris, 1989

Vlay, S. C., *Lessons From the Past and Reflections on the Cardiac Arrhythmia Suppression Trial*, Amer J Card, 65, 1/1990

Wallwork, J., Stepney, R., *Heart Disease*, Basil Blackwell, 1987

Wolfe, S., et al, *Worst Pills Best Pills*, Public Citizen Health Research Group,1988

Zamm, A.V., *Why Your House May Endanger Your Health*, Touchstone, 1980

INDEX

Aberg, Thorkel M.D., 8
ACAM, 162, 176, 179, 191, 195, 205, 260
Accuracy in Media, 13
Aetna Life and Casualty Company, 170
Aging, forestalling, 343
AHA
objections to chelation therapy, 165-168
see: American Heart Association
Ahrens, Edward, 286
AIDS, 89
Air filters, 231
Albin, Maurice, 8
Allen, George, 213
Allicin, 307
Alpern, Harvey L., 291
Alzheimer's Disease, 39, 132
and free radicals, 101
Amalgam fillings, 242
American Society of Dental Surgeons, 245
Americal Journal of Clinical Nutrition, 259
American Academy of Pediatrics, 289
American Cancer Society, 16
American Heart Association, 8, 16, 18, 54, 288
American Holistic Medical Association, 300
American Home Products, 173
American Journal of Cardiology, 60, 168, 189, 265
American Journal of Clinical Nutrition, 303
American Journal of Diseases in Children, 290
American Journal of Public Health, 215, 280
American Medical Association, 58, 165, 195
American Quack Association, 198
AMPS
see: ACAM
Anesthesia, risks, 5
Angina, 102
Angina
drugs for, 67-69
Angina pain
treatments, 57
Angiograms
innaccurate readings, 55, 103
risks, discomforts, 47, 55
Angioplasty, 47, 53
failures, 111
risks, 50
unjustified, 56

Antiarrhythmic drugs, 70
Anticoagulants, 61, 73
Antihyperlipidemics, 76
Antihypertensives, 78
Antioxidant supplementation, 264, 267, 273
Antioxidants
in foods, 308, 309
in herbs, 275
Arrhythmias
causes, 86-87, 90-91, 93
drug induced, 77
drugs for, 72
Arteriogram
see: Angiograms
Arteriosclerosis, 102
history, 45
treatments, 45
Artery-cleansing foods, 305
Arthritis, and free radicals, 101
Asai, Kazuhiko, 244
Ascorbic acid
see: Vitamin C
Aspirin, 53, 74, 75, 79
adverse reactions, 74
Atherosclerosis, 61, 92, 104, 106-107, 110, 259
over-stated dangers, 59
pain relief, 63
relation to smoking, 238
reversal by diet, 205
symptoms, 1
treatments, 57
see also: arteriosclerosis
Atkins, Robert C., 291
Atrial fibrillation, 88

Balanced Nutrition, 287
Bananas, 272
Barr, Roseanne, 224
Beans and legumes, 305
Benny, Jack, 344
Berlin Wall, 18
Beta blockers, 62, 68
Beta carotene, 309
Beta III , the super carrot, 309
Bible, diet, 305
Bigger, Thomas, J., 86
Biotin, 258
Bland, Jeffrey, 254
Blood platelet aggregation, 94
Blue Cross/Blue Shield, 169
Blumer, W. and Reich T., 141
Born, Grant, 181-182
Bottled water
purity of, 234-2355
substitutes, 236

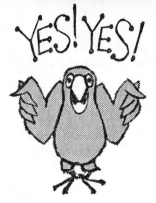

YES, the barriers to the free exchange of health-related information can be bypassed!
YES, there is a better way to learn about your health care options than relying on mass media!
YES, you can discover what others know about the power of natural healing!

INTRODUCING .....

ALTERNATIVE MEDICINE CONNECTION

Want to learn more about non-toxic remedies and natural medicine? About chelation therapy and other health-promoting remedies? Want to get the latest news on the science and politics of alternative medicine and learn how current happenings impact on your health?

To visit the world's only full service Website devoted exclusively to information about medical alternatives, set your Web Browser to: http://arxc.com.

FREE access to MedSearch™, the Holistic Health Providers directory (12,000+ names), files, forums, status of medical freedom legislation, discussion groups involving citizen activist groups, low cost natural remedies, Chapter One™ (browse health books OnLine), PIE-in-the-Sky™ (Patient Information Exchange) and much, much more.

Two words for computer dodos - TRUST US!!!!
You don't have to be a computer whiz to enjoy all the unique features of the ARxC Website. You do need a telephone, computer, modem and Internet connection. Isn't it about time?

FORTY-SOMETHING FOREVER
Now Available on Audio Tape

For individuals traumatized by the need to make an urgent decision; or people who have difficulty reading or don't have the patience to wade through a book; and for countless others who simply want fast, easy to digest, reliable information — here's a book that can be listened to.

Scripted and narrated by noted medical journalists Arline and Harold Brecher, this one-hour tape covers the essential information contained in their book, Forty-Something Forever.

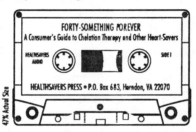

BOLSTER YOUR RESOLVE
TO LIVE A MORE HEALTHFUL
LIFE WITH THIS UNIQUE
HEALTH-BOOSTING AUDIO TAPE

SIDE 1 – 1/2 HOUR

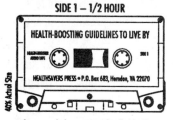

SIDE 2 – 1/2 HOUR

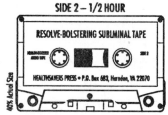

Side one of this tape is loaded with no-nonsense, health-saving tips, rules and guidelines to live by. No hype, hoopla or hyperbole. You get all you want and need to know to get your health back on course. Included in this tape, are spirited suggestions designed to motivate you to improve your diet and to get you moving both physically and mentally.

The second side bolsters your resolve with subliminal health-building messages you can't "consciously" hear. You do, however, hear beautiful and relaxing easy-to-listen-to music that camouflages subliminal messages which reach your subconscious and ease the pain of breaking entrenched health-destroying habits. (Subliminal message printout included)

HEALTHSAVERS PRESS • P.O. BOX 683, HERNDON, VA 22070

Please send _____ Health-Booster Audio Tape(s) to the address below.
Cassettes are $13.45 each ($11.95 plus $1.50 to cover postage and handling).
Credit Card, check or money order. Sorry, no cash or C.O.D.'s please.

Credit Card: Visa ☐   MasterCard ☐

Card Number_____ Exp. Date _____

Signature _____

Mr/Mrs/Miss/Ms_____

Address _____

City _____ State/Zip _____

Mail to: Above address ☐ or

Mr/Mrs/Miss/Ms_____

Address _____

City _____ State/Zip _____

Virginia residents add 4¹/2% tax ($13.99).
NOTE: Should you wish to include a note, enclose it with your order.

For the most coveted gift of all
– the gift of youthfulness –
send FORTY-SOMETHING FOREVER
to people dear to you.

**FOR INFORMATION ON QUANTITY DISCOUNTS
(10 UNITS OR MORE)
ON HEALTHSAVERS PRESS PRODUCTS
CALL 1-800-638-8807**